ADOLESCENTS, ALCOHOL, AND SUBSTANCE ABUSE

Adolescents, Alcohol, and Substance Abuse
Reaching Teens through Brief Interventions

Edited by
PETER M. MONTI
SUZANNE M. COLBY
TRACY A. O'LEARY

Foreword by William R. Miller

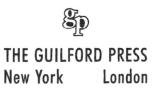

THE GUILFORD PRESS
New York   London

©2001 The Guilford Press
A Division of Guilford Publications, Inc.
72 Spring Street, New York, NY 10012
www.guilford.com

Printed in the United States of America

This book is printed on acid-free paper.

Last digit is print number: 9 8 7 6 5 4 3

Library of Congress Cataloging-in-Publication Data

Adolescents, alcohol, and substance abuse : reaching teens through brief
interventions / edited by Peter M. Monti, Suzanne M. Colby, Tracy A. O'Leary.
    p. cm.
  Includes bibliographical references and index.
  ISBN-10: 1-57230-658-0 ISBN-13: 978-1-57230-658-5 (hardcover)
  ISBN-10: 1-59385-090-5 ISBN-13: 978-1-59385-090-6 (pbk.)
    1. Teenagers—Substance use. 2. Teenagers—Alcohol use. 3. Substance
abuse—Prevention. 4. Alcoholism—Prevention. 5. Brief psychotherapy for
teenagers. 6. Teenagers—Counseling of. I. Monti, Peter M. II. Colby,
Suzanne M. III. O'Leary, Tracy A.

RJ506.D78 .A365 2001
616.86'00835—dc21   2001023784

For Christopher (at 24), Caroline (at 21),
Roseanne (at 19), and Alexandra (at 16)
—P. M. M.

For Paul and Timmy McCormick
—S. M. C.

For Joseph Tevyaw
—T. A. O'L.

About the Editors

Peter M. Monti, PhD, is Professor of Medical Science and Director of the Center for Alcohol and Addiction Studies and the Clinical Psychology Training Consortium at Brown University, in Providence, Rhode Island. His research is supported by a Senior Research Scientist Award from the Department of Veterans Affairs and he holds research grants from the National Institute on Alcohol Abuse and Alcoholism (NIAAA), the National Institute on Drug Abuse (NIDA), and the Department of Veterans Affairs. Widely published, Dr. Monti is coauthor of *Treating Alcohol Dependence: A Coping Skills Training Guide* (1989; Guilford Press) and coeditor of *Social Skills Training: A Practical Handbook for Assessment and Treatment* (1982; New York University Press). He is a Fellow of the American Psychological Society and the American Psychological Association.

Suzanne M. Colby, PhD, is Assistant Professor (Research) in Psychiatry and Human Behavior at Brown University, in Providence, Rhode Island. She joined the Center for Alcohol and Addiction Studies in 1988, received her PhD in Experimental Psychology from the University of Rhode Island in 1996, and joined the Center faculty in 1998. Currently, she is Principal Investigator on a National Cancer Institute research grant designed to study teen smoking and quitting and Co-Principal Investigator on two major research grants from NIAAA and NIDA that study motivational interventions with adolescents. Dr. Colby is also a member of several national panels and committees established to enhance research and treatment development for adolescent substance use. Her recent publications on adolescents have focused on nicotine dependence among youth, adolescent substance use prevalence and diagnosis, and innovative brief interventions.

Tracy A. O'Leary, PhD, is Assistant Professor (Research) in the Department of Psychiatry and Human Behavior at Brown University, in Providence, Rhode Island. She received her PhD in Clinical Psychology from the University at Albany, State University of New York, in 1997. She joined the Center for Alcohol and Addiction Studies in 1993 as a predoctoral intern and joined the Center faculty in 2000. Currently, Dr. O'Leary is studying college student drinking and is Project Director on a research grant from NIDA to test the efficacy of a brief, individual motivational interview for reducing rates and prevalence of adolescent smoking. Dr. O'Leary's recent publications have focused on anxiety and cocaine abuse, and predictors of motivation to change drinking in adolescents.

Contributors

David B. Abrams, PhD, Center for Behavioral and Preventive Medicine, Miriam Hospital, Providence, Rhode Island

Ana Abrantes, BA, Department of Psychology, University of California at San Diego, La Jolla, California

Kristen G. Anderson, MEd, MS, Department of Psychology, University of Kentucky, Lexington, Kentucky

Nancy P. Barnett, PhD, Center for Alcohol and Addiction Studies, Brown University, Providence, Rhode Island

Janet L. Brody, PhD, Department of Psychology, University of New Mexico, Albuquerque, New Mexico

Larry K. Brown, MD, Department of Child Psychiatry, Rhode Island Hospital and Brown University, Providence, Rhode Island

Sandra A. Brown, PhD, Department of Psychology, University of California at San Diego, La Jolla, California

Shawn Chirrey, MA, MHSc, Public Health Sciences/Centre for Health Promotion, University of Toronto, Toronto, Ontario, Canada

Richard R. Clayton, PhD, Kentucky School of Public Health, University of Kentucky, Lexington, Kentucky

Suzanne M. Colby, PhD, Center for Alcohol and Addiction Studies, Brown University, Providence, Rhode Island

Jason R. Kilmer, PhD, Evergreen State College, Olympia, Washington

Eleanor L. Kim, PhD, Psychology Service, VA Boston Healthcare System, Boston, Massachusetts

Kevin J. Lourie, PhD, Department of Child and Family Psychiatry, Brown University School of Medicine, Providence, Rhode Island

Jennifer L. Maggs, PhD, Department of Family Studies and Human Development, University of Arizona, Tucson, Arizona

Oonagh Maley, MISt, Department of Public Health Sciences and Graduate Department of Community Health, University of Toronto, Toronto, Ontario, Canada

G. Alan Marlatt, PhD, Department of Psychology, University of Washington, Seattle, Washington

Elizabeth T. Miller, PhD, DatStat.com, Inc., Seattle, Washington

Peter M. Monti, PhD, Center for Alcohol and Addiction Studies, Brown University, Providence, Rhode Island

Meg Morrison, MEd, Internet Strategy and Evalutation, The Inspire Foundation, Rozelle, New South Wales, Australia

Mark G. Myers, PhD, Department of Psychology, VA San Diego Healthcare System, San Diego, California

Tracy A. O'Leary, PhD, Center for Alcohol and Addiction Studies, Brown University, Providence, Rhode Island

John Schulenberg, PhD, Department of Psychology, University of Michigan, Ann Arbor, Michigan

Harvey Skinner, PhD, Department of Public Health Sciences and Graduate Department of Community Health, University of Toronto, Toronto, Ontario, Canada

Natasha Slesnick, PhD, Center for Family and Adolescent Research, Albuquerque, New Mexico

Gregory T. Smith, PhD, Department of Psychology, University of Kentucky, Lexington, Kentucky

Louise Smith, BA, Department of Public Health Sciences and Graduate Department of Community Health, University of Toronto, Toronto, Ontario, Canada

Kenneth J. Steinman, PhD, MPH, Division of Health Behavior and Health Promotion, Ohio State University School of Public Health, Columbus, Ohio

Susan Tate, PhD, Department of Psychiatry, University of California at San Francisco, San Francisco, California

Kristin Tomlinson, BS, Department of Psychology, University of California at San Diego, La Jolla, California

Aaron P. Turner, MS, Department of Psychology, University of Washington, Seattle, Washington

Holly Barrett Waldron, PhD, Department of Psychology, University of New Mexico, Albuquerque, New Mexico

Kenneth R. Weingardt, PhD, Here2Listen.com, San Mateo, California

Ken C. Winters, PhD, Department of Psychiatry, University of Minnesota, Minneapolis, Minnesota

Robert A. Zucker, PhD, Department of Psychiatry and Alcohol Research Center, University of Michigan, Ann Arbor, Michigan

Foreword

It has always been a puzzle to me how we in the United States fell into the particular ideological model that so dominated the treatment of substance use disorders for much of the latter half of the 20th century. There is, of course, the familiar debate as to whether these behavioral disorders are properly characterized as a "disease," but that is not really the crux of the matter. One would be hard pressed to find any other condition in either the *International Classification of Diseases* or the *Diagnostic and Statistical Manual of Mental Disorders* for which such peculiar methods have been accepted as standard and indicated treatment.

Central to most U.S. addiction treatment programs from the 1960s until the 1990s was the notion of *confrontation*. It was assumed, implicitly or explicitly, that people with these disorders were somehow uniquely incapable of comprehending or accepting the nature of their condition, that they were literally unable to see reality. The psychodynamic concept of *denial* as an unconscious ego-defense mechanism was invoked to explain this incapacity, and it was widely accepted that pathological denial was inherent in, and even diagnostic of, alcoholism and drug addiction. Indeed, this innate denial came to be viewed as the principal obstacle to treatment and recovery.

Once this premise was accepted, it followed that the principal task of treatment would be to break through the layers of denial and other defenses, laying bare the person's pathology and forcing him or her to face up to reality. The *Wall Street Journal* carried on its front page an admiring account of a medical director who "came down hard" in confronting an alcoholic executive during a surprise group meeting, shouting in the executive's face, "Shut up and listen! Alcoholics are liars, and we don't want to hear what you have to say!" Synanon promoted still greater excesses in allegedly therapeutic confrontation, becoming a formative influence in the therapeutic community movement to "tear them down in order to build them up." The "attack therapy" hot seat, therapeutic boot camps, and Scared Straight programs followed logically, as did bizarre methods of humiliation such as shaving the head of newcomers or obliging the noncompliant patient to wear diapers, a dunce cap, or a toilet seat. Such extremes, if not commonplace, were at least consistent enough with the U.S. treatment ethos to be regarded as falling within the range of acceptable practice rather than constituting professional abuse and malpractice.

How did this state of affairs come to be? For what other medical or mental disorder would such "treatment" even be tolerated, let alone prescribed, published, and praised? Somehow aggressive confrontation came to be regarded as justifiable and necessary for these particular people and disorders. For other disorders, professionals are expected to treat patients with reasonable respect, patience, and kindness. Yet somehow such harsh treatment was regarded not only as acceptable but as proper, necessary, and *good for* these particular patients. Alcoholics and addicts were, in essence, regarded as fundamentally different from other human beings by virtue of their disorder and therefore warranted and required such otherwise unconventional treatment. Consistent with this view, U.S. treatment programs commonly combined core elements intended to address the unique deficits of knowledge, awareness, and insight presumed to characterize addiction. Educational lectures and films became a mainstay of addiction treatment. Confrontation, to break down defenses and promote insight, was pursued through various kinds of psychotherapy, most often in groups but also in individual or family therapy.

These beliefs and behaviors created an approach in which patients were in a decidedly disadvantaged, one-down position, assumed to be out of touch with reality and in need of education, awakening, and enlightenment. This power differential is evident in the language that was used to describe what patients were expected to do: admit defeat, surrender, accept personal powerlessness, and ask for help. Healing was presumed to occur through the patient's contact with treatment professionals who imparted the reality, knowledge, and insight necessary to overcome denial. The longer the amount of time spent in contact with such professionals or programs, the greater the presumed benefit.

It was a house of cards. There is not and never has been scientific evidence to support the belief that people with substance use disorders show abnormally high levels of primitive defense mechanisms such as denial. Studies instead reveal a heterogeneity of personality that parallels the general population. Prevention and treatment approaches based on education and confrontation have an abysmal track record when it comes to behavior change. Randomized clinical trials show little benefit from increasing the length or intensity of such treatment. If anything, confrontational tactics tend to elicit defensiveness, increase resistance, and decrease the likelihood of retention and constructive behavior change.

Nowhere is this more true than with troubled adolescents, whose response to an authoritarian, one-up, confrontational style of communication is quite predictable. Any parent of teenagers can write the adolescent's lines in this script. Squaring off for a power struggle does not overcome an adolescent's oppositional style. It *is* the troubled adolescent's style.

To be sure, the urgency of behavior change can be great. Until a person reaches at least the age of 30, the leading causes of death are acute events that are often related to drugs, particularly alcohol. Life-threatening infectious diseases, some of them currently untreatable, can be contracted by young people through activities related to intoxication and drug use. A misstep can permanently alter or end a young life. It is understandable, then, to feel an urgency to help adolescents change their risky behavior. The stakes are high and can lead one to contemplate heroic and confrontational measures.

Within this frame of reference, it bends the mind a bit to think about brief interventions for substance abuse among adolescents. It's a serious problem, after all, so doesn't it require a serious response? Talking about brief interventions can connote a watered-down, minimalist approach. In the end, the data tell the story. Research is already clarifying the promise and limitations of brief intervention, and in the meantime there are some persuasive reasons to take seriously the subject matter of this book.

First of all, the opportunities for brief intervention are many. Although admission to a specialist treatment program is a relatively rare and typically expensive event, troubled adolescents regularly come into contact with schools, health care, and the Internet, as well as justice and social service agencies. In these contexts, contacts between adolescents and potential helping agents tend to be relatively brief, but they are numerous. This book offers a variety of creative ideas for how troubled adolescents can be reached through such opportunities.

Second, there is good evidence that certain kinds of relatively brief interventions can and do suppress substance use and abuse in both adolescents and adults. Some of that evidence is summarized in this volume. Brevity is by no means a synonym for ineffectiveness. In fact, turning points in life are often brief encounters. What and how we communicate can be more influential than the length of time we take to do it. It may even be that effective brief interventions are *better* suited to the nature and needs of adolescents.

Brevity can also focus us on the right issues. Substance use is fundamentally a motivational issue. The pharmacology of drugs of abuse involves motivation, but adolescent substance use does not occur in a vacuum. Adolescent drinking and drug use happen within a social and environmental context. There are limitations to treating such behavioral problems by prolonged removal, as in a hospital or residential program, which suggests that something is being done to repair the individual. Brief interventions leave the person in his or her natural environment, emphasize communication, and explicitly or implicitly acknowledge the individual's choice and responsibility. Autonomy is not complete among most adolescents, but it is a salient and growing issue. It is difficult to motivate change in volitional behavior without somehow acknowledging and dealing with autonomy.

In any event, I am delighted to see this book. Its chapters challenge us to think in new and broader ways about the helping process. Opportunities for brief intervention are many, and the promise is great. We are just beginning to understand what may constitute the necessary and critical elements of effective brief intervention to trigger behavior change, but clearly it is possible. The work reflected in this volume may pave the way for more effective approaches to help not only adolescents but also their elders.

WILLIAM R. MILLER, PhD
Distinguished Professor of Psychology and Psychiatry
The University of New Mexico

Preface

Contributors to this volume were invited to participate in a multidisciplinary conference, the purpose of which was to explore adolescent substance use, abuse, and early intervention. The Robert Wood Johnson Foundation, with the guidance of C. Tracy Orleans, generously provided support for the meeting, which was held in Newport, Rhode Island, in October 1998. Participants were leaders in adolescent and young adult substance abuse research, and each was asked to prepare a manuscript based on his or her presentation. The chapters of this volume represent elaborations of these manuscripts based on the fruitful discussions that followed each presentation. As significant gaps were identified, additional chapters were added. Specifically, invited chapters by Myers and colleagues on comorbidity and brief intervention and by Abrams and Clayton on how transdisciplinary research might improve brief interventions for adolescent substance abuse served to bridge those gaps and to complement the major themes of the book.

As organizers of the conference and editors of this volume, we are grateful to our contributors for their enthusiasm and sharing of knowledge and to William Miller for his thoughtful foreword. In addition, we thank Rebecca Lebeau-Craven, Jennifer Ziegler, Susan Storti, Ann Reid, and the many other staff members at the Brown University Center for Alcohol and Addiction Studies who worked tirelessly and graciously to make the conference happen. Special thanks go to Kathleen Bennett, whose perseverance, caring, and professionalism helped make the conference a pleasure and the preparation of this book a reality. Her dedication and disposition are sincerely appreciated.

Contents

PART II. EMPIRICAL ILLUSTRATIONS LINKED TO PART I/ CLINICAL APPLICATIONS OF BRIEF INTERVENTIONS

PART III. FUTURE DIRECTIONS

Introduction

PETER M. MONTI, SUZANNE M. COLBY,
and TRACY A. O'LEARY

Are adolescent substance abusers merely a younger version of adult sub-stance abusers, or are there important differences? Considering the com-plexity of adolescence and the potential severity of abuse and its conse-quences for teens, is intensive treatment always necessary? This book is motivated by and grounded in the notion that substance abuse and depend-ence in teens is different from that in adults and, further, that there is a place for brief motivational intervention for teen substance abuse. To this end, the chapters in the first section of the book support the premise that development and thorough assessment matter in treatment planning for ad-olescents; the chapters in the second section of the book demonstrate that certain brief interventions can be effective in a variety of contexts, particu-larly when delivered at a teachable moment. The final chapter considers how implications from transdisciplinary research could improve brief inter-ventions for adolescent substance abuse. In this introduction, we briefly discuss pertinent epidemiological data and racial and cultural consider-ations, as well as several overriding themes that include the stages of change model, the notion of harm reduction, the emerging role of pharm-acotherapy, and the elements of brief treatment.

PREVALENCE

Despite 2 decades of the "war on drugs" in the United States, adolescent substance abuse remains a major health and safety problem. The Moni-toring the Future Study, a long-term survey of the behaviors, attitudes, and

1

values of American secondary school students, college students, and young adults, has been tracking rates of alcohol and other substance use among youth for the past 25 years. The most recent figures from that study indicate that 80% of adolescents have consumed alcohol by their senior year in high school, with over one half having done so by the eighth grade (Johnston, O'Malley, & Bachman, 1999). More than 50% of high school seniors report getting drunk at least once (Johnston et al., 1999). Sixty-five percent have smoked cigarettes by their senior year of high school, and 35% are current smokers (Johnston et al., 1999). Up to 38% of high school seniors have used marijuana at least once in the previous 12 months, a substantial increase from the 22% who reported using marijuana in the early 1990s (Johnston et al., 1999). Evidence also indicates that adolescents who are not planning to attend college are at significantly higher risk for illicit drug use, hazardous drinking, and cigarette smoking than college-bound students (Johnston et al., 1999).

High school seniors are also reporting earlier age of onset for experiencing alcohol-related problems than in past years, suggesting increasingly younger ages of first alcohol use (Barnes, Farrell, & Dintcheff, 1997). Indeed, the percentage of college students who report binge drinking in high school rose from 69.7% in 1993 to 73.9% in 1999 (Wechsler, Lee, Kuo, & Lee, 2000). In the National Comorbidity Study, an age cohort effect was found for early onset of alcohol use, with a narrowing of the "gender gap," in that both men and women in younger cohorts are reporting earlier ages of first alcohol use (Nelson, Heath, & Kessler, 1998). The increase in symptom onset of alcohol problems during adolescence appears to be the root cause of increasing prevalence rates of alcohol dependence in recent cohorts (Nelson et al., 1998; Nelson, Little, Heath, & Kessler, 1996). These findings are consistent with another large survey study showing that 47% of adult respondents who reported first using alcohol at age 13 met *DSM-IV* diagnostic criteria for lifetime alcohol dependence versus 11% of those reporting first alcohol use at age 20 (Grant & Dawson, 1997). There is also some evidence that adolescent females are at higher risk for dependence than any other age group of women (Kandel, Chen, Warner, Kessler, & Grant, 1997). Robust risk factors for alcohol misuse, such as parent drinking, peer alcohol use, and ethnicity, appear to be mediated by age of alcohol initiation, underscoring the seriousness of early alcohol use among teens (Hawkins et al., 1997).

Moreover, the transition of students from high school to freshman year of college is associated with substantial increases in alcohol use (Baer, Kivlahan, & Marlatt, 1995). Excessive alcohol use that extends into later adolescence and young adulthood is also a cause for concern (Miller, Turner, & Marlatt, Chapter 2, this volume). Up to 81% of college students report using alcohol at least once in the past year (Wechsler et al., 2000), and 39%–44% are classified as heavy drinkers (Johnston, O'Malley, & Bachman, 1997; Presley, Meilman, & Cashin, 1996). The 1999 Harvard School of Public Health College Alcohol Study reported that, although the prevalence of binge drinking among college students has remained the same since 1993 (44%), the prevalence of frequent binge drinking, defined as binge drinking three or more times in a 2-week period, has increased to 23%. Over 21% of students report binge drinking one to two times in a 2-week period, bringing the total percentage of students who report binge drinking to 44% (Wechsler et al., 2000). Both occasional and frequent binge drinkers were significantly more likely to report experiencing alcohol-related problems than non-binge drinkers or abstainers (Wechsler et al., 2000). Prevalence rates for a *DSM-IV* diagnosis of lifetime alcohol dependence among 18- to 24-year-olds are high, with 25% of males and 14% of females meeting diagnostic criteria (Grant & Dawson, 1997). Overall, young adults consistently show the highest prevalence rates for alcohol dependence and alcohol-related problems (Nelson et al., 1998; Warner, Kessler, Hughes, Anthony, & Nelson, 1995).

Young adult college students who binge drink are significantly more likely to experience a host of negative consequences, including damaging property, getting in trouble with the police, sustaining injuries, driving after drinking, engaging in unplanned and unprotected sexual activity, and suffering impaired academic performance (Wechsler et al., 2000). Binge drinking also affects those who choose not to drink: 77% of college students report experiencing secondhand effects of other students' binge drinking, such as being awakened at night or interrupted while studying, having to take care of a drunken fellow student, or being insulted or humiliated (Wechsler et al., 2000). In spite of this, students tend to accept higher drinking levels than experts do in terms of defining a drinking problem in a peer (Posavac, 1993) and to report feeling in control of their drinking even after acknowledging excessive alcohol use (Burrell, 1992). Thus alcohol misuse and abuse among college-age individuals is a serious problem affecting not only those individuals but also their college campuses, neighborhoods, and social networks (Midanik & Clark, 1995).

It also appears that substance abuse predisposes adolescents to experience elevated prevalence rates of psychopathology (Myers, Brown, Tate, Abrantes, & Tomlinson, Chapter 9, this volume). For instance, 7% of a community sample of non-treatment-seeking adolescents received a *DSM-III-R* diagnosis of an alcohol or other substance use disorder, and 90% of those who received an alcohol or other substance use disorder diagnosis received an additional *DSM-III-R* diagnosis (Keller et al., 1992). In most cases, the onset of psychiatric disorders tends to occur prior to the onset of the substance use disorder (Hovens, Cantwell, & Kiriakos, 1994; Kessler et al., 1997; Wilens, Biederman, Mick, Faraone, & Spencer, 1997), suggesting that adolescents who develop alcohol and other substance use problems may have a preexisting vulnerability to psychopathology, which in turn intensifies the risk of subsequent alcohol and other substance use problems (Myers et al., Chapter 9, this volume; Winters, Chapter 3, this volume).

The implications of early and hazardous alcohol use, namely, its pernicious impact on successful developmental transitions during adolescence and adulthood (Schulenberg, Maggs, Steinman, & Zucker, Chapter 1, this volume), touch at the heart of this book. In addition to a higher risk of alcohol dependence in adulthood (Grant & Dawson, 1997), adolescent substance misuse is associated with earlier sexual maturation and activity (Brown & Lourie, Chapter 8, this volume; Krohn, Lizotte, & Perez, 1997; Millstein & Igra, 1995; Tschann et al., 1994), increased risk of dropping out of school (Gomberg, 1997; Mensch & Kandel, 1988), and living independently from parents or guardians prematurely (Fergusson, Horwood, & Lynskey, 1994; Krohn et al., 1997). These risks are in turn associated with other life problems, such as marital difficulties (Gomberg, 1986) and lower occupational status due to leaving school at earlier ages (Gomberg, 1997). For those adolescents who do not "grow out" of their early alcohol use, then, there may be effects that reach well into adulthood.

STAGES OF CHANGE

Because authors in this volume frequently refer to the stages of change model, also called the transtheoretical model of change (TMC; Prochaska & DiClemente, 1983; Prochaska, DiClemente, & Norcross, 1992), a brief introduction of this model is warranted. Approximately 2 decades ago, psychologists sought to understand how individuals successfully changed health risk behaviors on their own. What kinds of strategies did people use? What stages did they go through? What predicted success? The rationale for this line of research was this: If we could learn how people change their own behavior, perhaps we could help others apply similar strategies and achieve success as well. Although early thinking on the TMC did not explicitly focus on adolescents, the utility of the model for teens is apparent in this book.

Researchers gained several early insights from studying successful self-changers. First, they realized that the dichotomous distinction between those engaging in a healthy versus an unhealthy behavior pattern (e.g., smoker vs. nonsmoker; sedentary vs. active; binge drinker vs. moderate drinker) that was typically relied on for evaluating treatment outcomes masked some important differences within these two groups. Prospective research determined that individuals pass through a series of *stages of change* rather than shifting from user to nonuser and back again (for example). The stages include *precontemplation*, at which an individual does not identify a behavior as problematic and/or has no intention of changing it; *contemplation*, at which an individual begins to consider behavior change but has no immediate plans to make a change; *preparation*, at which an individual is ready to make a change and begins to take steps toward healthier behavior; *action*, at which an individual has changed his or her behavior but is still in the early stages of maintaining that change; and *maintenance*, at which an individual has successfully changed the behavior and maintained the change for a prolonged period of time (Prochaska & DiClemente, 1983). Progress toward successful behavior change occurs with each step forward along this continuum. This fact reframed the concept of success for professionals who were attempting to change health behaviors.

Second, researchers saw that individuals use different strategies at different points along the stage continuum. These strategies were termed *processes of change*, and they could be categorized into two higher order groups: experiential processes (e.g., restructuring thoughts), relied on more heavily in the early stages of change, and behavioral processes (e.g., cutting down on use), employed during later stages of change. This insight was important because it highlighted the fact that traditional treatments were action oriented and therefore inappropriate for those in the earliest stage of change. Thus, until individuals were committed to change, they were alienated from traditional interventions.

Third, researchers realized that change is a dynamic process and that people undertaking behavior change often relapse to unhealthy behavior patterns several times before ultimately succeeding. This knowledge enabled professionals to reframe the concept of relapse from one of failure to one of progress. People can learn from relapse, using the experience to identify their high-risk situations, to discover current strategies for change that are not working, and to come up with new plans that might work better for them.

The TMC has been successfully applied to a dozen different health behaviors (e.g., obesity, smoking, sun exposure) in adults, and more recently empirical support has been provided for its applicability to adolescents (Pallonen, Prochaska, Velicer, Prokhorov, & Smith, 1998; Stern, Prochaska, Velicer, & Elder, 1987). In this book, we endorse the use of the stages of change model with adolescents and emphasize interventions that can be used across the full range of teens who are engaging in behaviors risky to health. A particular strength of brief interventions is that the threshold for participation is low; that is, even adolescents not particularly interested in change may be willing to participate because an ultimate commitment to lifelong change is not required up front.

HARM REDUCTION

As will become evident in several chapters throughout this book (e.g., Chapters 2, 5, 6, 8, and 11), the prevention and treatment of adolescent substance abuse problems has been increasingly influenced by the concept of harm reduction. This concept is characterized by five basic principles, according to Marlatt (1998). First, harm reduction is an alternative to the moral, criminal, and disease models of substance abuse. It is more compatible with a public health perspective in that its proponents focus on the consequences of addiction rather than on drug use per se. Second, harm reduction accepts alternatives to total abstinence when abstinence is not a realistic goal. Marlatt (1998) sees abstinence as an ideal end point along a continuum that ranges from excessively harmful to less harmful consequences. As lifelong abstinence can be a particularly difficult concept for many adolescents to embrace, harm reduction is usually more appealing to teens. Third, compared with a "top down" policy (i.e., one that originates from authorities) promoted by drug policy makers, harm reduction has emerged as a "bottom up" approach (i.e., one that originates from consumers). This is yet another aspect of harm reduction that makes it likely to appeal to teens.

The fourth principle that characterizes harm reduction is that, as an alternative to high-threshold approaches to services, harm reduction promotes easier access to treatment. One illustration, as noted by Marlatt (1998), is that rather than setting abstinence as a precondition for receiving treatment, advocates are willing to settle for a reduction in harm to make it more acceptable for individuals to initiate treatment. The fifth characteristic is that harm reduction arose out of the dichotomy of compassionate pragmatism versus moralistic idealism. As Marlatt points out, harmful behavior happens—it always has and always will. After accepting this fact, the question becomes, What can be done for both the individual and society?

There are some clear advantages of a harm reduction approach when compared with more traditional models of abstinence, particularly when dealing with youth. There is increasing evidence that alcohol problems, rather than necessarily being "progressive and fatal," are intermittent and may remit without formal treatment (Sobell et al., 1996; Tucker & King, 1999). Thus Larimer and colleagues (1998) argue that viewing such problems as being on a continuum and having an intermittent course can direct resources from expensive "one-size-fits-all" abstinence-focused treatments for severe dependence toward a broader range of treatment services along a "stepped care" approach. Such an approach has recently been articulated by Sobell and Sobell (2000) and is described further in Chapter 11 in this volume. This latter approach takes people as they are and does not insist that they be totally abstinent—a condition that many young individuals simply will not buy. Indeed, as Larimer and colleagues (1998) note, if abstinence is not viable and no other options seem available, then there is little motivation to make any change in consumption whatsoever. The brief intervention program outlined by Monti and colleagues in Chapter 5 (this volume) illustrates how offering a low-threshold strategy in the emergency room can help get teens to attend to their problematic drinking without turning them off. Similarly, nearly all the clinical approaches described in the following chapters are both brief and consistent with a harm reduction perspective.

RACE AND CULTURE

This book does not cover race and culture considerations in as much depth as the field needs. We simply know less about the impact of brief interventions on individuals of different ethnic and cultural backgrounds. Similarly, we know little about the influence of gender on the efficacy and effectiveness of brief interventions. One obvious reason lies in the relatively recent emergence of brief interventions in clinical outcome trials. Fine-grained analyses of brief interventions with adolescent females and with individuals of different ethnic backgrounds are still in progress.

Another factor contributing to the lack of knowledge about racial and cultural issues in brief interventions lies in the fact that, by and large, the prevalence estimates of substance use and misuse among youth of color are lower than those for white youth (see Waldron, Brody, & Slesnick, Chapter 7, this volume). Additionally, the majority of adolescents who misuse and abuse substances are males (Hawkins et al., 1997), although there is increasing evidence that substance use and misuse among females is approaching the same levels as those among males (Nelson, Heath, & Kessler, 1998). Much of the work done in brief interventions with youth has focused on college campus settings, in which students of ethnic minority status are typically outnumbered by white students and who again demonstrate lower substance use and misuse rates in general.

There is some evidence that ethnicity may operate as a protective factor against adolescent substance use and abuse, depending on the adolescent's level of acculturation into American society. Felix-Ortiz and Newcomb (1995) found that Mexican American adolescents who were highly involved in ethnic activities and reported higher levels of ethnic pride also reported lower levels of substance use. One explanation for this is that high acculturation of Hispanic youth is related to higher levels of substance use in that Hispanic youth who are highly immersed in American culture are at greater risk (see Vega, Gil, & Wagner, 1998, for a review). Some interesting findings suggest that low acculturation is protective against substance use in immigrant youth but is not for those born in the United States (Vega et al., 1998). Thus identification with American values, beliefs, and attitudes appears to place ethnic minority youth at higher risk for substance use, possibly due to the support that American adolescents receive in behavior experimentation and in limit testing as part of their identity formation (Vega et al., 1998). As ethnic minority populations grow and shift, it will be important to track changes in adolescent substance use.

Still another reason for the lack of discussion on youth of color is the overall lack of concerted effort to recruit ethnic and racial minority youth into large-scale clinical outcome trials for brief interventions. Moreover, because of the lower prevalence rates of substance use among ethnic minority adolescents, many researchers are not able to analyze ethnicity separately as a risk or protective factor in larger treatment outcome trials. However, there have been a few notable exceptions. For example, Robinson and colleagues (Robinson, Klesges, Levy, & Zbikowski, 1999), with extensive curriculum development and piloting, developed a smoking prevention program that was tailored to African American youth. The program content emphasized a greater role for families and parents in the intervention due to reports in the literature that African American youth are far more susceptible to parental than to peer modeling of smoking behavior in terms of showing greater risk for future smoking (Robinson et al., 1999). Rather than blindly applying an existing intervention to minority adolescents, Robinson and colleagues incorporated sociocultural features and risk factors specific to African American adolescents into the intervention. Resnicow and colleagues have also developed culturally sensitive smoking cessation interventions for African Americans with promising results (Resnicow, Royce, Vaughan, Orlandi, & Smith, 1997; Resnicow, Vaughan, et al., 1997). Yet, as they point out, research is still needed to examine the effectiveness of culturally sensitive interventions (Resnicow, Baranowski, Ahluwalia, & Braithwaite, 1999).

Of course, any discussion about ethnicity as a factor in brief interventions must also look to other factors that may be more prevalent in ethnic groups and that may overshadow intervention efforts. Poverty status has long been a risk factor that overwhelms ethnicity and predisposes individuals to substance abuse and other social morbidities (see, e.g., Jenkins & Parron, 1995; Jones-Webb, Snowden, Herd, Short, & Hannan, 1997; Oetting, Donnermeyer, & Deffenbacher, 1998). However, focusing on ethnicity while ignoring socioeconomic status misrepresents the role of ethnicity in substance use and misuse. For example, Earls and Buka (1997) have convincingly demonstrated that neighborhood accounts for more of the variance in adolescent smoking than does ethnic or racial background.

In addition, researchers in the field debate the value and conceptual underpinnings of ethnically tailored interventions. For example, because there is so much heterogeneity within ethnic groups, many argue that collapsing ethnic groups together under the general categories of "Asian," "black," "white," and "Hispanic" results in gross misrepresentations of differences within, as well as between, ethnic groups and puts the validity of ethnic categorization of studies into question (see, e.g., Dakis & Rubin, 1998). In addition, ethnicity is insufficient as a proxy measure for an individual's family background (Hauser, 1994).

In light of these considerations, we offer the following suggestions for researchers and clinicians using brief interventions with adolescents:

1. Increase the cultural sensitivity of assessment and intervention tools by conducting focus groups and piloting material with minority youth.
2. Recruit adolescents at sites with high ethnic minority concentrations. For example, Brown and Lourie (Chapter 8, this volume) discuss using a brief intervention in a hospital setting, in which ethnic minority adolescents are more likely to receive general medical care.
3. Tailor social normative feedback for each individual teen and base it on samples specific to the teen's ethnicity and gender, particularly with respect to giving feedback to ethnic minority teens on how their substance use compares with prevalence rates in their own racial or ethnic group (part of the motivational intervention described in Monti et al., Chapter 5, this volume).
4. Cast a wider net into the community with such recruitment methods as intervening with neighborhood churches and church groups, using the "word of mouth" method to recruit friends and family members of ethnic minority adolescents, and targeting high schools in ethnically diverse neighborhoods.

PHARMACOTHERAPY

Another issue that is underdeveloped in this volume is pharmacotherapy with adolescents. A major reason for this is that pharmacotherapy usually necessitates more than brief intervention. Nevertheless, because there has been increasing interest in the use of pharmacotherapy for adolescent substance abuse problems, it warrants brief discussion here. The rationale for pharmacotherapy with teens follows the same basic strategies as its use with adults: (1) make drug use aversive; (2) substitute a similar drug for prolonged maintenance; (3) block the reinforcing effects of the drug; (4) relieve craving; and (5) treat withdrawal effects (Bukstein et al., 1997; Kaminer, 1992). Medications used to treat comorbid psychiatric disorders (e.g., depression, anxiety) in substance-abusing adolescents are widely accepted and are discussed by Myers and colleagues (Chapter 9, this volume).

To date, most adolescent pharmacotherapy trials for substance abuse have been case studies or open-label trials, and findings are ambiguous. But because alcohol and other substance use is a major source of morbidity and mortality, further research into pharmacotherapy may be warranted to increase treatment options, particularly for substance-dependent adolescents with chronic heavy use who have not benefited from other forms of treatment.

Disulfiram has long been used with adults as an aversive agent in the treatment of severe and chronic alcoholism (Larson, Olincy, Rummans, & Morse, 1991), but its use with adolescents is rare (Bukstein et al., 1997). Problems with safety and compliance are particular concerns, and caution is advised for its applications with youth (Myers, Donahue, & Goldstein, 1994). Indeed, Myers and colleagues (1994) recommended restricting disulfiram to use with older, alcohol-dependent adolescents.

Substitution therapies, such as use of methadone for heroin abuse, are used infrequently with adolescents and often are prohibited by law (Bukstein et al., 1997). Nicotine substitution approaches (e.g., nicotine gum or patch) are more commonly used with adolescents, despite the fact that the two published trials to date yielded very discouraging results (Hurt et al., 2000; Smith et al., 1996). Because sporadic use patterns are particularly characteristic of adolescents, substitution approaches risk iatrogenically increasing exposure levels (and possibly tolerance) to substances such as nicotine beyond the adolescent's pretreatment levels. Therefore, these approaches are recommended only for the most chronic substance abusers among adolescents.

Evidence for the efficacy of pharmacotherapy with adolescents to reduce or block the reinforcing effects of a drug is suggestive at best (Bukstein et al., 1997). A few case studies have reported positive results, including Kaminer's (1992) report of desipramine use with a cocaine-dependent adolescent and Lifrak and colleagues' (Lifrak, Alterman, O'Brien, & Volpicelli, 1997) use of naltrexone with alcohol-dependent adolescents. However, findings are far too preliminary to draw any firm conclusions.

Clinically significant substance use withdrawal syndromes are rare among adolescents (Chung et al., 2000; Martin, Kaczynski, Maisto, Bukstein, & Moss, 1995); thus pharmacotherapy to treat them should also be rare. Most of what we know about adolescent withdrawal symptoms is based on retrospective self-reported recall by adolescents, which has not been validated prospectively (Colby, Tiffany, Shiffman, & Niaura, 2000). Therefore, use of pharmacotherapy to relieve withdrawal should proceed only when an adolescent's quantity and frequency of substance use is sufficient to produce a withdrawal syndrome, for example, daily use for a month or longer (American Psychiatric Association, 1994).

Based on the state of the existing literature, we urge therapists to proceed cautiously in the area of pharmacotherapy for adolescent substance use. The following guidelines are recommended:

1. Clearly identify which pharmacotherapy strategy is being targeted and why it is appropriate for each adolescent on a case-by-case basis.
2. Carefully evaluate the potential risks versus benefits of pharmacotherapy. Ensure that parents and teens understand the nature and effects of the medications and the dangers of concurrent use of other drugs.
3. Psychiatric comorbidity, other medications, and potential interactions and polysubstance use must be thoroughly assessed and considered prior to prescribing any medication for an adolescent with a substance use disorder (Bukstein et al., 1997).
4. Until more is known, pharmacotherapy should occur only in the context of a comprehensive treatment program with adequate family support and motivation and compliance on the part of the adolescent (Bukstein et al., 1997). Close monitoring of medication tolerance and effects is needed on an ongoing basis.

For these reasons, use of pharmacotherapy in the context of brief interventions is not recommended.

BRIEF TREATMENT

As implied in the title of this volume, most of the approaches described in this book are brief. Thus a concise discussion of what we mean by "brief intervention" seems appropriate. Based on a review of brief interventions for alcohol problems, Miller and Sanchez (1994) outline six elements that are commonly included in effective brief interventions. These are summarized by the acronym FRAMES and include: (1) personalized Feedback or assessment results that usually take 2 to 3 hours to relay to a client; (2) emphasizing personal Responsibility for change; (3) Advice, or explicit direction to change; (4) a Menu offering a variety of change options; (5) Empathy, emphasizing a warm, reflective, and understanding approach; and (6) Self-efficacy, emphasizing optimism regarding the possibility of change. Each of the approaches outlined in this book includes these elements. Clearly, brief intervention is not merely traditional treatment done in a shortened time frame.

Interventions that range from one to five sessions are typically considered brief (Bien, Miller, & Tonigan, 1993). Although most of the approaches discussed in this book entail fewer than five sessions, two exceptions are discussed by Waldron and colleagues (Chapter 7) and Skinner, Maley, Smith, Chirrey, and Morrison (Chapter 10). Although they are not as brief, the approaches reflected in these chapters have been included because of their innovation and reliance on a FRAMES type of strategy with adolescents.

REFERENCES

American Psychiatric Association. (1997). *Diagnostic and Statistical Manual of mental disorders* (4th ed.). Washington, DC: Author.

Baer, J. S., Kivlahan, D. R., & Marlatt, G. A. (1995). High-risk drinking across the transition from high school to college. *Alcoholism: Clinical and Experimental Research, 19*, 54–61.

Barnes, G. M., Farrell, M. P., & Dintcheff, B. A. (1997). Family socialization effects on alcohol abuse and related problem behaviors among female and male adolescents. In R. W. Wilsnack & S. C. Wilsnack (Eds.), *Gender and alcohol: Individual and social perspectives* (pp. 156–175). New Brunswick, NJ: Rutgers Center of Alcohol Studies.

Bien, T. H., Miller, W. R., & Tonigan, J. S. (1993). Brief interventions for alcohol problems: A review. *Addiction, 88*, 315–336.

Bukstein, O., Dunne, J. E., Ayres, W., Arnold, V., Benedek, E., Benson, R. S., Bernet, W., Bernstein, G., Gross, R. L., King, R., Kinlan, J., Leonard, H., Licamele, W., McClellan, J., & Shaw, K. (1997). Practice parameters for the assessment and treatment of children and adolescents with substance use disorders. *Journal of the American Academy of Child and Adolescent Psychiatry, 36*, 140S–156S.

Burrell, L. F. (1992). Student perceptions of alcohol consumption. *Journal of Alcohol and Drug Education, 37*, 107–113.

Chung, T., Colby, S. M., Barnett, N. P., Rohsenow, D. J., Monti, P. M., & Spirito, A. (2000). Screening adolescents for problem drinking: ·Performance of brief screens against *DSM-IV* alcohol diagnoses. *Journal of Studies on Alcohol, 61,* 579–587.

Colby, S. M., Tiffany, S., Shiffman, S., & Niaura, R. S. (2000). Are adolescent smokers dependent on nicotine? A review of the evidence. *Journal of Drug and Alcohol Dependence, 59*, S83–S95.

Dakis, P., & Rubin, L. (1998). Obstruction of valid race/ethnicity data acquisition by current data collection instruments. *Methods of Information in Medicine, 37*, 188–191.

Earls, F., & Buka, S. L. (1997). *The project on human development in Chicago neighborhoods*. Washington, DC: National Institute of Justice.

Felix-Ortiz, M., & Newcomb, M. D. (1995). Cultural identity and drug use among Latino and Latina adolescents. In G. J. Botvin, S. Schinke, & M. A. Orlandi

(Eds.), *Drug use prevention with multiethnic youth* (pp. 147–165). Thousand Oaks, CA: Sage.

Fergusson, D. M., Horwood, L. J., & Lynskey, M. T. (1994). Parental separation, adolescent psychopathology, and problem behaviors. *Journal of the American Academy of Child and Adolescent Psychiatry, 33*, 1122–1131.

Gomberg, E. S. (1986). Women: Alcohol and other drugs. *Drugs and Society, 1*, 75–109.

Gomberg, E. S. (1997). Alcohol abuse: Age and gender differences. In R. W. Wilsnack & S. C. Wilsnack (Eds.), *Gender and alcohol: Individual and social perspectives* (pp. 225–244). New Brunswick, NJ: Rutgers Center of Alcohol Studies.

Grant, B. F., & Dawson, D. A. (1997). Age at onset of alcohol use and its association with *DSM-IV* alcohol abuse and dependence: Results from the National Longitudinal Alcohol Epidemiologic Survey. *Journal of Substance Abuse, 9*, 103–110.

Hauser, R. M. (1994). Measuring socioeconomic status in studies of child development. *Child Development, 65*, 1541–1545.

Hawkins, J. D., Graham, J. W., Maguin, E., Abbott, R., Hill, K. G., & Catalano, R. F. (1997). Exploring the effects of age of alcohol use initiation and psychosocial risk factors on subsequent alcohol misuse. *Journal of Studies on Alcohol, 58*, 280–290.

Hovens, J. G., Cantwell, D. P., & Kiriakos, R. (1994). Psychiatric comorbidity in hospitalized adolescent substance abusers. *Journal of the American Academy of Child and Adolescent Psychiatry, 33*, 476–483.

Hurt, R. D., Croghan, G. A., Beede, S. D., Wolter, T. D., Croghan, I. T., & Patten, C. A. (2000). Nicotine patch therapy in 101 adolescent smokers. *Archives of Pediatric Adolescent Medicine, 154*, 31–37.

Jenkins, R. R., & Parron, D. (1995). Guidelines for adolescent health research: Issues of race and class. *Journal of Adolescent Health, 17*, 314–322.

Johnston, L. D., O'Malley, P. M., & Bachman, J. G. (1997). *National survey results on drug use from the Monitoring the Future Study, 1975–1995* (Vol. 2) (NIH Publication No. 98-4140). Washington, DC: U.S. Government Printing Office.

Johnston, L. D., O'Malley, P. M., & Bachman, J. G. (1999). *National survey results on drug use from the Monitoring the Future Study, 1975–97*. Rockville, MD: National Institute on Drug Abuse.

Jones-Webb, R., Snowden, L., Herd, D., Short, B., & Hannan, P. (1997). Alcohol-related problems among black, Hispanic and white men: The contribution of neighborhood poverty. *Journal of Studies on Alcohol, 58*, 539–545.

Kaminer, Y. A. (1992). Desipramine facilitation of cocaine abstinence in an adolescent. *Journal of the American Academy of Child and Adolescent Psychiatry, 31*, 312–317.

Kandel, D., Chen, K., Warner, L. A., Kessler, R. C., & Grant, B. (1997). Prevalence of demographic correlates of symptoms of last year dependence on alcohol, nicotine, marijuana and cocaine in the U.S. population. *Drug and Alcohol Dependence, 44*, 11–29.

Keller, M. B., Lavori, P. W., Beardslee, W., Wunder, J., Drs, D. L., & Hasin, D. (1992). Clinical course and outcome of substance abuse disorders in adolescents. *Journal of Substance Abuse Treatment, 9*, 9–14.

Kessler, R. C., Crum, R. M., Warner, L. A., Nelson, C. B., Schulenberg, J., & Anthony, J. C. (1997). Lifetime co-occurrence of *DSM-III-R* alcohol abuse and dependence with other psychiatric disorders in the National Comorbidity Study. *Archives of General Psychiatry, 54,* 313–321.

Krohn, M. D., Lizotte, A. J., & Perez, C. M. (1997). The interrelationship between substance use and precocious transitions to adult statuses. *Journal of Health and Social Behavior, 38,* 87–103.

Larimer, M. E., Marlatt, G. A., Baer, J. S., Quigley, L. A., Blume, A. W., & Hawkins, E. H. (1998). Harm reduction for alcohol problems: Expanding access to and acceptability of prevention and treatment services. In G. A. Marlatt (Ed.), *Harm reduction: Pragmatic strategies for managing high-risk behaviors* (pp. 69–121). New York: Guilford Press.

Larson, E. W., Olincy, A., Rummans, T. A., & Morse, R. M. (1991). Disulfiram treatment of patients with both alcohol dependence and other psychiatric disorders: A review. *Alcoholism, 16,* 125–130.

Lifrak, P. D., Alterman, A. I., O'Brien, C. P., & Volpicelli, J. R. (1997). Naltrexone for alcoholic adolescents. *American Journal of Psychiatry, 154,* 439–441.

Marlatt, G. A. (1998). Basic principles and strategies of harm reduction. In G. A. Marlatt (Ed.), *Harm reduction: Pragmatic strategies for managing high-risk behaviors* (pp. 49–66). New York: Guilford Press.

Martin, C. S., Kaczynski, N. A., Maisto, S. A., Bukstein, O. G., & Moss, H. B. (1995). Patterns of alcohol abuse and dependence symptoms in adolescent drinkers. *Journal of Studies on Alcohol, 56,* 672–680.

Mensch, B. S., & Kandel, D. B. (1988). Dropping out of high school and drug involvement. *Sociology of Education, 61,* 95–113.

Midanik, L. T., & Clark, W. B. (1995). Drinking-related problems in the United States: Description and trends, 1984–1990. *Journal of Studies on Alcohol, 56,* 395–402.

Miller, W. R., & Sanchez, V. C. (1994). Motivating young adults for treatment and lifestyle change. In G. Howard (Ed.), *Issues in alcohol use and misuse by young adults* (pp. 55–81). Notre Dame, IN: University of Notre Dame Press.

Millstein, S. G., & Igra, V. (1995). Theoretical models of adolescent risk-taking behavior. In J. L. Wallander & L. J. Siegel (Eds.), *Adolescent health problems: Behavioral perspectives* (pp. 52–71). New York: Guilford Press.

Myers, W. C., Donahue, J. E., & Goldstein, M. R. (1994). Disulfiram for alcohol use disorders in adolescents. *Journal of the American Academy of Child and Adolescent Psychiatry, 33,* 484–489.

Nelson, C. B., Heath, A. C., & Kessler, R. C. (1998). Temporal progression of alcohol dependence symptoms in the U. S. household population: Results from the National Comorbidity Survey. *Journal of Consulting and Clinical Psychology, 66,* 474–483.

Nelson, C. B., Little, R. J. A., Heath, A. C., & Kessler, R. C. (1996). Patterns of *DSM-III-R* alcohol dependence symptom progression in a general population survey. *Psychological Medicine, 26,* 449–460.

Oetting, E. R., Donnermeyer, J. F., & Deffenbacher, J. L. (1998). Primary socialization theory: The influence of the community on drug use and deviance. *Substance Use and Misuse, 33,* 1629–1665.

Pallonen, U. E., Prochaska, J. O., Velicer, W. F., Prokhorov, A. V., & Smith, N. F. (1998). Stages of acquisition and cessation for adolescent smoking: An empirical integration. *Addictive Behaviors, 23,* 303–324.

Posavac, E. J. (1993). College students' views of excessive drinking and the university's role. *Journal of Drug Education, 23,* 237–245.

Presley, C. A., Meilman, P. W., & Cashin, J. R. (1996). *Alcohol and drugs on American college campuses: Use, consequences, and perceptions of the campus environment: Vol. 4. 1992–94.* Carbondale: Southern Illinois University at Carbondale, Core Institute.

Prochaska, J. O., & DiClemente, C. C. (1983). *The transtheoretical approach: Crossing traditional boundaries of change.* Homewood, IL: Dow Jones-Irving.

Prochaska, J. O., DiClemente, C. C., & Norcross, J. C. (1992). In search of how people change: Applications to addictive behaviors. *American Psychologist, 47*(9), 1102–1114.

Resnicow, K., Baranowski, T., Ahluwalia, J. S., & Braithwaite, R. L. (1999). Cultural sensitivity in public health: Defined and demystified. *Ethnicity and Disease, 9,* 10–21.

Resnicow, K., Royce, J., Vaughan, R., Orlandi, M. A., & Smith, M. (1997). Analysis of a multicomponent smoking cessation project: What worked and why. *Preventive Medicine, 26,* 373–381.

Resnicow, K., Vaughan, R., Weston, R. E., Royce, J., Parms, C., Hearn, M. D., Smith, M., Freeman, H. P., & Orlandi, M. A. (1997). A self-help smoking cessation program for inner-city African Americans: Results from the Harlem Health Connection Project. *Health Education and Behavior, 24,* 201–217.

Robinson, L. A., Klesges, R. C., Levy, M. C., & Zbikowski, S. M. (1999). Preventing cigarette use in a bi-ethnic population: Results of the Memphis Smoking Prevention Program. *Cognitive and Behavioral Practice, 6,* 136–143.

Smith, T. A., House, R. F., Croghan, I. T., Gauvin, T. R., Colligan, R. C., Offord, K. P., Gomez-Dahl, L. C., & Hurt, R. D. (1996). Nicotine patch therapy in adolescent smokers. *Pediatrics, 98,* 659–667.

Sobell, L. C., Cunningham, J. A., Sobell, M. B., Agrawal, S., Gavin, D. R., Leo, G. I., & Singh, K. N. (1996). Fostering self-change among problem drinkers: A proactive community intervention. *Addictive Behaviors, 21,* 817–833.

Sobell, M. B., & Sobell, L. C. (2000). Stepped care as a heuristic approach to the treatment of alcohol problems. *Journal of Consulting and Clinical Psychology, 68,* 573–579.

Stern, R. A., Prochaska, J. O., Velicer, W. F., & Elder, J. P. (1987). Stages of adolescent smoking acquisition: Measurement and sample profiles. *Addictive Behaviors, 12,* 319–329.

Tschann, J. M., Adler, N. E., Irwin, C. E., Jr., Millstein, S. G., Turner, R. A., & Kegeles, S. M. (1994). Initiation of substance use in early adolescence: The roles of pubertal timing and emotional distress. *Health Psychology, 13,* 326–333.

Tucker, J. A., & King, M. P. (1999). Resolving alcohol and drug problems: Influences on addictive behavior change and help-seeking processes. In J. A. Tucker, D. M. Donovan, & G. A. Marlatt (Eds.), *Changing addictive behavior: Bridging clinical and public health strategies* (pp. 97–126). New York: Guilford Press.

Vega, W. A., Gil, A. G., & Wagner, E. (1998). Cultural adjustment and Hispanic adolescent drug use. In W. A. Vega & A. G. Gil (Eds.), *Drug use and ethnicity in early adolescence* (pp. 125–148). New York: Plenum Press.

Warner, L. A., Kessler, R. C., Hughes, M., Anthony, J. C., & Nelson, C. B. (1995). Prevalence and correlates of drug use and dependence in the United States: Results from the National Comorbidity Survey. *Archives of General Psychiatry, 52,* 219–229.

Wechsler, H., Lee, J., Kuo, M., & Lee, H. (2000). College binge drinking in the 1990s: A continuing problem—Results of the Harvard School of Public Health 1999 College Alcohol Study. *Journal of American College Health, 48,* 199–210.

Wilens, T. E., Biederman, J., Mick, E., Faraone, S. V., & Spencer, T. (1997). Attention deficit hyperactivity disorder (ADHD) is associated with early onset substance use disorders. *Journal of Nervous and Mental Disease, 185,* 475–482.

I

Background and Context: Theory, Developmental, and Measurement Considerations

1

Development Matters

Taking the Long View on Substance Abuse Etiology and Intervention during Adolescence

JOHN SCHULENBERG, JENNIFER L. MAGGS,
KENNETH J. STEINMAN, and ROBERT A. ZUCKER

It would be difficult to argue against taking a developmental perspective on adolescent substance use. To do so would be to attempt to assert, for example, that age and other markers of developmental status (e.g., pubertal status, acquisition of adult roles) do not contribute importantly to our understanding of the onset and course of substance use, either directly or as moderators of risk factors. But what exactly does it mean to take a developmental perspective on the etiology and prevention of substance use during adolescence? And what are some advantages of doing so for research and intervention? We address these and related questions in this chapter.

To set the stage, consider Figure 1.1, a lithograph from 1895 entitled "The Smokers," by K. Wilkowski. On the surface, this is simply a nostalgic illustration of two boys who are about to light up, one a cigarette and the other a little corncob pipe (presumably containing tobacco). At another level, this shared experience can be seen as advancing the friendship between these two boys. Indeed, it appears that this is a first-time experience for the younger one on the right, with the tentative look and short pants. Perhaps the older one, who is lighting the match, is initiating his younger friend. According to Sullivan (1947), forming a "chumship" during early adolescence is critical for continued social and identity development (see also Berndt, 1982), and young adolescents clearly understand the social

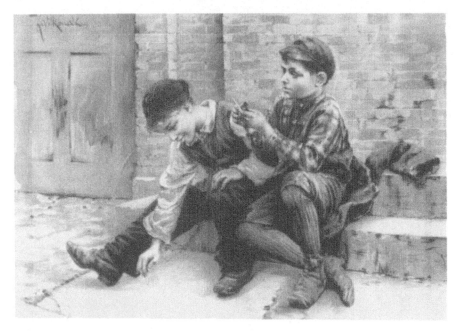

FIGURE 1.1. "The Smokers."

purposes of substance use (Johnson & Johnson, 1996). Thus, in this illustration, a consequential "bonding experience" is occurring for which substance use is a catalyst, despite the likely sequelae of negative health outcomes.

This example illustrates one of the key features of a developmental perspective, that is, to understand substance use in relation to adolescents' various developmental tasks and transitions (Schulenberg, Maggs, & Hurrelmann, 1997a). The second key feature is to examine individual courses of change over time in substance use and abuse and related risk factors. The single snapshot of "The Smokers" leaves us wondering what led up to this moment and what happened next. What individual and contextual characteristics set the stage for these two young people to use tobacco? How did this shared moment fit into the underlying course of their friendship and substance use? How did this and subsequent substance use influence future health and well-being? In this chapter, we expand on these two key and interrelated features of a developmental perspective on substance use during adolescence and discuss the implications of this developmental perspective for understanding risk and protective factors and for conceptualizing interventions.

SUBSTANCE USE IN RELATION TO ADOLESCENTS' CHANGING LIVES

In this section we offer an overview of adolescent development and consider the ways in which substance use can be viewed in relation to the numerous changes that typically occur during adolescence. It is not possible to consider these topics in a comprehensive manner here, so our approach is to be illustrative. We begin with a brief and selective overview of the study of adolescence, followed by a discussion of the pivotal importance of the adolescent years in the lifespan. We then consider the fundamental changes and major domains of transitions during adolescence and conclude this section with a consideration of conceptual models for linking substance use (and risks to health and well-being more generally) to the various normative and nonnormative developmental transitions during adolescence.

The Study of Adolescence

G. Stanley Hall, the founder of the scientific study of adolescence (Muuss, 1996), gave us the enduring image of adolescence as a time of unavoidable "storm and stress." According to Hall's biologically based theory, individual development (ontogeny) recapitulates species development (phylogeny), with adolescence reflecting the turbulent transition in human history from savagery to civilization (Hall, 1916). Nothing can be done to ease adolescents' pain because developmental maturation is controlled by biology and thus unaffected by culture or context. A century later, Hall's mythical image of the adolescent is still strongly reflected in popular culture, if not in the scientific literature.

Of course, Hall was not alone in his beliefs on this subject. Most prominently, Sigmund Freud's psychoanalytic theory viewed turmoil as an unavoidable and even essential component of adolescence. According to Freud, puberty brings on the genital stage of psychosexual development, during which the strengthening of sexual desire and the necessity of severing emotional dependence on parents leads to inner and interpersonal turmoil (Freud, 1958). Other psychoanalytic theorists (see, e.g., Blos, 1970; Erikson, 1950; Sullivan, 1947) also highlighted the inevitability of adolescent turmoil, although they emphasized different causes.

In addition to these organismic and psychoanalytic roots of current images of adolescence, there are mechanistic and contextual roots as well (cf. Pepper, 1942). Margaret Mead (1950) and Ruth Benedict (1950) argued that "storm and stress" is primarily a cultural phenomenon caused by the discontinuity in roles and responsibilities between childhood and adulthood in modern societies. Kurt Lewin (1939) attributed adolescent difficulties to adolescents' ambiguous life space rather than to their individual characteristics. Robert Havighurst (1952) identified culturally defined developmental tasks that individuals needed to accomplish during certain age ranges. He viewed difficulties that arose during adolescence in terms of inability or unwillingness to accomplish the necessary tasks.

Although some diversity in present-day scientific images of adolescence remains, reflecting strong roots in biology and culture, the notion that adolescence is *necessarily* a time of storm and stress has received little empirical support (Arnett, 1999; Offer, Ostrov, & Howard, 1981; Rutter, Graham, Chadwick, & Yule, 1976; Schlegel & Barry, 1991). Notions of stages and developmental determinism have given way to probabilistic conceptualizations of person–context interactions (Gottlieb, 1991; Jessor, 1993; Lerner, 1985; Lerner, Ostrom, & Freel, 1997; Sameroff, 1987). Consistent with life-span and ecological perspectives (Baltes, Cornelius, & Nesselroade, 1979; Bronfenbrenner & Crouter, 1982; Elder, 1974; Featherman, 1983; Schaie, 1965), the typical answer from those who study adolescence to any question about the impact of some characteristic or event on adolescent development has become "it depends." A common view now is "adolescence is characterized by change, and is challenging, but it need not be tumultuous and problematic unless societal conditions prompt it" (Petersen & Leffert, 1995, p. 3).

It is important to note that there is not one unified, agreed-upon developmental theory or conceptual framework. Indeed, developmental scientists often disagree about the very meaning of development, and this disagreement stems from differences in philosophical assumptions about humans and their nature and nurture. The developmental perspective we offer in this chapter is consistent with a developmental–contextual framework that emphasizes multidimensional and multidirectional development across the life span, with stability and change occurring as a function of the dynamic interaction between individuals and their contexts (Baltes, 1987; Lerner, 1985; Sameroff, 1987; Windle & Davies, 1999; Zucker, in press; Zucker, Fitzgerald, & Moses, 1995). Although genetic and other organismic factors certainly play a primary role in development, they do so in conjunction with contextual forces. Even physical maturation, which is heavily driven by biological factors, is partially regulated by the context structure that enhances and dampens the organism's basic genetic template, as well as assigns developmental and social meaning to the physical changes (Silbereisen & Kracke, 1997). In relation to the etiology of substance use, developmental stability and change are viewed clearly as dynamic interactions between individual and context. Not only does the etiology depend on individual characteristics that are given to developmental change, but it also depends on features of the context (e.g., availability of a given drug, regulatory and expectancy structures that govern its use), as well as on the strong and ongoing interactions between the two.

Why Focus on Adolescence?

When asked why he robbed banks, Willie Sutton allegedly answered, "because that's where the money is." Likewise, when considering substance use etiology and interventions, one obvious reason to focus on adolescence is "because that's where the drugs are." Very rarely is substance use initiated prior to or after the 2nd decade of life (Johnston, O'Malley, & Bachman, 1998). For some young people, the various psychosocial changes of adolescence set the stage for the manifestation of risky trajectories rooted in childhood (or earlier); for others, the many transitions of adolescence contribute to some (statistically) normative venturing into problem behaviors in general and into experimentation with substance use in particular (Jessor & Jessor, 1977; Rose, 1998).

There is no other time in the life span at which both individual and contextual changes are as rapid and pervasive as they are during adolescence. Although the rates of physical and cognitive growth are more rapid during infancy than during adolescence, unlike infants, adolescents are keenly aware of their physical and cognitive changes (Silbereisen & Kracke, 1997). For some young people, the immediacy and simultaneity of these changes may contribute to decreased health and well-being. Likewise, the varying tempo and timing of these changes also can threaten the health and well-being of adolescents (Brooks-Gunn & Reiter, 1990). For instance, once they are physically able, many young people engage in sexual intercourse before they acquire the motivations and skills to protect themselves and their partners (Brooks-Gunn & Paikoff, 1993). Similarly, they may gain access to automobiles or firearms without appreciating their own limited experience or the dangers involved. Such discrepancies between adolescents' repertoire of behaviors and their cognitive, emotional, and social development result in some disturbing outcomes (Moffitt, 1993). Indeed, the prevalence of traffic accidents, homicides, and sexually transmitted diseases is proportionally highest among adolescents (Millstein, Petersen, & Nightingale, 1993). Alcohol and other drug use begins amidst the biological, cognitive, emotional, and social changes of adolescence. The onset and escalation of substance use likely amplify other concurrent threats to health and well-being.

One of the most compelling reasons to focus on adolescents is that successful interventions are likely to have long-term benefits across the life span (Baer, 1993; Hamburg, Millstein, Mortimer, Nightingale, & Petersen, 1993; Susman, Feagans, & Ray, 1992). The primary causes of mortality and morbidity during adolescence are related to preventable social, environmental, and behavioral factors (Crockett, 1997; Irwin & Millstein, 1986, 1992; Millstein et al., 1993; U.S. Congress, 1991). Many physical and mental health problems of adulthood have their origin in habits that are formed during adolescence (e.g., smoking, exercise, eating habits; Friedman, 1993; Jessor, 1984), as well as in maladaptive coping styles that are consolidated during this time (Compas, 1993, 1995; Kazdin, 1993; Nurmi, 1997; Petersen, Leffert, Graham, Alwin, & Ding, 1997). In addition, during adolescence and young adulthood, many consequential life decisions are made concerning educational attainment, occupational choices, relationship and family formation, and lifestyle options, making this a formative period in regard to health and well-being across the life span. Thus adolescence can be viewed as a sensitive period for interventions that can have lifelong impact (Maggs, Schulenberg, & Hurrelmann, 1997).

Developmental Transitions during Adolescence

Many obvious developmental transitions occur during adolescence, such as puberty and moving from elementary school to junior high. Many more developmental transitions are less obvious but still important in defining the transformation from child to adult: cognitive shifts that set the stage for more abstract identities and future orientations, changes in parent–child relationships such that the adolescent gains more privacy and freedom, and heightened peer group involvement followed by individualized friendships and dating relationships. These developmental transitions are "the paths that connect us to transformed physical, mental, and social selves" (Schulenberg, Maggs, & Hurrelmann, 1997b, p. 1). They offer young people opportunities to compound or disrupt the strengths and difficulties acquired earlier in life and thus represent both continuity and discontinuity in functioning and adjustment (Caspi & Moffitt, 1993; Rutter, 1996). The challenge is how to influence young people's negotiations of developmental transitions such that health-enhancing characteristics of the individual and surrounding context are maintained and strengthened across adolescence and health-compromising characteristics are diminished.

The meaning of developmental transitions originates in the interaction of physical maturational processes, cultural influences and expectations, and personal values and goals. Individuals shape their own developmental transitions as they act on and are acted on by the social and physical environment (Gottlieb, 1991; Lerner, 1982; Scarr & McCartney, 1983). As with other developmental processes, these transitions are embedded in a sociocultural context, and therefore may vary by gender, class, culture, and historical period. Culturally based age-related expectations shape developmental transitions in that they provide a normative social timetable for role transitions (e.g., employment, parenthood). There are also significant interindividual variations in the order and importance of the various transitions, depending on personal goals and life situations (Nurmi, 1993, 1997).

Developmental transitions can be grouped into the following categories: (1) fundamental changes of pubertal and cognitive development, (2) affiliative transitions (e.g., changes in relationships with parents, peers, romantic partners), (3) achievement transitions (e.g., school and work transitions), and (4) identity transitions (e.g., changes in self-definition, increased self-regulation; Schulenberg et al., 1997a, 1997b).

Models Relating Developmental Transitions to Substance Use

Obviously, health risks increase during adolescence. Yet these risks do not accrue automatically with age but rather as direct and indirect functions of the numerous developmental transitions. There are several ways in which various developmental transitions during adolescence relate to risks to health and well-being and specifically to substance use (see, e.g., Graber, Brooks-Gunn, & Galen, 1998). We summarize five relevant conceptual models, the first four of which are based on Schulenberg and colleagues (1997b). Note that these models are not mutually exclusive: Given the multiplicity of developmental transitions, as well as of health risks and opportunities, all five models are likely to operate across individuals in a given population and within individuals over time. As we briefly discuss, each of these models has implications regarding substance abuse interventions (see also Maggs et al., 1997).

Overload Model

In the first model, health risks are viewed as a potential but not inevitable result of experiencing developmental transitions. When developmental transitions overwhelm current coping capabilities, health and well-being are likely to suffer, and health-risk behaviors (such as substance use) may become an alternative strategy for coping (Damphousse & Kaplan, 1998). This in turn may undermine other, more effective, coping strategies (Pandina, Labouvie, Johnson, & White, 1990; Wills & Hirky, 1996). Given the major and multiple transitions that occur during adolescence, existing coping strategies may be challenged (Mechanic, 1983). This view is consistent with Coleman's (1978) focal theory, in which he argues that decrements in well-being during adolescence result not from hormone-induced "storm and stress" but instead from the multiple and simultaneous transitions that occur in a relatively short period of time. Potential interventions based on this model include attempting to increase adolescents' coping capacities (Compas, 1995; Nurmi, 1997; Petersen et al., 1997), as well as attempting to stagger the timing of various transitions (Brooks-Gunn & Paikoff, 1997; Eccles, Lord, Roeser, Barber, & Jozefowicz, 1997), helping, for instance, most youth to avoid changing schools during the very years they are entering puberty.

Developmental Mismatch Model

In the second model, health risks and opportunities are viewed as a result of the impact of developmental transitions on the developmental match (Eccles et al., 1993, 1997; Galambos & Ehrenberg, 1997) or goodness of fit (Lerner, 1982; Lerner et al., 1997) between individuals and their contexts. In this model, developing individuals are embedded within changing ecological niches, and, therefore, the match between the individual's developmental needs and what the context provides is itself dynamic. Developmental transitions can serve to improve the match and thus provide health opportunities, or they can serve to lessen the match and thus adversely affect health.

Developmental mismatches can vary considerably across culture and history. Moffitt (1993), for example, partially attributes the growth in adolescent antisocial behavior in this century to social and economic reforms that have served to keep young people in school well into their teens rather than forcing or allowing them to enter the adult world with all of its responsibilities, expectations, and opportunities. As a result, the continued nurturing support and monitoring of parents and schools conflicts with adolescents' view of themselves as independent and valuable members of society. According to Moffitt, it is precisely this mismatch that leads many young people to use drugs as part of a quest to be taken seriously.

The mechanism for the developmental mismatch model could take many forms. For example, an increased mismatch, such as an adolescent with growing needs for independence and self-expression entering a junior high school that attempts to thwart such needs, could cause the young person to become "turned off" and go elsewhere to seek fulfillment and challenge in a compensatory context (e.g., deviant peer group) that ultimately may pose increased health risks (Eccles et al., 1993). On the other hand, an increased match could serve to provide the young person with developmentally appropriate challenges and experiences, feelings of competence, and increased well-being (Schulenberg, O'Malley, Bachman, & Johnston, 2000). To the extent that we can increase the synchrony between developmental needs and contextual affordances, we should be able to diminish health risks associated with developmental transitions.

Increased Heterogeneity Model

In this model, developmental transitions are viewed as moderators of ongoing health risk status. Developmental transitions can serve to increase interindividual variability in functioning and adjustment and in this way can be viewed as important junctures along one's health status trajectory. Evidence from a variety of studies indicates that divergence increases throughout adolescence between those who cope effectively with various stressors and those who do not (Kazdin, 1993; Petersen, 1993). For example, Eccles and colleagues (1993, 1997) provide evidence to suggest that the transition to junior high is worse for young people who are already experiencing difficulties with behavior problems and adjustment to school (see also Berndt & Mekos, 1995) and likewise that those who have difficulties with the transition are likely to have increasingly severe difficulties in high school. Evidence also indicates that psychopathology, including schizophrenia and major depression, tends to manifest first during adolescence and young adulthood, suggesting that one contributing factor is likely to be ongoing and escalating difficulties with negotiating developmental transitions (Kazdin, 1993; Petersen et al., 1993).

This "pathways" perspective (Cairns & Cairns, 1994; Caspi, Elder, & Bem, 1988; Crockett & Crouter, 1995) is consistent with Erikson's (1950, 1968) psychosocial theory of life course development, in which the individual's resolution of one developmental crisis (e.g., adolescent identity vs. identity confusion) is dependent on how he or she resolved previous crises (e.g., preadolescent industry vs. inferiority) and has implications for the resolution of subsequent crises (e.g., young adulthood intimacy vs. isolation; see also Havighurst, 1952; Sullivan, 1947). There are likely to be several mechanisms that serve to exacerbate a trajectory of ongoing health risks. According to Nurmi (1997), one mechanism is self-defeating cognitive styles. Another mechanism may be a lack of social support to alter, and an abundance of support to maintain, a trajectory of ongoing risky behaviors (Brown, Dolcini, & Leventhal, 1997; Caldwell & Antonucci, 1997). The prevention implications of this model include, for example, altering self-defeating coping strategies and enhancing social networks that discourage risky behavior for youth who are following worrisome trajectories (Eggert, Thompson, Herting, & Nicholas, 1994; Palinkas, Atkins, Miller, & Ferreira, 1996). Furthermore, as with the "mismatch" model discussed previously, interventions aimed at providing adolescents with alternative challenging experiences and opportunities for success are likely to have long-term beneficial health effects.

Transition Catalyst Model

According to the fourth model, substance use and risk taking in general can be viewed as important components of negotiating certain developmental transitions. The idea that a certain amount of adolescent risk taking is normative is supported by the high prevalence rates and by evidence that it often accompanies healthy personality development (Baumrind, 1987; Shedler & Block, 1990; Silbereisen, Eyferth, & Rudinger, 1986). According to Chassin, Presson, and Sherman (1989), risk taking and deviance can serve constructive, as well as destructive, functions in adolescents' health and development (see also Jessor & Jessor, 1977; Maggs, Almeida, & Galambos, 1995; Silbereisen & Noack, 1988; Zucker, 1989). For example, risk taking appears to be an important aspect of negotiating greater autonomy from parents (Irwin & Millstein, 1992). Likewise, as Maggs (1997) demonstrates, alcohol use and binge drinking during the transition to college may help adolescents achieve valued social goals, such as making friends in a new environment (although it also threatens their safety and short- and long-term health and well-being).

According to the identity literature, experimentation with alternative identities may involve some increased risk taking. Given that failing to explore options may lead to premature identity foreclosure (Erikson, 1968; Marcia, 1994), some risk taking can be viewed as an important component of developmental transitions associated with identity formation. This highlights an important dilemma with this model with respect to intervention implications. To the extent that risk taking plays an essential role in identity formation, as well as in negotiating peer-related and other developmental transitions (Brown et al., 1997; Chassin, Tetzloff, & Hershey, 1985), attempts to eliminate risk taking may in turn have adverse consequences for identity development in particular and optimal development in general (Baumrind, 1987).

Of course, health-enhancing behaviors may also be components of negotiating developmental transitions. For example, as Bachman, Wadsworth, O'Malley, Johnston, and Schulenberg (1997) demonstrate, reducing substance use is part of the transition to marriage (see also Leonard & Rothbard, 1999).

Heightened Vulnerability to Chance Events Model

The final model is based on the role of chance in altering the courses of individuals' lives. Random, unpredicted events or occurrences can include unexpected encounters with individuals, contexts, or situations. Bandura (1982), for example, points to the case of a young man who went to look for an acquaintance living outside Los Angeles. Not realizing his friend had moved, he knocked on the door of the house to find the new home of Charles Manson and company. Invited to join the party inside, he was soon drawn into a world of unrestrained sex, drug use, and even murder. No one could have predicted that his life would take such an abrupt turn in a single day. Less dramatic but equally powerful chance events are ubiquitous: Some people meet in an elevator and end up marrying, others die from freak accidents, and so on. Yet chance events, large and small, are often less random than they may first appear (Bandura, 1998). The couple who met in an elevator likely shared lifestyles, interests, or professions that led them both to be on that elevator at that time, and both were likely to be receptive to this chance meeting.

Just as there are individual differences in receptivity to chance events, there are also intraindividual changes in this receptivity, with certain periods during the life span being more conducive to chance effects. Major developmental transitions that involve new contexts, such as the transition to college, may be particularly conducive periods because they engender heightened sensitivity to and exploratory behavior of the new context and the self in relation to the new context. Young people undergoing such transitions may seek out and be open to the effects of novel experiences. As they explore their niche in the new context, chance events may take on special significance. Thus developmental transitions can increase one's contact with novel experiences and heighten one's vulnerability to the positive and negative effects of chance events. Just as there are likely to be unexpected salutary effects that result from these significant chance events and encounters, there are likely to be some health-compromising effects, including increased substance use and increased negative consequences of such use.

Intervening in such chance events and encounters typically is viewed as being beyond the ken of prevention efforts. Nevertheless, resiliency to some of the negative effects of chance events and encounters is possible. In particular, Rutter's (1990) and Garmezy's (1983) work concerning the beneficial effects of early but limited exposure to risks suggests that some adolescents can learn to better withstand insults to their health and well-being. Similarly, programs that aim to build basic social skills (e.g., Life Skills Training; Botvin & Tortu, 1988) also may enable young people to take advantage of promising opportunities that arise by chance.

EXAMINING THE COURSE OF SUBSTANCE USE AND RELATED FACTORS

As we illustrated in the previous section, one key feature of a developmental perspective on alcohol and other drug use is the consideration of substance use in relation to the numerous developmental transitions of adolescence. Examining change and stability in substance use and related factors within individuals over time is the second key feature of a developmental perspective. We start this section with a brief discussion of the necessity for and advantages of panel research. We then consider strategies for examining change over time and include illustrations from some of our etiological and intervention research.

Why Conduct Multiwave Panel Studies?

Multiwave panel studies (in which the same individuals are followed prospectively) are expensive in terms of funding and effort, complicated in
terms of measurement and analysis, and sometimes compromised by differential attrition. So why do we need them?

At a general level, panel designs are necessary for addressing the primary goals of developmental research: the description and explanation of
intraindividual developmental change and of interindividual differences
and similarities in intraindividual developmental change (Baltes, Reese &
Nesselroade, 1977; Cairns, Cairns, Rodkin, & Xie, 1998). Panel data permit the direct identification of within-person change at the individual
rather than the group level. Developmental change may occur in smooth or
abrupt quantitative increments; or it may involve discontinuous, qualitative
transformations in which one behavior is superseded by another; or it may
involve changes in patterns of relationships among variables. Although
cross-sectional data can be used to estimate age changes at the group level,
they are inadequate to determine precisely the nature, magnitude, and
structure of such changes. Furthermore, panel data provide information
about the determinants and consequences of intraindividual change and
about individual differences in these processes. Hypotheses about time-
ordered antecedents and consequences require the relevant variables to be
measured in the sequence in which they occur. Within-time correlations
among relevant variables may in fact reflect spurious associations that are
due to a third, shared, determining variable. With longitudinal data, it becomes possible to ask whether hypothesized causes precede their effects, as
well as to examine long-term treatment outcomes, discontinuous phenomena (e.g., sleeper effects), and multidirectional processes (Rutter, 1994;
Schaie & Hertzog, 1985).

To help us address the most important questions we face about substance use etiology and intervention, following the same individuals over
several points in time represents our best (and arguably our only) strategy
(Eddy, Dishion, & Stoolmiller, 1998; Kaplan, 1995). Particularly during
adolescence, when change is the backdrop, knowing a young person's substance use at only one point in time tells us very little about the likely
course, causes, and consequences of his or her substance use (Duncan,
Alpert, Duncan, & Hops, 1997; Newcomb, Scheier, & Bentler, 1993).

Although it is far better to have two waves of data than one, panel
data that span three or more waves are especially informative. Multiple
waves of data permit the consideration of more complex mediational and
reciprocal models aimed at understanding how relationships between risk
factors and substance use unfold (Sher & Wood, 1997). In addition, multiple waves of panel data make it possible to identify different trajectories of

substance use in terms of the timing of onset and pattern of change over time, information that is essential for determining the type and severity of substance abuse problems (Babor et al., 1992; Cloninger, 1987; Zucker, 1987).

Short-term multiwave panel data are useful for examining processes among temporally proximal risk factors and substance use, especially during major developmental transitions such as the transition to college (Maggs, 1997). Longer intervals between waves make it difficult to capture the sometimes rapid changes and influences that occur during these transitions, such as making new friends and escalating binge drinking. However, long-term multiwave panel data are essential for understanding how distal influences relate to proximal ones. In particular, early delinquent activity during adolescence is one of the strongest predictors of both the early onset of substance use and later problem substance use (Dishion, Capaldi, & Yoerger, 1999; Donovan & Jessor, 1985; Kandel, 1978), and long-term longitudinal studies suggest even earlier distal influences. For example, in a longitudinal study of alcohol-related symptomatology and alcohol dependence in late adolescence and early adulthood, Moffitt, Caspi, Dickson, Silva, and Stanton (1996) traced the source of the effect found between adolescent delinquency and substance use all the way back to differences in behavioral undercontrol that were observed at age 3. This long-term follow-up of preschool-age children suggests that adolescent delinquent activity serves less as a stand-alone causative agent and more as a mediator (or ongoing extension) of earlier behavior difficulties (see also Brook & Newcomb, 1995). Without long-term panel data, this distal causal connection would be overlooked, a meaningful oversight given the alternative intervention implications.

Perhaps one of the most compelling reasons for longitudinal studies on substance use is to identify why great numbers of individuals do not develop serious substance abuse problems despite exposure to significant risk factors and, likewise, why many individuals do develop problems despite little exposure to risk factors (Rutter, 1989). The concepts of equifinality and multifinality are relevant to this point (Cicchetti & Rogosch, 1996). Equifinality refers to the multiple pathways that can lead to a similar outcome. For example, Weber, Graham, Hansen, and Flay (1989) reported that among youth with high levels of substance use in midadolescence, some had a lengthy history of persistent and severe difficulties, whereas others had only recent and moderate behavioral difficulties. In this example, the trajectory of use and the ramifications of such difficulties are substantially different (Zucker, Fitzgerald, & Moses, 1995). Multifinality pertains to multiple alternative outcomes that stem from a given initial level of adaptation. Whereas some adolescents who misuse substances are likely to experience difficulty during the transition to early adulthood, many others

exhibit patterns of misuse that will subside with the onset of early adulthood (Jessor, Donovan & Costa, 1991). Clearly, as these examples show,
relying only on a "snapshot" at one point in time to capture the multiplicity of antecedent and consequent pathways of substance use during adolescence would be inadequate at best and very likely misleading.

Strategies for Studying Individual-Level Change and Stability

There has been a perennial tension in psychology between the nomothetic
goals of science (i.e., to find general laws of behavior that apply to all) and
the idiographic goals (i.e., to describe and explain a given individual's
behavior). More than 60 years ago, Gordon Allport (1937) argued for an
intermediate position:

> There is no reason why we should not learn from every generalization
> about human nature that we can. At the same time we need to be alert for
> concepts and methods that enable us to understand patterned individuality.
> (p. 12)

Similarly, nearly 30 years ago, Jack Block (1971) stated:

> [A] greater lawfulness may be discerned (when) what is general and undif-
> ferentiated is partitioned into smaller but more homogeneous classes for
> study. . . . [T]his conceptual recognition demands a respect for the possibil-
> ity of different courses of character evolution without a denial of what in-
> deed may be universal for all persons. (p. 11)

More recently, John Nesselroade (1992) stated:

> In the study of developmental phenomena, changes over the life-span,
> which . . . can be multidirectional and multidimensional and which are . . .
> temporally and culturally embedded, demand differential representations
> of individuals' lives while recognizing generalized trends or patterns of
> changes. (p. 265)

Finding and maintaining an appropriate balance between nomothetic and
idiographic perspectives should be an important goal for developmental
and clinical methodology. Recent methodological and statistical advances
have made it possible to approach this goal.

Figure 1.2 is an adaptation of Raymond Cattell's three-dimensional
data box (1988). This cube includes three key dimensions of psychosocial
research: Persons, Variables, and Occasions. The interrelatedness of these
three dimensions has general implications for how we collect and analyze
data, including how we define and sample from "the population." That is,

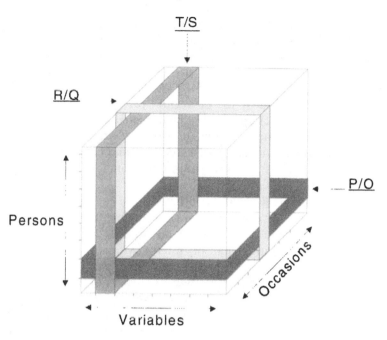

FIGURE 1.2. Adaptation of Cattell's original data box. From Cattell (1988). Copyright 1998 by Plenum Press. Adapted by permission.

populations should be thought of not only in terms of persons but also in terms of variables and occasions. This model also has specific implications for how we conceptualize and analyze individual-level change over time. These implications are considered below as we examine the three two-dimensional "slices" in Figure 1.2.

R/Q-Techniques

The R/Q slice represents a sample of variables collected from a sample of individuals at one occasion. The R-technique refers to aggregating variables across persons in order to examine interindividual differences and variability in the variables at one point in time (e.g., to examine the correlation between risk taking and substance use in a sample of adolescents). Because there is only one occasion of measurement, it is not possible to examine intraindividual change and stability prospectively over time. Nevertheless, much of what we as a field believe about the normative course of substance use and associated risk factors comes from cross-sectional R-technique studies that examine age and grade-level differences.

The Q-technique refers to aggregating persons across variables in order to identify types of people according to their common constellations of scores on variables at one point in time (e.g., to distinguish a subgroup of adolescents with high scores on both risk taking and substance use from a subgroup with high scores on risk taking and low scores on substance use). This strategy is illustrated by the powerful "person- or pattern-centered" (typically cluster analytic) approaches championed by Magnusson (Magnusson, 1997; Magnusson & Bergman, 1988), Cairns (Cairns & Cairns, 1994), and others. Nevertheless, as Nesselroade and Ghisletta (2000) indicate, this strategy results in static groupings of individuals, leaving open questions regarding intraindividual change.

Of course, multiple R/Q slices can be taken in an attempt to generalize over time or to explicitly examine change over time. However, in the case of multiwave R-technique, the focus is on stability and change in interindividual differences (rather than on interindividual differences in intraindividual change) and the static predictors of such change (e.g., in a cross-lag panel analysis). Even with more than two waves of data, the emphasis on change and stability is still in two-wave segments. In the case of multiwave Q-technique, change and stability in types or subgroups of individuals (based on constellations of scores) can be examined, for example, by conducting Q-technique analyses (e.g., cluster analyses) at two points in time and then linking the subgroups across time (Bergman, 2000). Despite a lack of emphasis on intraindividual change trajectories (see the subsequent discussion of T/S-techniques), such strategies are useful for examining types of individuals and tracking their change from one point in time to another.

P/O-Techniques

The P/O slice represents a sample of variables collected during a sample of multiple occasions (e.g., 100) from a single person. The P-technique refers to aggregating variables across occasions in order to examine how variables vary and covary over time in an individual (e.g., to examine the extent to which risk taking and substance use co-occur within a given individual), a strategy ideal for identifying moods, states, and other day-to-day changes (Nesselroade, 1992). The O-technique refers to aggregating occasions across variables in order to examine how occasions group together on variables within an individual (e.g., to examine what sorts of occasions or contexts elicit risk taking and substance use within a given individual). P/O-technique research is relatively rare in the relevant substance use literature, although Birkett and Cattell (1978) conducted a P-technique study to examine the day-to-day variability dimension in an alcohol-dependent patient. Clearly, P-technique strategies are idiographic, but they can also be made more nomothetic by conducting multiple P-technique studies and determining the extent of interindividual differences and similarities in the state dimensions (analogous steps could be taken with the O-technique). And to explicitly examine interindividual variation in intraindividual *directional* change, for instance, dynamic factor analysis (Molenaar, 1985) or pooled time-series analyses (Velicer & Colby, 1997) can be used (see also Nesselroade & Ghisletta, 2000).

T/S-Techniques

The T/S slice represents a single variable (or set of variables) collected from a sample of individuals across several occasions (a minimum of three waves, and preferably more). T- and S-techniques permit some blending of nomothetic and idiographic perspectives, providing an ideal balance between the two for many purposes.

The T-technique refers to aggregating occasions across persons in order to determine, for example, the average rate of change in the one variable (or set of variables) over time, as well as interindividual differences in the average rate of change (e.g., to examine the average trajectory of increased alcohol use during adolescence, as well as interindividual variations from the average trajectory). T-technique, as represented by growth curve modeling (Bryk & Raudenbush, 1987; Muthén & Curran, 1997; Raudenbush, in press; Willett & Sayer, 1994), allows researchers to focus on group-level and individual trajectories of change over time and to examine static and time-varying predictors of interindividual variations in the average trajectory of change (e.g., to determine whether initially high or increasing levels of risk taking contribute to a faster than average increase in substance use during adolescence). Latent transition analysis (Collins, Graham, Rousculp, & Hansen, 1997), also representative of T-technique analyses, allows for the consideration of normative qualitative (or structural level) trajectories of change over time and of interindividual variation from normative trajectories. As powerful as these T-technique strategies are for understanding group and individual trajectories of substance use and more generally the etiology and prevention of substance use (see also Curran & Muthén, 1999; Duncan et al., 1997; Maggs & Schulenberg, 1998; Sher & Wood, 1997), one important limitation from a developmental perspective is that such techniques tend to assume a single developmental "ideal" trajectory, with individual variations being viewed in terms of departures from the single developmental ideal trajectory (but see recent advances in growth mixture modeling, e.g., Muthén & Muthén, 1999).

In contrast, the S-technique assumes multiple developmental ideal trajectories. The S-technique refers to aggregating persons across occasions in order to examine what we call developmental typologies—that is, grouping individuals according to how they change over time on a developmentally important variable. By forming relatively few homogenous categories of individuals according to how they change over time, it is possible to obtain important information about distinctive patterns of change over time without becoming overwhelmed with the nearly infinite variations of individual-level change. Given this focus on grouping individuals, the S-technique is more appropriate with larger and representative samples of persons. S-technique research can be very useful when distinctly different developmental trajectories are expected, for example, in regard to theoretical groups that are hypothesized to differ in their course of substance use (Cloninger, 1987; Zucker, 1987). This strategy is also useful for examining developmental transitions when increased diversity in paths is expected (Schulenberg et al., 2000), as well as for examining longer term intervention effects in controlled experiments (Steinman & Schulenberg, 1999). Trajectory groups can be formed in a number of ways, including logical groupings, cluster analysis, and configural frequency analysis (von Eye, 1990). Recently, Nagin (Nagin & Tremblay, 1999) has advanced a semi-parametric mixture modeling procedure for locating homogenous groups (according to patterns of change in a given variable over time) and assigning individual probabilities of being in each of the groups.

The S-technique is gaining popularity in the substance-use literature (see, e.g., Barnes et al., 1998; Chassin, Presson, Sherman, & Edwards, 1991; Labouvie, Pandina, & Johnson, 1991; Schulenberg, O'Malley, Bachman, Wadsworth, & Johnston, 1996; Schulenberg, Wadsworth, O'Malley, Bachman, & Johnston, 1996; Steinman & Schulenberg, 1999; Stice, Myers, & Brown, 1998; Wills, McNamara, Vaccaro, & Hirky, 1996). To illustrate how it can be useful, we draw some examples from our own work. Using panel data from our large-scale Alcohol Misuse Prevention Study, Steinman and Schulenberg (1999) sought to identify patterns of alcohol use during early and middle adolescence (6th through 10th grades). Based on conceptual considerations and empirical analyses, they identified five trajectories of alcohol use (Figure 1.3), including early escalating use, nonescalating use, middle onset, high school onset, and rare use (some students did not exhibit a clear pattern of change over time). Similarly, based on the Monitoring the Future national panel data sets, Schulenberg and colleagues (Schulenberg, O'Malley, et al., 1996; Schulenberg, Wadsworth, et al., 1996) identified six distinct trajectories of binge drinking during the transition from adolescence to young adulthood. Five of these trajectories (chronic, decrease, increase, fling, and rare) are illustrated in Figure 1.4 (the "never" group [36%] is excluded from the figure, as well as the 10% of the sample that did not fit any trajectory group). Perhaps what is most striking in these two figures is how much infor-

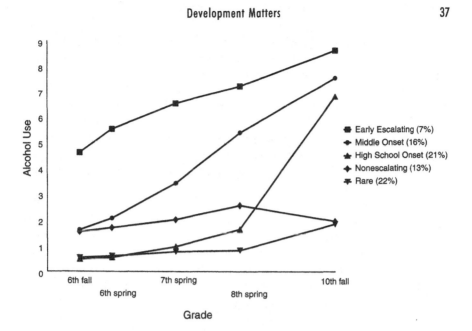

FIGURE 1.3. Alcohol use trajectories: Means at each grade. Note: *never* (14%) and *other* (8%) are not shown. Data from Steinman & Schulenberg (1999).

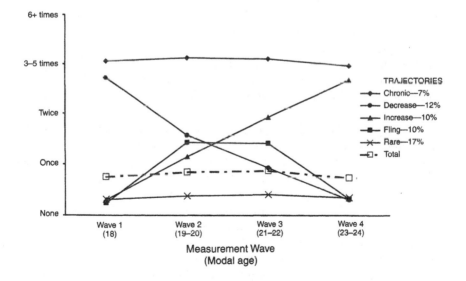

FIGURE 1.4. Mean score for 5+ drinks in a row in past 2 weeks by binge-drinking trajectory. Data from Schulenberg, O'Malley, et al. (1996).

mation is lost when considering only the normative trends of alcohol use and binge drinking during adolescence. In both figures, there are examples of equifinality (i.e., several pathways to a given outcome), including the three different pathways into heavy alcohol use at 10th grade (early escalating, middle escalating, and high school onset, Figure 1.3) and the three different pathways into low levels of binge drinking at age 24 (decrease, fling, and rare, Figure 1.4). Examples of multifinality (i.e., several alternative pathways originating from a given initial status) are also represented in many diverging trajectories (e.g., middle escalating and nonescalating in Figure 1.3; increase, fling, and rare in Figure 1.4).

Once trajectories or developmental typologies are identified, it is then possible to predict membership as a function of initial risk factors (especially among initially similar but subsequently diverging trajectories), as well as to predict from the different trajectories to various outcomes. For example, Steinman and Schulenberg (1999) found that among some of the trajectories, susceptibility to peer pressure was a stable individual characteristic that consistently distinguished different patterns of alcohol use, even prior to their divergence. Perceptions of peer alcohol use also were important across all the patterns, though only immediately prior to and after the onset of frequent drinking. Schulenberg, Wadsworth, and colleagues (1996) found that self-efficacy at Wave 1 (age 18) predicted subsequent divergence between the chronic (lower efficacy) and decrease (higher efficacy) trajectories. In addition, despite the general lack of Wave 1 predictors of the subsequent divergences among the increase, fling, and rare trajectories, the increase trajectory group was found to have more psychosocial difficulties at age 30 than the other two trajectories (Schulenberg, 1999). By using S-technique analyses, these findings offer insights into types of change patterns in alcohol use during adolescence (in contrast to a single normative change trajectory), as well as into the timing and robustness of various risk and protective mechanisms, that are not available via other analytic strategies.

As this illustrative discussion of the various techniques (along with a far-from-comprehensive list of available representative analytic strategies) shows, the data box can be a useful heuristic tool for developmentally minded researchers. Some of the distinctions drawn among the techniques may not always hold up, and, indeed, one would not want to restrict their focus to a single slice in the data box (but rather to gather data along all three dimensions). Nevertheless, the key to advancing our understanding of the etiology of and effective interventions for substance use during adolescence is a primary focus on individual trajectories of substance use, a focus that requires the inclusion of multiple occasions of data on individuals and effective analytic strategies that can move the field beyond a "two-wave at a time" view of change.

IMPLICATIONS FOR UNDERSTANDING RISK AND PROTECTIVE FACTORS

A more developmentally sensitive understanding of risk and protective factors will provide a stronger foundation for addressing fundamental questions about substance use etiology and intervention (Clayton, 1992). Much effort over the past few decades has gone into identifying and cataloguing risk and protective factors, and these successful efforts have yielded a useful, albeit overwhelming, array of relevant individual and contextual factors (Hawkins, Catalano, & Miller, 1992). Indeed, it is likely that the great majority of potential psychosocial risk or protective factors have been identified. Identifying and cataloguing salient dimensions and constructs is an essential first phase in the scientific process (Pepper, 1942). In the case of theory and research regarding risk and protective factors, the field has to continue to move to the second phase, which is specifying the processes that link risk and protective factors with substance use within individuals over time and across contexts. In this section, in an effort to assist the relevant literature in continuing to move from the first to the second phase, we offer a series of conceptual guideposts.

Antecedent–Consequent Conceptualizations of Causality

The first guidepost pertains to conceptualizations about causality in studies examining risk and protective factors.[1] Typically, correlational and quasi-experimental studies implicitly or explicitly view causality in terms of antecedent–consequent relations. That is, a causal direction (or at least temporal precedence) is either assumed in single-outcome analyses (e.g., multiple regressions in which multiple risk factors predict substance use controlling for prior substance use) or examined in cross-lagged panel analyses (e.g., in which Time 1 variables predict change over time in other variables). Often, the purpose of such analyses is to attempt to draw conclusions about the sequencing of risk factors and mediational relationships, a purpose consistent with understanding how risk and protective factors are linked over time. Yet it is important to recognize that this sequential view of causality (A causes B causes C) refers only to the normative sequence. Although it might describe what happens for most adolescents (e.g., that doing poorly in school contributes to onset of substance use), the opposite sequence is very likely to occur for some adolescents (e.g., that substance use onset contributes to drops in school performance). The failure to ac-

---

[1]Establishing causality is primarily an issue of research design, not statistical analysis. Although the randomized longitudinal experiment remains a gold standard, other designs often are necessary for practical and ethical considerations and can still yield valuable insight into causal processes.

knowledge such alternative sequences in our conceptualizations and practical implications concerning risk and protective factors can contribute to models that describe "everyone in general and no one in particular" (Lewin, 1931).

We are not suggesting that researchers abandon the role of temporal order in conceptualizations of causality. But alternative conceptualizations that focus on the diversity of causal connections deserve consideration (Cairns et al., 1998; Cloninger, Svrakic, & Svrakic, 1997; Magnusson, 1997), particularly ones that attend to reciprocal and co-occurrent relations. Indeed, determining that two variables "move together" within individuals over time may be a more powerful finding than determining that one variable seems to trigger the other in general, especially when we are focusing on risk and protective factors that are proximal to substance use.

For more distal risk and protective factors, the concepts of equifinality and multifinality are of particular importance (Cicchetti & Rogosch, 1996; Gjerde, 1995; Gottlieb, 1991). When considering how risk and protective factors might "cause" alcohol use, several different types of risk factors can lead to the same outcome (i.e., equifinality). For example, as discussed previously, among youth with high levels of binge drinking in high school, two likely pathways are represented by those with an early and enduring history of substance abuse and those who began drinking heavily in high school (Weber et al., 1989). Each of these histories reflect different developmental trajectories that involve two distinct constellations of risk and protective factors (Moffitt, 1993). With regard to multifinality, certain risk factors can also serve as protective factors for some individuals in some circumstances. A prime example of this is parental alcoholism, with children of alcoholics being at heightened risk for becoming alcoholic (Russell, 1990; Sher, 1991); nevertheless, they also have a higher than average chance of becoming abstainers. As these examples attest, efforts to design and model simple antecedent–consequent conceptions of causality may yield misleading results. That is, there may be several potential risk factors, but none are sufficient or necessary for given outcomes.

Relationship between Risk and Protective Factors

A second guidepost involves the relationship between risk and protective factors. One common approach is to view risk and protective factors as opposite ends of the same continuum. Thus a variable such as peer alcohol use can heighten one's risk for drinking if it is high or reduce one's risk if it is low. Labeling something either a risk or a protective factor merely depends on which end of the scale is emphasized. The benefit of this conceptualization is in its elegance and interpretability. It precludes the need to consider risk and protective factors separately and fits nicely into statistical models that assume linear relationships among continuous variables. Unfortunately, many studies of adolescent substance use employ these models without considering the limitations of this implicit conceptualization. Many variables—for example, depressed affect (Shedler & Block, 1990), parent–child bonding (Stein, Newcomb, & Bentler, 1987), and sociability (Chassin, Pillow, Curran, & Molina, 1993)—may have nonlinear relationships with substance use.

By describing how protective factors may moderate or buffer the effects of risk factors, Garmezy, Masten, and Tellegen (1984), Rutter (1990), Hawkins and colleagues (1992), and Brook and colleagues (1997) have offered an expanded view of the risk–protective factor relationship. According to their work, protective factors operate only in the presence of risk factors whose effects they moderate.[2] A supportive family environment, for example, might have a protective effect only in the presence of peer influences to use drugs. Without such peer influences, family environment may have no effect on an adolescent's propensity to use drugs because use is unlikely (Oetting & Beauvais, 1986).

Although this interactive model affords a more sophisticated theoretical description of risk, it is difficult to test empirically. Researchers typically rely on statistically significant interaction effects to demonstrate the moderating effects of protective factors. Yet such effects are often nonsignificant, or, when they are significant, they explain relatively little variance in the outcome (Luthar & Zigler, 1991). In addition, interaction effects in this area often fail to replicate across studies or even across subsamples within the same studies (Luthar, 1993). Rutter (1990) also warns that statistical interaction effects may not always capture the protective processes they are intended to represent. Protective factors, for instance, may not only moderate the effect of risk factors but may actually reduce the presence of risk factors to begin with. In other words, protective factors can be mediated by (as well as moderate) risk factors. So a supportive family environment, for instance, may not only lessen the effects of negative peer influences but may also reduce the presence of negative peer influences in the first place.

Robustness and Continuity of Risk and Protective Factors

Ideally, risk and protective factors predict a likely outcome in advance, providing us essential information about who is likely to encounter difficulties and who is not. Longitudinal panel studies from early childhood to young

---

[2]Garmezy and colleagues (1984) reserve the term "protective factors" for the interactive process described herein. They also account for the main effects of protective factors, but these they label as "compensatory." See Luthar (1993) for a discussion of the semantic confusion related to the inconsistent use of the term "protective factor" as either a main effect or an interactive process.

adulthood suggest that some risk and protective factors first appear during childhood or earlier, well before the onset of any substance use. Although such factors as early antisocial behavior or genetic susceptibility to substance use do not necessarily doom a child to a life of inebriation and failure (O'Connor & Rutter, 1996), they do offer researchers and clinicians early indicators of a child's heightened vulnerability. Either directly or indirectly, these factors continue to contribute to a young person's vulnerability despite the many transitions she or he will experience during adolescence and young adulthood (Moffitt, 1993).

Risk and protective factors can be grouped according to whether they are robust (i.e., predict current levels of and future changes in substance use), emergent (i.e., predict future changes in, but not current levels of, substance use), or concurrent (i.e., predict current levels of, but not changes in, substance use). For example, Schulenberg, Wadsworth, and colleagues (1996) found that gender (male) and the motivation of drinking "to get drunk" at age 18 were robust risk factors because both predicted current binge drinking, as well as increased binge drinking during the transition to young adulthood. In addition, they found that general self-efficacy at age 18 was an emergent protective factor because, although it did not predict current binge drinking, it did predict less drinking during the transition to young adulthood.

In longitudinal studies of substance use that spanned the transition to young adulthood, many risk and protective factors are found to be only concurrent (Bates & Labouvie, 1997; Gore, Aseltine, Colten, & Lin, 1997; Schulenberg, Wadsworth, et al., 1996), which is not surprising given the difficulties of predicting change over time and the fact that risk and protective factors also change over time. It is important to distinguish between two types of concurrent risk and protective factors. *Moving concurrent* risk and protective factors change in unison with changes in substance use and reflect the continuous association of these variables (Kandel & Raveis, 1989). For example, Schulenberg, Wadsworth, and colleagues (1996) found that risk taking is a moving concurrent risk factor for binge drinking during the transition to young adulthood; that is, risk taking is related to binge drinking throughout adolescence and young adulthood. Moving concurrent factors also may represent proximal influences on substance use that appear to be concurrent because the interval between waves of data collection is too long. *Developmentally limited* risk and protective factors cease to change or change independently from substance use. That is, they are of importance for only a limited time period. In Schulenberg, Wadsworth, and colleagues' (1996) study, for example, overt hostility was associated with binge drinking in high school but not during young adulthood, suggesting some discontinuity in the web of influences related to this behavior.

An important question concerning moving concurrent risk and protective factors is whether it is appropriate to term such variables "risk and protective factors" if they fail to precede substance use. We believe it is appropriate to the extent that these variables can be considered proximal to substance use, in other words, that they mediate the effects of more distal influences on substance use (cf. Petraitis, Flay, & Miller, 1995). Oetting and Beauvais (1986), for example, argue that virtually all risk factors for substance use operate by increasing an adolescent's likelihood of participating in a group of substance-using peers. Thus more distal influences, such as feeling alienated or suffering from an unsupportive family environment, may only increase substance use to the extent that they lead individuals to join and actively participate in peer groups who use drugs.

The constellation of risk and protective factors that move together over time with substance use also may reflect the reciprocal nature of their relationship. Just as high self-efficacy in refusal skills, for example, can protect against substance use, abstaining from substances may increase self-efficacy in refusal skills. The same phenomenon exists for more distal influences as well. Personality traits that contribute to the initiation and development of a pattern of substance abuse can be exacerbated once an individual begins using drugs (Shedler & Block, 1990). So long as these relationships remain intact, individuals likely will maintain a developmental trajectory that continues to elicit substance use.

INTERVENTION IMPLICATIONS OF DEVELOPMENTAL PERSPECTIVE

From a developmental perspective, two primary goals of intervention are to (1) redirect potentially risky trajectories, such that unhealthy behavioral patterns are replaced by more positive ones; and (2) alter the web of influence, such that initial risk factors lose their impact and do not inevitably lead to undesirable outcomes (Maggs et al., 1997; Schulenberg & Maggs, 1999).

To achieve these two goals, universal, targeted, and selected interventions may be employed. At the population level, it is essential to reduce risky behaviors that become widely prevalent during the adolescent years, such as binge drinking, unprotected sex, and unsafe driving. However, in addition to undertaking universal interventions that aim to promote healthy behaviors among all adolescents, we should give particular attention to those individuals who are already manifesting signs of problematic behavioral trajectories. Targeted and selected interventions may be necessary to assist adolescents to quit smoking, to successfully parent an unplanned child, or to finish high school after dropping out.

Strategically, developmental transitions may provide opportune windows for successful intervention. As noted earlier in this chapter, developmental transitions can be stressful due to powerful needs to adapt to changes in the environment, in the individual, and in their interaction. Thus these periods in the life course represent potential times of vulnerability. At the same time, change and discontinuity represent opportunities for individuals to develop new healthy habits, skills, and relationships. For example, the move from high school to college may allow an adolescent who was a frequent binge drinker to make new friends who have more healthful and balanced social interactions. In this way, developmental transitions may be sensitive periods for intervention; programmers can take advantage of these naturally occurring windows of disequilibrium.

A developmental perspective also reminds us of the importance of taking the long view on intervention and health promotion. Positive short-term effects of preventive or clinical efforts are certainly of consequence, particularly as they relate to avoiding immediate health risks. However, when such efforts produce enduring changes, the long-term impact is of a much greater magnitude (Eddy et al., 1998). It is also often the case that no measurable changes in behavior are visible immediately after the conclusion of a preventive intervention, for example, a middle school program to prevent escalations in substance use during adolescence (Dielman, 1994). However, minor alterations in the slope of a developmental trajectory can result in consequential changes as they accumulate over a period of years (Kellam & Rebok, 1992). This important long-term impact would be missed if data were collected only at the time of the program.

Finally, intervention research has much to offer developmental theory and research by providing opportunities to address fundamental questions about causal relationships in adolescent development in general and substance use in particular. Etiological theories can be put to rigorous test by attempts to alter the constellation of risk factors and observing whether hypothesized changes in targeted behaviors occur (Bronfenbrenner, 1979; Coie et al., 1993; Dishion, McCord, & Poulin, 1999; Flay & Petraitis, 1994; Kellam & Rebok, 1992; MacKinnon, 1994).

SUMMARY AND CONCLUSIONS

As we have discussed in this chapter, alcohol and other drug use among young people is embedded within the many developmental transitions that take place during adolescence and the transition to young adulthood. This makes it essential to examine substance use in relation to adolescents' changing lives and changing contexts, as well as to follow individuals over time. Developmental transitions during adolescence and young adulthood include the fundamental changes of pubertal and cognitive development, affiliative transitions, achievement transitions, and identity transitions. As we have argued, increased health risks, including substance use, are best understood in relation to these developmental transitions. We presented five interrelated conceptual models that consider the ways in which developmental transitions relate to increased health risks, including (1) the overload model (health risks are viewed as a potential but not inevitable result of experiencing multiple developmental transitions); (2) the developmental mismatch model (health risks and opportunities are viewed as a result of the impact of developmental transitions on the developmental match or goodness of fit between individuals and their contexts); (3) the increased heterogeneity model (developmental transitions are viewed as moderators of ongoing health risk status); (4) the transition catalyst model (substance use and risk taking in general can be viewed as important components of negotiating certain developmental transitions); and (5) the heightened vulnerability to chance events model (developmental transitions can increase effects of chance events).

The understanding of how substance use relates to developmental transitions, including how individual characteristics and contextual features serve to moderate these relationships, offers an important foundation for attempts to effect lasting change in young people. The many transitions that occur during adolescence represent windows of opportunity to intervene to change courses of behavior that are already changing. By redirecting potentially risky trajectories, successful developmental interventions can not only assist in the resolution of immediate difficulties but also set the stage for continued enhanced health and well-being across the life span. Furthermore, intervention research can assist in the understanding of basic developmental processes. By following the reverberations of interventions over time, we can gain a better understanding about what, in the naturally occurring environment, causes such reverberations.

Few scientists who conduct prevention research would argue that there exists a single "magic bullet" that can inoculate all young people against substance use. Instead, because there are several potential paths into substance use initiation and escalation, effective prevention programs are likely to be those that are prepared to block or alter as many of these potential paths as possible (Howard, Boyd, & Zucker, 1995; Maggs et al., 1997).

ACKNOWLEDGMENTS

This chapter is based on an invited paper presented by the first author at the National Conference on Adolescents, Alcohol, and Substance Abuse: Reaching Teens through Brief Intervention, sponsored by the Center for Alcohol and Addiction Studies, Brown University, held in Newport, Rhode Island, October 1998. Effort on this chapter was funded in part by a grant from the National Institute on Alcohol Abuse and Alcoholism (No. AA06324). We wish to thank Virginia Laetz and Tanya Hart for their assistance with this manuscript and the editors and reviewers for their helpful comments on previous drafts.

REFERENCES

Allport, G. W. (1937). *Pattern and growth in personality.* New York: Holt, Rinehart & Winston.

Arnett, J. J. (1999). Adolescent storm and stress, reconsidered. *American Psychologist, 54,* 317–326.

Babor, T. F., Hofmann, M., DelBoca, F. K., Hesselbrock, V. M., Meyer, R. E., Dolinsky, Z. S., & Rounsaville, B. (1992). Types of alcoholics: 1. Evidence for an empirically derived typology based on indicators of vulnerability and severity. *Archives of General Psychiatry, 49,* 599–608.

Bachman, J., Wadsworth, K. N., O'Malley, P. M., Johnston, L. D., & Schulenberg, J. (1997). *Smoking, drinking, and drug use in young adulthood: The impact of new freedoms and new responsibilities.* Mahwah, NJ: Erlbaum.

Baer, J. S. (1993). Etiology and secondary prevention of alcohol problems with young adults. In J. S. Baer, G. M. Marlatt, & R. J. McMahon (Eds.), *Addictive behaviors across the life span: Prevention, treatment, and policy issues* (pp. 111–137). Newbury Park, CA: Sage.

Baltes, P. B. (1987). Theoretical propositions of life-span developmental psychology: On the dynamics between growth and decline. *Developmental Psychology, 23,* 611–626.

Baltes, P. B., Cornelius, S. W., & Nesselroade, J. R. (1979). Cohort effects in developmental psychology. In J. R. Nesselroade & P. B. Baltes (Eds.), *Longitudinal research in the study of behavior and development* (pp. 61–88). New York: Academic Press.

Baltes, P. B., Reese, H. W., & Nesselroade, J. R. (1977). *Life-span developmental psychology: Introduction to research methods.* Hillsdale, NJ: Erlbaum.

Bandura, A. (1982). The psychology of chance encounters and life paths. *American Psychologist, 37,* 747–755.

Bandura, A. (1998). Exploration of fortuitous determinants of life paths. *Psychological Inquiry, 9,* 95–98.

Barnes, G. M., Hoffman, J. H., Dintcheff, B. A., Farrell, M. P., Uhteg, L., & Welte, J. (1998, June). *Predictors of alcohol use trajectories using six waves of data.* Paper presented at the Annual Scientific Meeting of the Research Society on Alcoholism, Hilton Head, SC.

Bates, M. E., & Labouvie, E. W. (1997). Adolescent risk factors and the prediction of persistent alcohol and drug use into adulthood. *Alcoholism: Clinical and Experimental Research, 21,* 944–950.

Baumrind, D. (1987). A developmental perspective on adolescent risk taking in contemporary America. In C. E. Irwin, Jr. (Ed.), *Adolescent social behavior and health* (pp. 93–125). San Francisco: Jossey-Bass.

Benedict, R. (1950). *Patterns of culture*. New York: New American Library.

Bergman, L. R. (2000). The application of a person-oriented approach: Types and clusters. In L. R. Bergman & R. B. Cairns (Eds.), *Developmental science and the holistic approach* (pp. 137–154). Mahwah, NJ: Erlbaum.

Berndt, T. J. (1982). The features and effects of friendship in early adolescence. *Child Development, 53*, 1447–1460.

Berndt, T. J., & Mekos, D. (1995). Adolescents' perceptions of the stressful and desirable aspects of the transition to junior high school. *Journal of Research on Adolescence, 5*, 123–142.

Birkett, H., & Cattell, R. B. (1978). Diagnosis of the dynamic roots of a clinical symptom by P-technique: A case of episodic alcoholism. *Multivariate Experimental Clinical Research, 3*, 173–194.

Block, J. (1971). *Lives through time*. Berkeley, CA: Bancroft Books.

Blos, P. (1970). *The young adolescent: Clinical studies*. New York: The Free Press.

Botvin, G. J., & Tortu, S. (1988). Preventing adolescent substance abuse through life skill training. In R. H. Price, E. I. Cowen, R. P. Lorion, & J. R McKay (Eds.), *Fourteen ounces of prevention: A casebook for practitioners* (pp. 98–110). Washington, DC: American Psychological Association.

Bronfenbrenner, U. (1979). *The ecology of human development: Experiments by nature and design*. Cambridge, MA: Harvard University Press.

Bronfenbrenner, U., & Crouter, A. C. (1982). Work and family through time and space. In S. B. Kamerman & C. D. Hayes (Eds.), *Families that work: Children in a changing world* (pp. 39–83). Washington, DC: National Academy of Sciences.

Brook, J. S., Balka, E. B., Gursen, M. D., Brook, D. W., Shapiro, J., & Cohen, P. (1997). Young adults' drug use: A 17-year longitudinal inquiry of antecedents. *Psychological Reports, 80*, 1235–1251.

Brook, J. S., & Newcomb, M. D. (1995). Childhood aggression and unconventionality: Impact on later academic achievement, drug use, and workforce involvement. *Journal of Genetic Psychology, 156*, 393–410.

Brooks-Gunn, J., & Paikoff, R. L. (1993). Sex is a gamble, kissing is a game: Adolescent sexuality and health promotion. In S. G. Millstein, A. C. Petersen, & E. O. Nightingale (Eds.), *Promoting the health of adolescents: New directions for the twenty-first century* (pp. 180–208). New York: Oxford University Press.

Brooks-Gunn, J., & Paikoff, R. L. (1997). Sexuality and developmental transitions during adolescence. In J. Schulenberg, J. Maggs, & K. Hurrelmann (Eds.), *Health risks and developmental transitions during adolescence* (pp. 190–219). New York: Cambridge University Press.

Brooks-Gunn, J., & Reiter, E. O. (1990). The role of pubertal processes. In S. S. Feldman & G. R. Elliott (Eds.), *At the threshold: The developing adolescent* (pp. 16–53). Cambridge, MA: Harvard University Press.

Brown, B. B., Dolcini, M. M., & Leventhal, A. (1997). Transformations in peer relationships at adolescence: Implications for health-related behavior. In J. Schulenberg, J. L. Maggs, & K. Hurrelmann (Eds.), *Health risks and developmental transitions during adolescence* (pp. 161–189). New York: Cambridge University Press.

Bryk, A. S., & Raudenbush, S. W. (1987). Application of hierarchical linear models to assessing change. *Psychological Bulletin, 101,* 147–158.

Cairns, R. B., & Cairns, B. D. (1994). *Lifelines and risks: Pathways of youth in our time.* New York: Cambridge University Press.

Cairns, R. B., Cairns, B. D., Rodkin, P., & Xie, H. (1998). New directions in developmental research: Models and methods. In R. Jessor (Ed.), *New perspectives on adolescent risk behavior* (pp. 13–40). New York: Cambridge University Press.

Caldwell, C. H., & Antonucci, T. C. (1997). Childbearing during adolescence: Mental health risks and opportunities. In J. Schulenberg, J. L. Maggs, & K. Hurrelmann (Eds.), *Health risks and developmental transitions during adolescence* (pp. 220–245). New York: Cambridge University Press.

Caspi, A., Elder, G. H., Jr., & Bem, D. J. (1988). Moving away from the world: Life-course patterns of shy children. *Developmental Psychology, 24,* 824–831.

Caspi, A., & Moffitt, T. E. (1993). When do individual differences matter? A paradoxical theory of personality coherence. *Psychological Inquiry, 4,* 247–271.

Cattell, R. B. (1988). The data box: Its ordering of total resources in terms of possible relational systems. In J. R. Nesselroade & R. B. Cattell (Eds.), *Handbook of multivariate experimental psychology* (2nd ed., pp. 69–130). New York: Plenum Press.

Chassin, L., Pillow, D. R., Curran, P. J., & Molina, B. S. (1993). Relation of parental alcoholism to early adolescent substance use: A test of three mediating mechanisms. *Journal of Abnormal Psychology, 102,* 3–19.

Chassin, L., Presson, C. C., & Sherman, S. J. (1989). "Constructive" vs. "destructive" deviance in adolescent heath-related behaviors. *Journal of Youth and Adolescence, 18,* 245–262.

Chassin, L., Presson, C. C., Sherman, S. J., & Edwards, D. A. (1991). Four pathways to young-adult smoking status: Adolescent social-psychological antecedents in a midwestern community sample. *Health Psychology, 10,* 409–418.

Chassin, L., Tetzloff, C., & Hershey, M. (1985). Self-image and social-image factors in adolescent alcohol use. *Journal of Studies on Alcohol, 46,* 39–47.

Cicchetti, D. & Rogosch, F. A. (1996). Equifinality and multifinality in developmental psychopathology. *Development and Psychopathology, 8,* 597–600.

Clayton, R. R. (1992). Transitions in drug use: Risk and protective factors. In M. D. Glantz & R. Pickens (Eds.), *Vulnerability to drug use* (pp. 15–51). Washington, DC: American Psychological Association.

Cloninger, C. R. (1987). Neurogenetic adaptive mechanisms and alcoholism. *Science, 236,* 410–416.

Cloninger, C. R., Svrakic, N. M., & Svrakic, D. M. (1997). Role of personality self-organization in development of mental order and disorder. *Development and Psychopathology, 9,* 881–906.

Coie, J. D., Watt, N. F., West, S. G., Hawkins, J. D., Asarnow, J. R., Markman, H. J., Ramey, S. L., Shure, M. B., & Long, B. (1993). The science of prevention: A conceptual framework and some directions for a national research program. *American Psychologist, 48,* 1013–1022.

Coleman, J. (1978). Current contradictions in adolescent theory. *Journal of Youth and Adolescence, 7,* 1–11.

Collins, L. M., Graham, J. W., Rousculp, S. S., & Hansen, W. B. (1997). Heavy caffeine use and the beginning of the substance use onset process: An illustration of latent transition analysis. In K. J. Bryant, M. Windle, & S. G. West (Eds.), *The science of prevention: Methodological advances from alcohol and substance abuse research* (pp. 79–99). Washington, DC: American Psychological Association.

Compas, B. E. (1993). Promoting positive mental health during adolescence. In S. G. Millstein, A. C. Petersen, & E. O. Nightingale (Eds.), *Promoting the health of adolescents: New directions for the twenty-first century* (pp. 159–179). New York: Oxford University Press.

Compas, B. E. (1995). Promoting successful competence during adolescence. In M. Rutter (Ed.), *Psychosocial disturbances in young people: Challenges for prevention* (pp. 247–273). New York: Cambridge University Press.

Crockett, L. J. (1997). Cultural, historical, and subcultural contexts of adolescence: Implications for health and development. In J. Schulenberg, J. L. Maggs, & K. Hurrelmann (Eds.), *Health risks and developmental transitions during adolescence* (pp. 23–53). New York: Cambridge University Press.

Crockett, L. J., & Crouter, A. C. (Eds.). (1995). *Pathways through adolescence: Individual development in relation to social contexts*. Mahwah, NJ: Erlbaum.

Curran, P. J., & Muthén, B. O. (1999). The application of latent curve analysis to testing developmental theories in intervention research. *American Journal of Community Psychology, 27*, 567–595.

Damphousse, K. R., & Kaplan, H. B. (1998). Intervening processes between adolescent drug use and psychological distress: An examination of the self-medication hypothesis. *Social Behavior and Personality, 26*, 115–130.

Dielman, T. E. (1994). School-based research on the prevention of adolescent alcohol use and misuse: Methodological issues and advances. *Journal of Research on Adolescence, 4*, 271–293.

Dishion, T. J., Capaldi, D. M., & Yoerger, K. (1999). Middle childhood antecedents to progressions in male adolescent substance use: An ecological analysis of risk and protection. *Journal of Adolescent Research, 14*, 175–205.

Dishion, T. J., McCord, J., & Poulin, F. (1999). When interventions harm: Peer groups and problem behavior. *American Psychologist, 54*, 755–764.

Donovan, J. E., & Jessor, R. (1985). Structure of problem behavior in adolescence and young adulthood. *Journal of Consulting and Clinical Psychology, 53*, 890–904.

Duncan, S. C., Alpert, A., Duncan, T. E., & Hops, H. (1997). Adolescent alcohol use development and young adult outcomes. *Drug and Alcohol Dependence, 49*, 39–48.

Eccles, J. S., Lord, S. E., Roeser, R. W., Barber, B. L., & Jozefowicz, D. M. H. (1997). The association of school transitions in early adolescence with developmental trajectories through high school. In J. Schulenberg, J. L. Maggs, & K. Hurrelmann (Eds.), *Health risks and developmental transitions during adolescence* (pp. 283–320). New York: Cambridge University Press.

Eccles, J. S., Midgley, C., Wigfield, A., Buchanan, C. M., Reuman, D., Flanagan, C., & Mac Iver, D. (1993). Development during adolescence: The impact of stage-environment fit on young adolescents' experiences in schools and in families. *American Psychologist, 48*, 90–101.

Eddy, J. M., Dishion, T. J., & Stoolmiller, M. (1998). The analysis of intervention change in children and families: Methodological and conceptual issues embedded in intervention studies. *Journal of Abnormal Child Psychology, 26,* 53–69.

Eggert, L. L., Thompson, E. A., Herting, J. R., & Nicholas, L. J. (1994). Preventing adolescent drug abuse and high school dropout through an intensive school-based social network development program. *American Journal of Health Promotion, 8,* 202–215.

Elder, G. H., Jr. (1974). *Children of the Great Depression: Social change life experience.* Chicago: University of Chicago Press.

Erikson, E. H. (1950). *Childhood and society.* New York: Norton.

Erikson, E. H. (1968). *Identity, youth and crisis.* New York: Norton.

Featherman, D. L. (1983). Life-span perspectives in social science research. In P. B. Baltes & O. G. Brim, Jr. (Eds.), *Life-span development and behavior* (Vol. 5, pp. 1–59). New York: Academic Press.

Flay, B., & Petraitis, J. (1994). The theory of triadic influence: A new theory of health behavior with implications for preventive interventions. *Advances in Medical Sociology, 4,* 19–44.

Freud, A. (1958). Adolescence. *Psychoanalytic Study of the Child, 13,* 255–278.

Friedman, H. L. (1993). Adolescent social development: A global perspective. *Journal of Adolescent Health, 14,* 588–594.

Galambos, N. L., & Ehrenberg, M. F. (1997). The family as health risk and opportunity: A focus on divorce and working families. In J. Schulenberg, J. L. Maggs, & K. Hurrelmann (Eds.), *Health risks and developmental transitions during adolescence* (pp. 139–160). New York: Cambridge University Press.

Garmezy, N. (1983). Stressors of childhood. In N. Garmezy & M. Rutter (Eds.), *Stress, coping, and development in children* (pp. 43–84). New York: McGraw-Hill.

Garmezy, N., Masten, A. S., & Tellegen, A. (1984). The study of stress and competence in children: A building block for developmental psychopathology. *Child Development, 55,* 97–111.

Gjerde, P. F. (1995). Alternative pathways to chronic depressive symptoms in young adults: Gender differences in developmental trajectories. *Child Development, 66,* 1277–1300.

Gore, S., Aseltine, R., Jr., Colten, M. E., & Lin, B. (1997). Life after high school: Development, stress, and well-being. In I. H. Gotlib (Ed.), *Stress and adversity over the life course: Trajectories and turning points* (pp. 197–214). New York: Cambridge University Press.

Gottlieb, G. (1991). Experiential canalization of behavioral development: Theory. *Developmental Psychology, 27,* 4–13.

Graber, J. A., Brooks-Gunn, J., & Galen, B. R. (1998). Betwixt and between: Sexuality in the context of adolescent transitions. In R. Jessor (Ed.), *New perspectives on adolescent risk behavior* (pp. 270–316). New York: Cambridge University Press.

Hall, G. S. (1916). *Adolescence* (Vols. 1–2). New York: Appleton.

Hamburg, D. A., Millstein, S. G., Mortimer, A. M., Nightingale, E. O., & Petersen, A. C. (1993). Adolescent health promotion in the twenty-first century: Current frontiers and new directions. In S. G. Millstein, A. C. Petersen, & E. O. Nightingale (Eds.), *Promoting the health of adolescents: New directions for the twenty-first century* (pp. 375–388). New York: Oxford University Press.

Havighurst, R. (1952). *Developmental tasks and education.* New York: McKay.

Hawkins, J. D., Catalano, R. F., & Miller, J. Y. (1992). Risk and protective factors for alcohol and other drug problems in adolescence and early adulthood: Implications for substance abuse prevention. *Psychological Bulletin, 112,* 64–105.

Howard, J., Boyd, G. M., & Zucker, R. A. (1995). An overview of the issues. In G. M. Boyd, J. Howard, & R. A. Zucker (Eds.), *Alcohol problems among adolescents: Current directions in prevention research* (pp. 1–12). Hillsdale, NJ: Erlbaum.

Irwin, C. E., Jr., & Millstein, S. G. (1986). Biopsychosocial correlates of risk-taking behaviors during adolescence. *Journal of Adolescent Health Care, 7,* 825–956.

Irwin, C. E., Jr., & Millstein, S. G. (1992). Risk-taking behaviors and biopsychosocial development during adolescence. In E. J. Susman, L. V. Feagans, & W. J. Ray (Eds.), *Emotion, cognition, health, and development in children and adolescents* (pp. 75–102). Hillsdale, NJ: Erlbaum.

Jessor, R. (1984). Adolescent development and behavioral health. In J. D. Matarazzo & C. L. Perry (Eds.), *Behavioral health: A handbook of health enhancement and disease prevention* (pp. 69–90). New York: Wiley.

Jessor, R. (1993). Successful adolescent development among youth in high-risk settings. *American Psychologist, 48,* 117–126.

Jessor, R., Donovan, J. E., & Costa, F. M. (1991). *Beyond adolescence: Problem behavior and young adult development.* New York: Cambridge University Press.

Jessor, R., & Jessor, S. L. (1977). *Problem behavior and psychological development: A longitudinal study of youth.* New York: Academic Press.

Johnson, P. B., & Johnson, H. L. (1996). Children's beliefs about the social consequences of drinking and refusing to drink. *Journal of Alcohol and Drug Education, 41,* 34–43.

Johnston, L. D., O'Malley, P. M., & Bachman, J. G. (1998). *National survey results on drug use from the Monitoring the Future Study, 1975–97.* Rockville, MD: National Institute on Drug Abuse.

Kandel, D. B. (1978). Homophily, selection, and socialization in adolescent friendships. *American Journal of Sociology, 84,* 427–436.

Kandel, D. B., & Raveis, V. H. (1989). Cessation of illicit drug use in young adulthood. *Archives of General Psychiatry, 46,* 109–116.

Kaplan, H. B. (1995). Contemporary themes and emerging directions in longitudinal research on deviant behavior. In H. B. Kaplan (Ed.), *Drugs, crime and other deviant adaptations: Longitudinal studies* (pp. 233–241). New York: Plenum Press.

Kazdin, A. E. (1993). Adolescent mental health: Prevention and treatment programs. *American Psychologist, 48,* 127–141.

Kellam, S. G., & Rebok, G. W. (1992). Building developmental and etiological theory through epidemiologically based preventive intervention trials. In J. McCord & R. E. Tremblay (Eds.), *Preventing antisocial behavior: Interventions from birth through adolescence* (pp. 162–195). New York: Guilford Press.

Labouvie, E. W., Pandina, R. J., & Johnson, V. (1991). Developmental trajectories of substance use in adolescence: Differences and predictors. *International Journal of Behavioral Development, 14,* 305–328.

Leonard, K. E., & Rothbard, J. C. (1999). Alcohol and the marriage effect. *Journal of Studies on Alcohol, 13,* 139–146.

Lerner, R. M. (1982). Children and adolescents as producers of their own development. *Developmental Review, 2,* 342–370.

Lerner, R. M. (1985). Individual and context in developmental psychology: Conceptual and theoretical issues. In J. R. Nesselroade & A. von Eye (Eds.), *Individual development and social change: Explanatory analysis* (pp. 155–187). New York: Academic Press.

Lerner, R. M., Ostrom, C. W., & Freel, M. A. (1997). Preventing health-compromising behaviors among youth and promoting their positive development: A developmental contextual perspective. In J. Schulenberg, J. L. Maggs, & K. Hurrelmann (Eds.), *Health risks and developmental transitions during adolescence* (pp. 498–521). New York: Cambridge University Press.

Lewin, K. (1931). Environmental forces. In C. Murchison (Ed.), *Handbook of child psychology* (2nd ed., pp. 590–625). Worcester, MA: Clark University Press.

Lewin, K. (1939). The field theory approach to adolescence. *American Journal of Sociology, 44,* 868–897.

Luthar, S. S. (1993). Annotation: Methodological and conceptual issues in research on childhood resilience. *Journal of Child Psychology and Psychiatry, 34,* 441–453.

Luthar, S. S., & Zigler, E. (1991). Vulnerability and competence: A review of the research on resilience in childhood. *American Journal of Orthopsychiatry, 61,* 6–22.

MacKinnon, D. P. (1994). Analysis of mediating variables in prevention and intervention research. In A. Cazeres & L. A. Beatty (Eds.), *Scientific methods for prevention research* (NIDA Monograph No. 139, pp. 127–154). Rockville, MD: National Institute on Drug Abuse.

Maggs, J. L. (1997). Alcohol use and binge drinking as goal-directed action during the transition to postsecondary education. In J. Schulenberg, J. L. Maggs, & K. Hurrelmann (Eds.), *Health risks and developmental transitions during adolescence* (pp. 345–371). New York: Cambridge University Press.

Maggs, J. L., Almeida, D. M., & Galambos, N. L. (1995). Risky business: The paradoxical meaning of problem behavior for young adolescents. *Journal of Early Adolescence, 15,* 339–357.

Maggs, J. L., & Schulenberg, J. (1998). Reasons to drink and not to drink: Altering trajectories of drinking through an alcohol misuse prevention program. *Applied Developmental Science, 2,* 48–60.

Maggs, J. L., Schulenberg, J., & Hurrelmann, K. (1997). Developmental transitions during adolescence: Health promotion implications. In J. Schulenberg, J. L. Maggs, & K. Hurrelmann (Eds.), *Health risks and developmental transitions during adolescence* (pp. 522–546). New York: Cambridge University Press.

Magnusson, D. (Ed.). (1997). *The lifespan development of individuals: Behavioral, neurobiological, and psychosocial perspectives: A synthesis.* New York: Cambridge University Press.

Magnusson, D., & Bergman, L. R. (1988). Individual and variable-based approaches to longitudinal research on early risk factors. In M. Rutter (Ed.), *Studies of psychosocial risk* (pp. 45–61). Cambridge, England: Cambridge University Press.

Marcia, J. (1994). Identity and psychotherapy. In S. L. Archer (Ed.), *Interventions for adolescent identity development* (pp. 29–46). Thousand Oaks, CA: Sage.

Mead, M. (1950). *Coming of age in Samoa.* New York: New American Library.

Mechanic, D. (1983). Adolescent health and illness behavior: Review of the literature and a new hypothesis for the study of stress. *Journal of Human Stress, 9*, 4–13.

Millstein, S. G., Petersen, A. C., & Nightingale, E. O. (Eds.). (1993). *Promoting the health of adolescents: New directions for the twenty-first century.* New York: Oxford University Press.

Moffitt, T. E. (1993). Adolescence-limited and life-course-persistent antisocial behavior: A developmental taxonomy. *Psychological Review, 100*, 674–701.

Moffitt, T. E., Caspi, A., Dickson, N., Silva, P., & Stanton, W. (1996). Childhood-onset versus adolescent-onset antisocial conduct problems in males: Natural history from ages 3 to 18 years. *Development and Psychopathology, 8*, 399–424.

Molenaar, P. C. M. (1985). A dynamic factor model for the analysis of multivariate time series. *Psychometrika, 50*, 181–202.

Muthén, B. O., & Curran, P. J. (1997). General longitudinal modeling of individual differences in experimental designs: A latent variable framework for analysis and power estimation. *Psychological Methods, 2*, 371–402.

Muthén, B., & Muthén, L. K. (1999). *Integrating person-centered and variable-centered analyses: Growth mixture modeling with latent trajectory classes.* Unpublished manuscript, University of California at Los Angeles.

Muuss, R. E. (1996). *Theories of adolescence* (6th ed.). New York: Random House.

Nagin, D. S., & Tremblay, R. E. (1999). Trajectories of boys' physical aggression, opposition, and hyperactivity on the path to physically violent and nonviolent juvenile delinquency. *Child Development, 70*, 1181–1196.

Nesselroade, J. R. (1992). Adult personality development: Issues in assessing constancy and change. In R. A. Zucker, A. I. Rabin, J. Aronoff, & S. Frank (Eds.), *Personality structure in the life course* (pp. 221–275). New York: Springer.

Nesselroade, J. R., & Ghisletta, P. (2000). Beyond static concepts in modeling behavior. In L. R. Bergman & R. B. Cairns (Eds.), *Developmental science and the holistic approach* (pp. 121–135). Mahwah, NJ: Erlbaum.

Newcomb, M. D., Scheier, L. M., & Bentler, P. M. (1993). Effects of adolescent drug use on adult mental health: A prospective study of a community sample. *Experimental and Clinical Psychopharmacology, 1*, 215–241.

Nurmi, J. E. (1993). Adolescent development in an age-graded context: The role of personal beliefs, goals, and strategies in the tackling of developmental tasks and standards. *International Journal of Behavioral Development, 16*, 169–189.

Nurmi, J. E. (1997). Self-definition and mental health during adolescence and young adulthood. In J. Schulenberg, J. L. Maggs, & K. Hurrelmann (Eds.), *Health risks and developmental transitions during adolescence* (pp. 395–419). New York: Cambridge University Press.

O'Connor, T. G., & Rutter, M. (1996). Risk mechanisms in development: Some conceptual and methodological considerations. *Developmental Psychology, 32*, 787–795.

Oetting, E. R., & Beauvais, F. (1986). Peer cluster theory: Drugs and the adolescent. *Journal of Counseling and Development, 65*, 17–22.

Offer, D., Ostrov, E., & Howard, K. I. (1981). *The adolescent: A psychological self-portrait.* New York: Basic Books.

Palinkas, L. A., Atkins, C. J., Miller, C., & Ferreira, D. (1996). Social skills training for drug prevention in high-risk female adolescents. *Preventive Medicine, 25,* 692–701.

Pandina, R. J., Labouvie, E. W., Johnson, V., & White, H. R. (1990). The relationship between alcohol and marijuana use and competence in adolescence. *Journal of Health and Social Policy, 1,* 89–108.

Pepper, S. C. (1942). *World hypotheses: A study of evidence.* Berkeley: University of California Press.

Petersen, A. C. (1993). Creating adolescents: The role of context and process in developmental trajectories. *Journal of Research on Adolescence, 3,* 1–18.

Petersen, A. C., Compas, B., Brooks-Gunn, J., Stemmler, M., Ey, S., & Grant, K. (1993). Depression in adolescence. *American Psychologist, 48,* 155–168.

Petersen, A. C., & Leffert, N. (1995). What is special about adolescence? In M. Rutter (Ed.), *Psychosocial disturbances in young people: Challenges for prevention* (pp. 3–36). New York: Cambridge University Press.

Petersen, A. C., Leffert, N., Graham, B., Alwin, J., & Ding, A. (1997). Promoting mental health during the transition to adolescence. In J. Schulenberg, J. L. Maggs, & K. Hurrelmann (Eds.), *Health risks and developmental transitions during adolescence* (pp. 471–497). New York: Cambridge University Press.

Petraitis, J., Flay, B. R., & Miller, T. Q. (1995). Reviewing theories of adolescent substance use: Organizing pieces of the puzzle. *Psychological Bulletin, 117,* 67–86.

Raudenbush, S. W. (in press). Toward a coherent framework for comparing trajectories of individual change. In L. M. Collins & A. G. Sayer (Eds.), *New methods for the analysis of change.* Washington, DC: American Psychological Association.

Rose, R. J. (1998). A developmental behavioral-genetic perspective on alcoholism risk. *Alcohol Health and Research World, 22,* 131–143.

Russell, M. (1990). Prevalence of alcoholism among children of alcoholics. In M. Windle & J. S. Searles (Eds.), *Children of alcoholics: Critical perspectives* (pp. 9–38). New York: Guilford Press.

Rutter, M. (1989). Isle of Wight revisited: Twenty-five years of child psychiatric epidemiology. *Journal of the American Academy of Child and Adolescent Psychiatry, 28,* 633–653.

Rutter, M. (1990). Psychosocial resilience and protective mechanisms. In J. Rolf, A. Mastern, D. Cicchetti, K. H. Nuechterlein, & S. Weintraub (Eds.), *Risk and protective factors in the development of psychopathology* (pp. 181–214). Cambridge, England: Cambridge University Press.

Rutter, M. (1994). Beyond longitudinal data: Causes, consequences, changes, and continuity. *Journal of Consulting and Clinical Psychology, 62,* 928–940.

Rutter, M. (1996). Transitions and turning points in developmental psychopathology: As applied to the age span between childhood and mid-adulthood. *International Journal of Behavioral Development, 19,* 603–626.

Rutter, M., Graham, P., Chadwick, O. F., & Yule, W. (1976). Adolescent turmoil: Fact or fiction? *Journal of Child Psychology and Psychiatry and Allied Disciplines, 17,* 35–56.

Sameroff, A. J. (1987). The social context of development. In N. Eisenberg (Ed.), *Contemporary topics in developmental psychology* (pp. 273–291). New York: Wiley.

Scarr, S., & McCartney, K. (1983). How people make their own environments: A theory of genotype-environment effects. *Child Development, 54,* 424–435.

Schaie, K. W. (1965). A general model for the study of developmental problems. *Psychological Bulletin, 64,* 92–107.

Schaie, K. W., & Hertzog, C. (1985). Measurement in the psychology of adulthood and aging. In J. E. Birren (Ed.), *Handbook of the psychology of aging* (2nd ed., pp. 61–92). New York: Van Nostrand Reinhold.

Schlegel, A., & Barry, H., III. (1991). *Adolescence: An anthropological inquiry.* New York: The Free Press.

Schulenberg, J. (1999, June). *Binge drinking trajectories before, during, and after college: More reasons to worry from a developmental perspective.* Paper presented at the preconference session, Adolescence and Alcohol: Implications for College Drinking, at the meeting of the American Psychological Society, Denver, CO.

Schulenberg, J., & Maggs, J. L. (1999). *Prevention as altering the course of development: Comparison of growth models of alcohol misuse and associated risk factors during adolescence.* Manuscript submitted for publication.

Schulenberg, J., Maggs, J. L., & Hurrelmann, K. (Eds.). (1997a). *Health risks and developmental transitions during adolescence.* New York: Cambridge University Press.

Schulenberg, J., Maggs, J. L., & Hurrelmann, K. (1997b). Negotiating developmental transitions during adolescence and young adulthood: Health risks and opportunities. In J. Schulenberg, J. L. Maggs, & K. Hurrelmann (Eds.), *Health risks and developmental transitions during adolescence* (pp. 1–19). New York: Cambridge University Press.

Schulenberg, J., O'Malley, P. M., Bachman, J. G., & Johnston, L. D. (2000). "Spread your wings and fly": The course of health and well-being during the transition to young adulthood. In L. J. Crockett & R. K. Silbereisen (Eds.), *Negotiating adolescence in times of social change* (pp. 224–255). New York: Cambridge University Press.

Schulenberg, J., O'Malley, P. M., Bachman, J. G., Wadsworth, K. N., & Johnston, L. D. (1996). Getting drunk and growing up: Trajectories of frequent binge drinking during the transition to young adulthood. *Journal of Studies on Alcohol, 57,* 289–304.

Schulenberg, J., Wadsworth, K. N., O'Malley, P. M., Bachman, J. G., & Johnston, L. D. (1996). Adolescent risk factors for binge drinking during the transition to young adulthood: Variable and pattern-centered approaches to change. *Developmental Psychology, 32,* 659–674.

Shedler, J., & Block, J. (1990). Adolescent drug use and psychological health: A longitudinal inquiry. *American Psychologist, 45*(5), 612–630.

Sher, K. J. (1991). *Children of alcoholics: A critical appraisal of theory and research.* Chicago: University of Chicago Press.

Sher, K. J., & Wood, P. K. (1997). Methodological issues in conducting prospective research on alcohol-related behavior: A report from the field. In K. J. Bryant, M. Windle, & S. G. West (Eds.), *The science of prevention: Methodological advances from alcohol and substance abuse research* (pp. 3–41). Washington, DC: American Psychological Association.

Silbereisen, R. K., Eyferth, K., & Rudinger, G. (Eds.). (1986). *Development as action in context: Problem behavior and normal youth development.* New York: Springer-Verlag.

Silbereisen, R. K., & Kracke, B. (1997). Self-reported maturational timing and adaptation in adolescence. In J. Schulenberg, J. L. Maggs, & K. Hurrelmann (Eds.), *Health risks and developmental transitions during adolescence* (pp. 85–109). New York: Cambridge University Press.

Silbereisen, R. K., & Noack, P. (1988). On the constructive role of problem behavior in adolescence. In N. Bolger, A. Caspi, G. Downey, & M. Moorehouse (Eds.), *Persons in context: Developmental processes* (pp. 152–180). Cambridge, England: Cambridge University Press.

Stein, J. A., Newcomb, M. D., & Bentler, P. M. (1987). Personality and drug use: Reciprocal effects across four years. *Personality and Individual Differences, 8,* 419–430.

Steinman, K. J., & Schulenberg, J. (1999, June). *Alcohol use in adolescence: A developmental approach to understanding etiology and prevention.* Paper presented at the annual conference of the Society for Prevention Research, New Orleans, LA.

Stice, E., Myers, M. G., & Brown, S. A. (1998). A longitudinal grouping analysis of adolescent substance use escalation and de-escalation. *Psychology of Addictive Behaviors, 12,* 14–27.

Sullivan, H. S. (1947). *Conceptions of modern psychiatry.* Washington, DC: William Alanson White Psychiatric Foundation.

Susman, E. J., Feagans, L. V., & Ray, W. J. (1992). Historical and theoretical perspectives on behavioral health in children and adolescents: An introduction. In E. J. Susman, L. V. Feagans, & W. J. Ray (Eds.), *Emotion, cognition, health, and development in children and adolescents* (pp. 1–8). Hillsdale, NJ: Erlbaum.

U.S. Congress, Office of Technology Assessment (1991). *Adolescent health: Vol. 1. Summary and policy options.* Washington, DC: U.S. Government Printing Office.

Velicer, W. F., & Colby, S. M. (1997). Time series analysis for prevention and treatment research. In K. J. Bryant, M. Windle, & S. G. West (Eds.), *The science of prevention: Methodological advances from alcohol and substance abuse research* (pp. 211–249). Washington, DC: American Psychological Association.

von Eye, A. (1990). *Introduction to configural frequency analysis: The search for types and antitypes in cross-classification.* New York: Cambridge University Press.

Weber, M. D., Graham, J. W., Hansen, B., & Flay, B. R. (1989). Evidence for two paths of alcohol use onset in adolescents. *Addictive Behaviors, 14,* 399–408.

Willett, J. B., & Sayer, A. G. (1994). Using covariance structure analysis to detect correlates and predictors of individual change over time. *Psychological Bulletin, 116,* 363–381.

Wills, T. A., & Hirky, A. E. (1996). Coping and substance abuse: A theoretical model and review of the evidence. In M. Zeidner (Ed.), *Handbook of coping: Theory, research, applications* (pp. 279–302). New York: Wiley.

Wills, T. A., McNamara, G., Vaccaro, D., & Hirky, A. E. (1996). Escalated substance use: A longitudinal grouping analysis from early to middle adolescence. *Journal of Abnormal Psychology, 105,* 166–180.

Windle, M., & Davies, P. T. (1999). Developmental theory and research. In K. E. Leonard & H. T. Blane (Eds.), *Psychological theories of drinking and alcoholism* (2nd ed., pp. 164–202). New York: Guilford Press.

Zucker, R. A. (1987) The four alcoholisms: A developmental account of the etiologic process. In P. C. Rivers (Ed.), *Nebraska Symposium on Motivation, 1987: Alcohol and addictive behavior* (pp. 27–83). Lincoln: University of Nebraska Press.

Zucker, R. A. (1989). Is risk of alcoholism predictable? A probabilistic approach to a developmental problem. *Drugs and Society, 3,* 69–93.

Zucker, R. A. (in press). Alcohol involvement over the life course. In National Institute on Alcohol Abuse and Alcoholism (Ed.), *Tenth special report to the U.S. Congress on Alcohol and Health* (AH10). Rockville, MD: U.S. Government Printing Office.

Zucker, R. A., Fitzgerald, H. E., & Moses, H. D. (1995). Emergence of alcohol problems and the several alcoholisms: A developmental perspective on etiologic theory and life course trajectory. In D. Cicchetti & D. J. Cohen (Eds.), *Developmental psychopathology: Vol. 2. Risk, disorder, and adaptation* (pp. 677–711). New York: Wiley.

2

The Harm Reduction Approach to the Secondary Prevention of Alcohol Problems in Adolescents and Young Adults

Considerations across a Developmental Spectrum

ELIZABETH T. MILLER, AARON P. TURNER,
and G. ALAN MARLATT

WHAT IS HARM REDUCTION?

Over the past 2 decades, the prevention and treatment of adolescent alcohol abuse has been increasingly influenced by principles grounded in the philosophy of harm reduction. Broadly defined, harm reduction consists of strategies focused on minimizing the consequences associated with drinking and other high-risk behaviors. Proponents of harm reduction contend that it represents a compassionate and pragmatic alternative to traditional moral and disease models of addiction and that it views alcohol abuse along a continuum of problem behavior and not simply as the presence or absence of a disease state or as a personal shortcoming. Harm reduction evaluates policy and treatment interventions from a practical perspective, holding abstinence and minimal harm as an ideal goal but recognizing that any behavior change that reduces harm can be considered a positive outcome.

The origins of the harm reduction movement can be traced to the international AIDS crisis of the early 1980s. In the Netherlands, organized groups of addicts advocated for policy changes designed to promote the safety and well-being of drug users unwilling to commit to traditional abstinence-based treatment programs. Addict groups lobbied to implement needle exchange programs to reduce the transmission of HIV among injection drug users, arguing that any reduction in the risk of disease associated with needle sharing was beneficial to public health. Dutch needle exchange programs provided the groundwork to view risk reduction as a legitimate focus of intervention efforts independent of reductions in drug use. More broadly, they set the stage to provide a new framework for evaluating prevention and treatment outcomes across a variety of behaviors, such as excessive drinking, drug use, overeating, and gambling.

Harm reduction programs for adolescents contain many common strategies that fall into two general categories: those centered on individuals and groups, and those centered on modifying social environments and public policies. Education is the primary focus of individual and group interventions. Unlike most prevention programs for youth that focus exclusively on abstinence and promote a zero-tolerance (i.e., "just say no") approach, programs based on harm reduction are designed to accommodate individuals who have already said "yes" when it comes to engaging in risky behavior. Such programs can be structured in group (e.g., prevention programs in schools) or individual (e.g., one-on-one feedback) settings to include frank and open discussions of the relative pros and cons of engaging in and refraining from a behavior such as alcohol or drug use. They typically require active involvement on the part of participants in the form of feedback or role playing to ensure a cooperative dialogue that emphasizes the importance of making healthy choices without dictating or imposing "correct" answers. Programs are geared to ensure effective self-management and often stress the practice of specific coping skills, such as rehearsing ways to refuse alcoholic beverages politely at a party. Consistent with the grassroots, advocacy-based history of harm reduction, adolescent interventions are developed from the "bottom up" and are often based on extensive input from youth rather than being implemented from the "top down" by adult experts. Most traditional alcohol and drug treatment strategies can be incorporated into a harm reduction program if they are presented from this perspective.

Linked to the goal of enhancing self-management is environmental and public policy change. The goal of reduced harm cannot be met unless the environmental means are accessible (Marlatt, 1998). Rideshare programs designed to keep drunk drivers off the roads and condom distribution programs designed to reduce teen pregnancy and the spread of sexually transmitted diseases are two examples of ways in which social environments can be modified to provide adolescents who engage in risky behavior with lower risk alternatives. Both strategies provide individuals with additional choices and potentially increase the likelihood that a safer lifestyle can be maintained. In many cases, however, public policy dictates what can and cannot be legally done to make harm reduction tools and techniques more widely available. Often risk-reducing strategies conflict with traditional moral and medical models that view behaviors such as underage alcohol and drug use as categorically unhealthy and unacceptable. The future success of harm reduction will depend largely on its ability to address the concerns of its critics that it "sends the wrong message" to young people by continuing to provide evidence that its cooperative and inclusive message succeeds where other programs have failed.

This chapter reviews alcohol use among college students, unique concerns regarding the development of interventions for this population, the advantages of adopting a harm reduction perspective for these interventions, and gives a description of several interventions developed in our laboratory at the University of Washington.

COLLEGE STUDENT DRINKING REPRESENTS PUBLIC HEALTH CONCERN

Alcohol use among adolescents and young adults continues to be an important public health issue. Given that drinking can be considered a primary "rite of passage" from adolescence to adulthood, it is ironic that the greatest health risks individuals aged 18–22 face are those problems associated with excessive alcohol use in the college community (Berkowitz & Perkins, 1986; Saltz & Elandt, 1986; Stenmark, Walfish, & Brennan, 1981).

Although in the United States it is illegal for individuals under the age of 21 to consume alcohol, adolescents and young adults experience alcohol-related negative consequences at alarming rates (Meilman, Stone, Gaylor, & Turco, 1990). In a recent national survey, nearly 85% of undergraduate college students reported drinking alcohol in the past year (Johnston, O'Malley, & Bachman, 1996; Presley, Meilman, & Lyerla, 1994), and as many as 62.5% had used alcohol in the past 30 days, with 3.6% reporting daily use (Johnston et al., 1996). In a comprehensive survey of more than 45,000 students across 87 U.S. undergraduate institutions, 27.3% of men and 13.9% of women used alcohol on at least three occasions weekly (Presley et al., 1994).

Of even greater concern are those students who drink in a heavy, hazardous fashion, consuming large quantities over a brief period of time, thereby putting themselves at risk for increased negative consequences. For example, Presley and colleagues reported that 21% of the sample drank 2 to 5 drinks weekly, 9% reported consuming 10 to 15 drinks weekly, and 4.1% consumed more than 20 drinks weekly (Presley et al., 1994). Wechsler and colleagues surveyed 17,592 students at 140 universities and found that 44% engaged in "binge" drinking (e.g., five or more drinks in a row for men and four or more drinks in a row for women on at least one occasion in the past 2 weeks; Wechsler, Davenport, Dowdall, Moeykens, & Castillo, 1994; Wechsler & Isaac, 1992). Astonishingly, 19% reported three or more binge episodes in the preceding 2 weeks. Most alarming is the finding that alcohol-related accidents and injuries are the leading cause of death in this age group (Institute of Medicine, 1990; National Institute on Alcohol Abuse and Alcoholism, 1992; Johnston et al., 1996).

College communities feel the effects of hazardous drinking practices in a profound sense, according to Anderson and Gadaleto (1997). College students are at great risk for excessive alcohol consumption (Baer, Kivlahan, & Marlatt, 1995; Meilman et al., 1990; Pope, Ionescu, Aizley, & Varma, 1990) and related problems, including academic failure (Presley et al., 1994); relationship difficulties, sexual aggression, and acquaintance rape (Berkowitz & Perkins, 1986; Engs & Hanson, 1985; Koss, Gidycz, & Wisniewsli, 1987; Norris, Nurius, & Dimeff, 1996); sexually transmitted diseases (Donovan & McEwan, 1995; Strunin & Hingson, 1992); vandalism and violence (Engs & Hanson, 1990); and motor vehicle accidents and fatalities (Campbell, Zobeck, & Bertolucci, 1995; McGinnis & Foege, 1993; National Highway Traffic Safety Administration, 1994). Not surprisingly, these physical, psychological, and behavioral consequences associated with hazardous drinking are of concern to college administrators, parents, university communities, and the media (Hanson & Engs, 1995; Wechsler, 1996; Wechsler & Isaac, 1992; Wechsler et al., 1994; Winerip, 1998).

UNIQUE FEATURES OF COLLEGE STUDENT DRINKING

Entrance to college represents a developmental transition and encompasses a unique window of risk for older adolescents. The varied pattern of alcohol use among adolescents suggests that not all drinking is problematic and that engaging in problematic alcohol use is frequently not chronic (Samson-Herman, Maxwell, & Doyle, 1989). Distinguishing between alcohol abuse, dependence, problem use, and nonproblem use remains unclear and depends on several factors: normative environmental drinking patterns, sociocultural drinking norms, and the continuum of negative consequences encountered. Baer, McLean, and Marlatt (1998) state that knowing whether an adolescent drinks alcohol or drinks alcohol heavily does not offer much information about the presence or absence of negative consequences or related problems. For this reason, it is important to take current developmental challenges and environmental factors into consideration when categorizing adolescent alcohol use and considering intervention strategies. The prevalence of alcohol use on the typical college campus may be considered normative, and therefore problem use should be contextually and situationally defined.

Patterns of alcohol use among adolescents differ from those of adults in several important ways: (1) they engage in more episodic drinking, (2) alcohol-related problems associated with adolescence are not usually those associated with chronic conditions of adult alcohol dependence, and (3) the types of drinking patterns associated with negative consequences for adults are different than for adolescents (Bailey & Rachal, 1993; Kilty, 1990). This pattern of intermittent alcohol use is consistent with the categorization of most adolescent users as "infrequent" (88%; Gutierres, Molof, & Ungerleider, 1994), "experimental" (50%; Shedler & Block, 1990), or "nonproblem" (85%; Donovan & Jessor, 1978) drinkers. However, the negative consequences associated with heavy alcohol use primarily occur during these "infrequent" binge episodes. Students engaging in hazardous alcohol use are doing so in an episodic manner that appears to be maximally contingent on the university environment.

In a comprehensive review of the literature, Baer and colleagues (1998) reviewed several longitudinal adolescent alcohol and substance use studies and highlight two general themes across studies: (1) Alcohol use begins in adolescence and declines substantially with the transition to adulthood, suggesting that some adolescent alcohol abuse patterns are part of a "stage"; and (2) the alcohol use problems that are maintained into adulthood are predicted by adolescent problem behavior and nonconformity and not by amount of alcohol consumed nor by patterns of alcohol consumption. These findings suggest that prevention efforts aimed at expediting adolescents and young adults through this risky "stage" unscathed would be highly beneficial. However, despite the increase in prevention efforts and policies aimed at decreasing alcohol use on high school and college campuses (Anderson & Gadaleto, 1997; Wechsler, Moeykens, Davenport, Castillo, & Hansen, 1995), students continue to engage in harmful and hazardous drinking (Baer, 1993). Prevention programs and interventions with an abstinence-only message fail to resonate with this population (Baer, 1993).

In summary, use and abuse of alcohol by young people is different from that by adults and therefore should be responded to in a different manner. The normative-developmental perspective asserts that some degree of alcohol use is a normal part of adolescent exploration of adult behaviors (Dusenbury & Botvin, 1992; Hillman & Sawilowsky, 1992; Schulenberg, Maggs, Steinman, & Zucker, Chapter 1, this volume). Several researchers assert that in order to accurately examine alcohol use among young adults, a developmental framework should be considered (Newcomb & Bentler, 1988; Tarter & Vanyukov, 1994; Zucker, 1986).

Very few adolescents and young adults meet *DSM-IV* criteria for alcohol dependence (Baer et al., 1995). For most students, heavy drinking tends to decline as students progress through college, assume increased responsibilities, and learn their limits (Fillmore, 1988; Jessor, Donovan, & Costa, 1991; Zucker, Fitzgerald, & Moses, 1995). Therefore, many students are faced with negotiating through this "developmentally limited" high-risk period during their college career. Given the realities of college student drinking, one universal goal for prevention programming may be to expedite students through this risky developmental period unscathed as opposed to attempting to eliminate alcohol use altogether (Dimeff, 1997).

ADVANTAGES OF HARM REDUCTION FOR COLLEGE STUDENT POPULATION

Harm reduction represents a new approach to reducing alcohol problems among the adolescent population. At first glance, harm reduction appears to offer a number of advantages and potential strengths as an alternative to traditional, abstinence-only programs. On the other hand, because harm reduction is still such a new and largely untested approach, considerable controversy exists regarding the question of whether it helps or hurts the adolescent drinker. In this section we first address the potential strengths of harm reduction, then briefly discuss its potential ethical problems.

As a first advantage, harm reduction is "user friendly" and has the potential of engaging young high-risk drinkers and motivating them to participate in programs designed to minimize the negative consequences of heavy, episodic alcohol consumption. Issues of personal autonomy and the need for independence predominate for most adolescents. When told by adult authorities what to do (or what *not* to do), many teens experience reactance and resistance to the extent that oppositional behavior (including heavy drinking) may increase. Such "top down" programs targeted to a teen audience may backfire, thereby increasing the risk of dangerous drinking. The harm reduction message is likely to be more attractive to active drinkers in this age range, simply because it meets teens who are willing to "come as you are" (Marlatt, 1996). In contrast, they are more likely to resist being told that "this is the way you *should* be" by adults who insist on abstinence and zero tolerance for underage drinkers.

Additional advantages of the harm reduction model include the focus on low-threshold access to prevention and treatment programs (teens are welcome even if they are still drinking), as well as the lack of stigmatization and moral criticism that are often associated with abstinence-only programs. Adolescents may find the harm reduction message more appealing because of its greater emphasis on active learning principles, such as acquiring safer drinking skills. The focus on active learning is congruent with the way in which teens are taught safe driving skills in their "driver's education" courses.

A final potential strength of the harm reduction approach concerns the developmental course of alcohol problems in adolescence. As summarized in the recent developmental literature (cf. Baer, McLean, & Marlatt, 1998), most adolescents show reductions in alcohol consumption and related problems as they grow older. The majority appear to "mature out" of problem drinking as they acquire the responsibilities of adult life, such as establishing a career and building a family. Others, however, will continue to drink heavily, and some will become alcohol dependent over time. Because this group represents a minority in terms of the number of adolescents who qualify for the diagnosis of alcohol dependence, the majority of teen drinkers may be significantly more responsive to harm reduction than they would be to an approach that focuses extensively on an increasingly negative trajectory of drinking and drinking problems. Also, to the extent that teens are involved as partners in the development and implementation of harm reduction prevention programs (e.g., peer-based education), their "stakeholder" status is enhanced. As stakeholders in program development, their allegiance and adherence are likely to increase.

Despite these potential advantages, the harm reduction approach is not without controversy. The essential goals of harm reduction, to reduce hazardous drinking and to minimize negative consequences, run counter to the goal of total abstinence in a disease model. The clash occurs between the legal requirement of abstinence prior to age 21 and the public health reality that many teens are actively engaged in drinking behavior that may put them at high risk for injury or even death. A seemingly parallel moral and practical dilemma can arise in the debate over sex education for teens. Proponents of premarital sexual abstinence for adolescents decry any attempt to provide information about safe sexual practices or the distribution of condoms to sexually active teens. Often the opposition is based on the fear that this approach will "send the wrong message" and increase the risk of teen pregnancy because of its "permission-giving" stance.

For both drinking and sexual activity, the debate continues between those who insist on a "Just Say No" message and those who would rather endorse a "Just Say *Know*" alternative. For those in the former camp, the provision of knowledge and skills about safer sex or safer drinking may be a dangerous undertaking, especially when directed at teens who are currently abstinent. For those in the latter camp, however, information and skills are important to know because of their safety value. Here the rationale is similar to the one that underlies society's emphasis on requiring fire drills or other emergency procedures. Even for teens who do not drink, the harm reduction information may come in handy when helping friends who have had too much to drink (e.g., serving as a designated driver). Ultimately, the argument boils down to one of moralism versus pragmatism. Continued research efforts are needed to elucidate what approach works and for whom it works better. The ultimate goal of harm reduction is to reduce the risk of injury and save lives. It remains an empirical question as to whether the harm reduction approach to adolescent drinking best serves this goal.

Prevention and treatment programs based on harm reduction principles provide an important addition to existing efforts to reduce alcohol abuse among college students. In many instances, intervention strategies focused on minimizing the risks associated with drinking offer distinct advantages over more traditional programs based on moral and disease models of addiction. Unlike the disease model, harm reduction recognizes that alcohol misuse among college students represents a broad spectrum of problems. Students who experience negative consequences as a result of their drinking may not necessarily suffer from a lifelong progressive illness. Instead, considerable evidence suggests that their difficulties are most often time-limited and highly situation specific (Alterman, Bridges, & Tarter 1986; Vaillant, 1996). Harm reduction asserts that all potentially risky behavior, including alcohol use, can be placed on a continuum and that behavior change strategies are intended to move individuals from higher to lower levels of risk. Although abstinence is desirable in that it represents the point of lowest risk for harm, any reduction in consequences is considered to be a positive outcome within a harm reduction model.

Viewing excessive drinking as more than the presence or absence of a disease state allows for a more flexible approach to assessment and opens the door to a wider range of treatment and prevention options. Instead of focusing expensive, specialized treatments on a small subset of college students who qualify as alcohol dependent, emphasis is placed on reducing the harm associated with drinking at any point along the continuum of risk (Larimer et al., 1998). Expanded options for prevention and treatment allow for a greater opportunity to match appropriate interventions to the specific needs that individuals present. Programs based on the traditional disease model of addiction are often limited to treatment strategies that promote abstinence. For college students who do not have long and problematic histories of alcohol use, who do not identify with the disease model, who are unwilling to quit drinking, or who would like simply to learn skills to use alcohol in a less risky manner, harm reduction programs offer an attractive, alternative context for engaging in behavior change.

Harm reduction also offers advantages over the moral model of addiction (Brickman et al., 1982). Based in compassionate pragmatism, harm reduction recognizes the reality that the majority of college students drink and that most perceive it to be a normal behavior (Larimer et al., 1998). By refraining from labeling and stigmatizing drinking, harm reduction interventions attempt to meet students "where they are" and minimize the possibility that they will alienate their audience. Such strategies lower the likelihood that students will resist these interventions because they do not believe themselves to be at risk and can help to increase overall rates of participation.

Meeting students "where they are" implies that there is not only a continuum of use but also a continuum for changing use. Prochaska and DiClemente refer to this as the stages of change model (1986) and assert that behavior change, such as reducing hazardous alcohol use, occurs along a temporal dimension. Marcus and Simkin (1994) assert that each stage of change can be viewed as a representation of both traits and states. Whereas traits are considered to be relatively stable and fixed, stages are open to change and are somewhat unstable. This approach implies that both behavior and behavioral intention contribute to an individual's progression from one stage to another (Marcus & Simkin, 1994). Here behavior is defined as the act of behaving in a particular manner, whereas behavioral intention is the serious intent to engage in a particular behavior in the very near future—a mindful commitment to adopt a new behavior. It is hypothesized that as individuals decrease hazardous alcohol use, they move through certain stages in a cyclical fashion, with periods of progression and regression (Prochaska & DiClemente, 1986). Recent research suggests the importance of the following five-stage model rather than the four-stage model (Prochaska, DiClemente, & Norcross, 1992). In the *precontemplation* stage, there is no intention to change behavior in the foreseeable future. In the *contemplation* stage, people are aware that a problem exists and have begun to consider overcoming that problem but have not yet made a commitment to take action. Individuals in the *preparation* stage have been unsuccessful in their attempts to take action in the past year but intend to take action in the next month. It is while in the *action* stage that individuals modify their behavior, experiences, or environment in order to overcome their problems. During the *maintenance* stage, people work to prevent relapse and to sustain the changes made in the action stage (Prochaska et al., 1992).

Consistent with the stages of change perspective is the practice of matching interventions with individuals and the clinical implications of utilizing a multistage process (Marlatt & Baer, 1988). Specifically, the level and the intensity of the intervention effort are important considerations, particularly when directed at individuals (Keller, Bennett, McCrady, Paulus, & Frankenstein, 1994). For example, students contemplating decreasing their alcohol use may be open to discussions related to examining the pros and cons of drinking within a didactic framework. This type of intervention could be delivered in brief group settings. On the other hand, a one-on-one meeting that includes personalized feedback about the individual's attempts to quit might be more relevant and worthwhile for the student who is actively engaged in trying to remain abstinent.

The Institute of Medicine (IOM; 1990) recommends a sequential stepped approach to developing prevention interventions for persons such as college students who are at risk for alcohol-related negative consequences but who may never develop alcohol dependence. Therefore, initial efforts should be focused on brief preventive interventions so as to minimize unnecessary resource expenditures.

RATIONALE FOR BRIEF INTERVENTIONS

In 1990 the IOM released an influential report asserting that nationwide research and clinical efforts should be expanded to include wider definitions of alcohol problems and appropriate interventions. Although the report highlights alcohol use in the general population, its message is also relevant to college student communities. Arguments for "broadening the base of alcohol treatment" are illustrated in a diagram that has been reprinted here as Figure 2.1.

The triangle in this figure represents a continuous distribution of alcohol problems in the general population. The left side of the triangle, corresponding to the largest segment of society, contains individuals who either do not drink or do not experience problems as a result of their alcohol use. Primary prevention programs aimed at reducing initiation into risky drinking behavior are considered appropriate interventions for this group. The middle section of the triangle contains individuals who experience mild or moderate alcohol problems. Brief interventions designed to change drinking behavior and decrease resulting consequences are recommended for this group. The far right side of the triangle is composed of individuals who suffer from significant, severe alcohol problems and who most likely meet criteria for alcohol dependence. Specialized group and individual treatment programs have long existed for this segment of society.

Overall, as one moves from left to right across Figure 2.1, the number of drinkers decreases but the acuity of drinking problems increases. Individuals in the far right corner of the triangle are few in number but suffer from the most severe alcohol problems. College student drinking appears to conform to this general pattern as well. Despite rates of binge drinking that are higher than those found in adult populations, the majority of students engage in sporadic and experimental alcohol use. A smaller segment of college students experience significant consequences as a result of their drink-

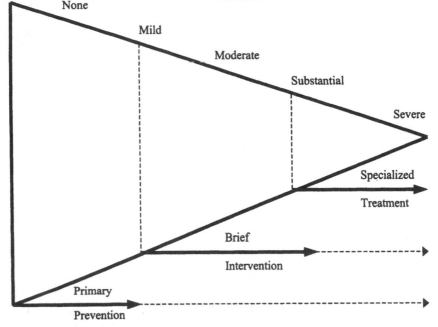

FIGURE 2.1. A spectrum of responses to alcohol problems. The triangle represents the population of the United States, with the spectrum of alcohol problems experienced by the population shown along the upper side. Responses to the problems are shown along the lower side (based on Skinner, 1988). In general, specialized treatment is indicated for persons with substantial or severe alcohol problems; brief intervention is indicated for persons with mild or moderate alcohol problems; and primary prevention is indicated for persons who have not had alcohol problems but are at risk of developing them. The dotted lines extending the arrows suggest that both primary prevention and brief intervention may have effects beyond their principal target populations. The prevalence of categories of alcohol problems in the population is represented by the area of the triangle occupied; most people have no alcohol problems, many people have a few alcohol problems, and some people have many alcohol problems. From the Institute of Medicine (1990, p. 212). Copyright 1990 by the National Academy of Sciences. Reprinted by permission.

ing, and only a small minority qualify as alcohol dependent. Historically, the great majority of clinical and research attention has been focused on this final smallest segment of the drinking population. Over the past decade, there has been increasing recognition that individuals with mild and moderate difficulties with alcohol, those found in the middle of the triangle, are the least likely to receive attention (Kreitman, 1986; Larimer et al. 1998). The IOM report asserts that this substantial group should not be neglected by treatment services:

If the alcohol problems experienced by the population are to be reduced significantly, the distribution of these problems in the population suggests that a principal focus of intervention should be on persons with mild or moderate alcohol problems. . . . The implications of this analysis are clear. There is a need for a spectrum of interventions that matches the spectrum of alcohol problems. (1990, p. 215)

Harm reduction approaches to problem drinking, which seek to lower the risk of harm associated with drinking across all levels of alcohol use, are sympathetic to the Institute of Medicine's public health argument. As a result of the recognized need to expand the scope of alcohol interventions on college campuses, brief programs have been developed that specifically address the difficulties faced by students who experience only mild or moderate alcohol problems.

BRIEF INTERVENTIONS

Research suggests that the majority of college students will mature out of the "developmentally limited" pattern of hazardous alcohol use and alcohol problems on their own and without treatment (Baer, Stacy, & Larimer, 1991; Fillmore, 1988). However, numerous risks are associated with passing through this stage. This situation creates a conundrum for university officials across the nation entrusted with the care of millions of college students each year.

To date, most universities typically focus their efforts on designing comprehensive campus-wide interventions aimed at managing the campus environment (e.g., creating a drug-free campus, sponsoring alternative alcohol-free activities), integrating alcohol education and prevention programs into existing curricula (e.g., course lectures), or teaching skills for handling risky party situations (Anderson & Milgram, 1996). Outcome research has been conducted on some prevention efforts that include educational programs designed to increase student awareness of the risks of alcohol problems (see, e.g., Goodstadt & Caleekal, 1984) and/or to develop alternative nonalcoholic recreational activities (Botvin, 1991). Community-based programs that attempt to modify the campus environment as a whole (cf. Wagenaar & Perry, 1995) or to influence drinking rates at the policy level by raising the price of alcohol, decreasing availability of alcohol to underage youth (Grossman, Chaloupka, Saffer, & Laixuthai, 1995), or raising the legal drinking age (O'Malley & Wagenaar, 1991) have also been studied. However, there is little empirical evidence to support the effectiveness of these campus-based programs in reducing hazardous alcohol use among college students. Additionally, increasing knowledge regarding alcohol (Mills & McCarty, 1983; Nathan, 1983) or changing attitudes toward alcohol use (Kraft, 1984; Mills & McCarty, 1983; Nathan, 1983) do not appear to independently affect changes in alcohol consumption.

At the University of Washington, Marlatt and colleagues have developed and empirically validated several early intervention programs for college students who have already initiated heavy or hazardous drinking patterns. Rather than focus on abstinence as the exclusive goal, these interventions are based on harm reduction principles (cf. Marlatt et al., 1998). Initial programs focused on cognitive–behavioral principles and incorporated self-management techniques (Baer et al., 1992; Kivlahan, Marlatt, Fromme, Coppel, & Williams, 1990). These interventions were delivered in a classroom setting and incorporated various behavior change strategies, such as didactic presentations about the effects of alcohol (e.g., defining the physiological and psychological influences of alcohol use), cognitive modification (e.g., challenging irrational or erroneous beliefs regarding tolerance), skills training (e.g., setting and observing drinking limits, estimating blood alcohol level, practicing drink refusal techniques, developing self-monitoring skills), and social learning and peer influence (e.g., providing feedback regarding normative alcohol use among college students). Results from this program, called the Alcohol Skills Training Program (ASTP), revealed that the original 8-week course and the subsequent 6-week course were efficacious in reducing hazardous alcohol use and related problems (Dimeff, Baer, Kivlahan, & Marlatt, 1999).

A follow-up trial was conducted in order to evaluate the effectiveness of the program content presented in different formats (Baer et al., 1992). Participants were randomly assigned to one of three conditions: a classroom group program (a shorter six-session version of the original ASTP), a "correspondence course" (a six-lesson self-help manual based on the ASTP program content), or a single one-on-one session of "professional advice" consisting of individualized feedback and advice given directly to the participant. Previous studies had indicated that even a single session of advice or motivational enhancement can have a significant impact on decreasing subsequent drinking behavior, including those with more problematic alcohol use (Edwards et al., 1977; Miller & Rollnick, 1991). All study participants significantly reduced their alcohol consumption by the end of the intervention period and maintained their reduced consumption at 2-year follow-up. Of considerable interest was the finding that students who received the single session of professional advice did not differ significantly from those who attended the more extensive programs.

These findings spurred a third study (Marlatt et al., 1998) that used a brief version of the ASTP with high-risk college student drinkers. The content of the individualized feedback intervention was developed based on the contents described earlier (see also Baer et al., 1992) and was delivered using principles of motivational interviewing (Miller & Rollnick, 1991). This approach assumes that individuals are in a natural state of ambivalence regarding their own alcohol use and must arrive at their own decision regarding whether to change their drinking habits (see Marlatt et al., 1998, for a review). Participants engaged in a 60-minute personalized feedback interview and were provided with alcohol consumption monitoring cards and asked to keep track of their drinking on a daily basis for 2 weeks prior to their scheduled interview (see Marlatt et al., 1998, for a review). Although on average all students in both the intervention and control conditions drank less and reported fewer alcohol-related problems at the 2-year follow-up, participants who received the brief intervention showed a significant decrease in drinking rates, alcohol-related problems, and alcohol dependency compared with the participants in the control group (Marlatt et al., 1998; Roberts, Neal, Kivlahan, Baer, & Marlatt, 2000).

Marlatt and colleagues recently investigated the efficacy of a brief motivational intervention that was based on the content of the aforementioned programs condensed into two 50-minute sessions (Dimeff et al., 1999). The Brief Alcohol Screening and Intervention for College Students (BASICS) incorporates many of the same cognitive–behavioral skills and motivational techniques as mentioned previously. Outcome data support the efficacy of this individualized one-on-one indicated prevention approach in reducing alcohol use and related problems among college students who are heavy or hazardous drinkers (Dimeff et al., 1999). Although one-on-one programs have shown some efficacy in decreasing alcohol abuse and reducing the associated negative consequences, the immediate and short-term cost of implementing this type of intervention may be prohibitive at many universities.

Reis and her colleagues at the University of Illinois at Urbana–Champaign (Reis, Riley, Lokman, & Baer, in press) pilot tested a cognitive–behavioral skills-based interactive CD-ROM intervention (Alcohol 101 CD-ROM) in an effort to provide a more cost-effective alternative to universities. The interactive software of the CD-ROM integrates theories of behavioral change used in the health promotion and prevention field (Bandura, 1977; Fishbein & Ajzen, 1975; Prochaska et al., 1992). The CD-ROM presents users with several video, text, music, and graphic animation elements related to three content areas that were found in school-based substance use programs to be relevant and interesting to adolescents (Hansen, 1992). The three content areas of the Alcohol 101 CD-ROM program—perceived norms, expectancies, and life skills—are divided into several modules.

The Alcohol 101 CD-ROM was compared with an alternative alcohol education condition and a no-alcohol education condition with university students to determine the short-term impact of the CD-ROM as a preventative alcohol education program for young adults. Evaluation of the pre-post self-report measures of intentions to use revealed that students who used the interactive software program learned more about dose–response and ways to intervene with friends in peril (Reis et al., in press). However, it is unclear whether utilization of the Alcohol 101 CD-ROM is effective in reducing the rates of alcohol abuse and alcohol-related negative consequences.

Despite the fact that using mental health professionals to deliver normative feedback and information about the risks of heavy drinking has proven effective in reducing drinking rates and consequences (Agostinelli, Brown, & Miller, 1995; Botvin, Tortu, Baker, & Dusenbury, 1990; Hansen, Graham, Wolkenstein, & Rohrbach, 1991; Kivlahan et al., 1990; Marlatt, Baer, & Larimer, 1995; Marlatt et al., 1998; Sanchez-Craig, Wilkinson, & Walker, 1987; Weinstein & Klein, 1995), the costs of implementing such programs is often prohibitive (Dimeff, 1997).

With this in mind, Miller and colleagues at the University of Washington tested the efficacious components of the ASTP in a group setting facilitated by college-age peers, as compared with the Alcohol 101 CD-ROM and two assessment-only control groups. The study was designed to test the effectiveness of the ASTP and CD-ROM programs as group interventions in reducing alcohol abuse and alcohol-related problems and to evaluate the feasibility and cost efficiency of conducting longitudinal survey research utilizing the Internet. The overall pattern of results suggests that college students who complete an assessment of drinking behaviors and consequences upon entrance to college, followed by a brief intervention and/or subsequent assessments during their freshman year, show significantly less alcohol consumption and fewer harmful consequences than students in a no-intervention control condition who completed only a single assessment at the end of the freshman year (Miller, 2000). Additionally, Internet-based data collection methods[1] of assessing alcohol use in college students appear to be more rapid, cost effective, and free of data entry errors than traditional paper-and-pencil surveys (Miller et al., in press).

CONCLUSIONS

The movement toward conceptualizing alcohol and other high-risk behaviors along a continuum rather than as a dichotomous issue has been advantageous to the substance abuse field. Alternative treatment and intervention techniques allow for a broader array of services for those seeking to change harmful drinking patterns. The idea of a "one size" drinker (Institute of

---

[1]DatStat.com, Inc., a Web-based data collection, management, and analysis service provider. *http://www.datstat.com.*

Medicine, 1990) has not been supported, and therefore recognizing that not all adolescents and young adults who use alcohol need, desire, or benefit from formal treatment interventions (Dawson, 1996; Sobell et al., 1996) allows for the development of a broader public health goal. Adopting harm reduction principles in this effort has resulted in clarifying previous alcohol treatment advances and directing future research and intervention approaches (Larimer et al., 1998).

Adolescents and young adults represent an unparalleled segment of the population. This "stage" of development brings with it a set of unique challenges, particularly those associated with navigating through situations involving "sex, drugs, and rock'n'roll." It is evident that an alternative approach is necessary in order to have an impact on the adolescent and young adult population; the "just say no" approach has not been successful. Those programs oriented toward decreasing alcohol consumption and reducing harmful effects appear to be the most promising (Baer, 1993; Kivlahan et al., 1990; Larimer et al., 1994), suggesting that the ideal goal for prevention programming may be to expedite students through this risky developmental period undamaged. However, because this cannot be guaranteed, adopting a harm reduction perspective as opposed to attempting to eliminate alcohol use altogether is a more realistic goal (Marlatt et al., 1995).

Harm reduction strategies are not limited to treatment and intervention programs. The physical and social environment can be altered (Plant, Single, & Stockwell, 1997), as can policies surrounding alcohol and other high-risk behaviors (Single, 1996). Furthermore, although the ideal goal is the experience of nominal negative consequences due to alcohol consumption through the practice of abstinence, any behavior change that reduces harm is considered a positive outcome (e.g., moderation and decrease of negative consequences). Even if abstinence is the goal of the intervention program, harm reduction can be applied to reduce the frequency or intensity of negative consequences encountered along the way.

Harm reduction is well suited to the secondary prevention of alcohol problems through moderation goals. Rather than requiring abstinence as the only acceptable first step, harm reduction encourages a gradual reduction of negative consequences associated with heavy and hazardous alcohol use. Incremental change encourages people to continue pursuing the ultimate goal, be it moderation or abstinence. The harm reduction approach encourages individuals to set their own personal goals rather than trying to fit into a "one-size-fits-all" category, and this characteristic may be particularly appealing to adolescents and young adults. Harm reduction promotes uniqueness and flexibility, important considerations not just across the developmental spectrum in general but specifically to the phenomenon of adolescence.

ACKNOWLEDGMENTS

Special thanks to Jessica Cronce and Rebekka Palmer for their editorial assistance. Preparation of this chapter was supported by a grant from the National Institute on Alcohol Abuse and Alcoholism (No. 5R3A AA05591) awarded to G. Alan Marlatt.

REFERENCES

Agostinelli, G., Brown, J. M., & Miller, W. R. (1995). Effects of normative feedback on consumption among heavy drinking college students. *Journal of Drug Education, 25*(1), 31–40.

Alterman, A. I., Bridges, K. R., & Tarter, R. E. (1986). Drinking behavior of high-risk college men: Contradictory preliminary findings. *Alcoholism: Clinical and Experimental Research, 10,* 305–310.

Anderson, D. S., & Gadaleto, A. F. (1997). *1997 college alcohol survey.* Fairfax, VA: George Mason University.

Anderson, D. S., & Milgram, G. G. (1996). *Promising practices sourcebook: Campus alcohol strategies.* Fairfax, VA: George Mason University.

Baer, J. S. (1993). Etiology and secondary prevention of alcohol problems with young adults. In J. S. Baer, G. A. Marlatt, & R. J. McMahon (Eds.), *Addictive behaviors across the life span: Prevention, treatment, and policy issues* (pp. 111–137). Newbury Park, CA: Sage.

Baer, J. S., Kivlahan, D. R., & Marlatt, G. A. (1995). High-risk drinking across the transition from high school to college. *Alcoholism: Clinical and Experimental Research, 19,* 54–61.

Baer, J. S., Marlatt, G. A., Kivlahan, D. R., Fromme, K., Larimer, M. E., & Williams, E. (1992). An experimental test of three methods of alcohol risk reduction in young adults. *Journal of Consulting and Clinical Psychology, 60*(6), 974–979.

Baer, J. S., McLean, M. G., & Marlatt, G. A. (1998). Linking etiology and treatment for adolescent substance abuse: Toward a better match. In R. Jessor (Ed.), *New perspectives on adolescent risk behaviors* (pp. 182–220). Cambridge: Cambridge University Press.

Baer, J. S., Stacy, A., & Larimer, M. E. (1991). Biases in the perception of drinking norms among college students. *Journal of Studies on Alcohol, 52*(6), 580–586.

Bailey, S. L., & Rachal, J. V. (1993). Dimensions of adolescent problem drinking. *Journal of Studies on Alcohol, 54,* 555–565.

Bandura, A. (1977). Self-efficacy: Toward a unifying theory of behavioral change. *Psychological Review, 84*(2), 191–215.

Berkowitz, A. D., & Perkins, H. W. (1986). Problem drinking among college students: A review and recent research. *College Health, 35,* 21–28.

Botvin, E. M. (1991). Stress, coping and substance use among adolescents: Predictors of substance use and the impact of school transition. *Dissertation Abstracts International, 52*(4-B), 2350.

Botvin, G. J., Tortu, S., Baker, E., & Dusenbury, L. (1990). Preventing adolescent cigarette smoking: Resistance skills training and development of the life skills. *Special Services in the Schools, 6*(1–2), 37–61.

Brickman, P., Rabinowitz, V. C., Karuza, J., Coates, D., Cohn, E., & Kidder, L. (1982). Models of helping and coping. *American Psychologist, 37,* 368–384.

Campbell, K. E., Zobeck, T. S. & Bertolucci, D. (1995). *Trends in alcohol-related fatal traffic crashes, United States, 1977–1993* (Surveillance Report #34). Rockville, MD: U.S. Department of Health and Human Services.

Dawson, D. A. (1996). Correlates of past-year status among treated and untreated persons with former alcohol dependence: United States, 1992. *Alcoholism: Clinical and Experimental Research, 20,* 771–779.

Dimeff, L. A. (1997). *Brief intervention for heavy and hazardous college drinkers in a student primary health care setting.* Unpublished doctoral dissertation, University of Washington, Seattle.

Dimeff, L. A, Baer, J. S., Kivlahan, D. R., & Marlatt, G. A. (1999). *Brief Alcohol Screening and Intervention for College Students (BASICS): A harm reduction approach.* New York: Guilford Press.

Donovan, C., & McEwan, R. (1995). A review of the literature examining the relationship between alcohol use and HIV-related sexual risk-taking in young people. *Addiction, 90*(3), 319–328.

Donovan, J. E., & Jessor, R. (1978). Adolescent problem drinking: Psychosocial correlates in a national sample study. *Journal of Studies on Alcohol, 39*(9), 1506–1524.

Dusenbury, L., & Botvin, G. J. (1992). Applying the competency enhancement model to substance abuse prevention. In M. Kessler, S. E. Goldston, & M. J. Joffe (Eds.), *The present and future of prevention: In honor of George W. Albee* (pp. 182–195). Newbury Park, CA: Sage.

Edwards, G., Orford, J., Egert, S., Guthrie, S., Hawker, A., Hensmen, C., Mitcheson, M., Oppenheimer, E., & Taylor, C. (1977). Alcoholism: A control-led trial of "treatment" and "advice." *Journal of Studies on Alcohol, 38,* 1004–1031.

Engs, R. C., & Hanson, D. J. (1985). Drinking patterns and problems of college students. *Journal of Alcohol and Drug Education, 31,* 65–82.

Engs, R. C., & Hanson, D. J. (1990). Gender differences in drinking patterns and problems among college students: A review of the literature. *Journal of Alcohol and Drug Education, 35,* 36–47

Fillmore, M. (1988). *Alcohol use across the life course.* Toronto, Ontario, Canada: Alcoholism and Drug Addiction Research Foundation.

Fishbein, M., & Ajzen, I. (1975). *Belief, attitude, intention and behavior: An Introduction to theory and research.* Reading, MA: Addison-Wesley.

Goodstadt, M., & Caleekal, J. (1984). Alcohol education programs for university students: A review of their effectiveness. *International Journal of the Addictions, 19*(7), 721–741.

Grossman, M., Chaloupka, F. J., Saffer, H., & Laixuthai, A. (1995). Effects of alcohol price policy on youth: A summary of economic research. In G. M. Boyd, J. Howard, & R. Zucker (Eds.), *Alcohol problems among adolescents: Current directions in prevention research* (pp. 225–242). Hillsdale, NJ: Erlbaum.

Gutierres, S. E., Molof, M., & Ungerleider, S. (1994). Relationship of "risk" factors to teen substance use: A comparison of abstainers, infrequent users, and frequent users. *International Journal of Addictions, 29,* 1559–1579.

Hansen, W. B. (1992). School-based substance abuse prevention: A review of the state of the art in curriculum, 1980–1990. *Health Education Research*, 7(3), 403–430.

Hansen, W. B., Graham, J. W., Wolkenstein, B. H., & Rohrbach, L. A. (1991). Program integrity as a moderator of prevention program effectiveness: Results for fifth-grade students in the adolescent alcohol prevention trial. *Journal of Studies on Alcohol*, 52(6), 568–579.

Hanson, D., & Engs, R. (1995). Collegiate drinking: Administrator perceptions, campus policies, and student behaviors. *NASPA Journal*, 32(2), 106–114.

Hillman, S. B., & Sawilowsky, S. S. (1992). A comparison of two grouping methods in distinguishing levels of substance use. *Journal of Clinical Child Psychology*, 21, 348–353.

Institute of Medicine. (1990). *Broadening the base of treatment for alcohol problems.* Washington, DC: National Academy Press.

Jessor, R., Donovan, J. E., & Costa, F. M. (1991). *Beyond adolescence: Problem behavior and young adult development.* Cambridge: Cambridge University Press.

Johnston, L. D., O'Malley, P. M., & Bachman, J. G. (1996). *National survey results on drug use from the Monitoring the Future Study, 1975–1994: Vol. II. College students and young adults.* Rockville, MD: U.S. Department of Health and Human Services.

Keller, D. S., Bennett, M. E., McCrady, B. S., Paulus, M. D., & Frankenstein, W. (1994). Treating college substance abusers: The New Jersey collegiate substance abuse program. *Journal of Substance Abuse Treatment*, 11, 569–581.

Kilty, K. M. (1990). Drinking styles of adolescents and young adults. *Journal of Studies on Alcohol*, 51, 556–564.

Kivlahan, D. R., Marlatt, G. A., Fromme, K., Coppel, D. B., & Williams, E. (1990). Secondary prevention with college drinkers: Evaluation of an alcohol skills training program. *Journal of Consulting and Clinical Psychology*, 58(6), 805–810.

Koss, M. P., Gidycz, C. A., & Wisniewsli, N. (1987). The scope of rape: Incidence and prevalence of sexual aggression and victimization in a national sample of higher education students. *Journal of Consulting and Clinical Psychology*, 55(2), 162–170.

Kraft, D. P. (1984). A comprehensive prevention program for college students. In P. M. Miller & T. D. Nirenberg (Eds.), *Prevention of alcohol abuse* (pp. 327–369). New York: Plenum Press.

Kreitman, N. (1986). Alcohol consumption and the preventive paradox. *British Journal of Addiction*, 88, 591–595.

Larimer, M. E., Kilmer, J. R., Dimeff, L. A., Quigley, L., Williams, E., Baer, J. S., & Marlatt, G. A. (1994). The chapter lifestyle choices project: Initial assessment and description of a motivational alcohol prevention program for fraternities and sororities. *Alcoholism: Clinical and Experimental Research*, 2, 467–497

Larimer, M. E., Marlatt, G. A., Baer, J. S., Quigley, L. A., Blume, A. W., & Hawkins, E. H. (1998). Harm reduction for alcohol problems: Expanding access to and acceptability of prevention and treatment services. In G. A. Marlatt (Ed.), *Harm reduction: Pragmatic strategies for managing high-risk behaviors* (pp. 69–121). New York: Guilford Press.

Marcus, B. H., & Simkin, L. R. (1994). The transtheoretical model: Applications to exercise behavior. *Medicine and Science in Sports and Exercise, 26*(11), 1400–1404.

Marlatt, G. A. (1996). Harm reduction: Come as you are. *Addictive Behaviors, 21,* 779–788.

Marlatt, G. A. (1998). Basic principles and strategies of harm reduction. In G. A. Marlatt (Ed.), *Harm reduction: Pragmatic strategies for managing high-risk behaviors* (pp. 49–66). New York: Guilford Press.

Marlatt, G. A., & Baer, J. S. (1988). Addictive behaviors: Etiology and treatment. *Annual Review of Psychology, 39,* 223–252.

Marlatt, G. A., Baer, J. S., Kivlahan, D. R., Dimeff, L. A., Larimer, M. E., Quigley, L. A., Somers, J. M., & Williams, E. (1998). Screening and brief intervention for high-risk college student drinkers: Results from a two-year follow-up assessment. *Journal of Consulting and Clinical Psychology, 66*(4), 604–615.

Marlatt, G. A., Baer, J. S., & Larimer, M. E. (1995). Preventing alcohol abuse in college students: A harm-reduction approach. In G. Boyd, J. Howard, & R. Zucker (Eds.), *Alcohol problems among adolescents: Current directions in prevention research* (pp. 147–172). Hillsdale, NJ: Erlbaum.

McGinnis, J. M., & Foege, W. (1993). The role of patient education in achieving national health objectives. *Patient Education and Counseling, 21*(1–2), 1–3.

Meilman, P. W., Stone, J. E., Gaylor, M. S., & Turco, J. H. (1990). Alcohol consumption by college undergraduates: Current use and 10-year trends. *Journal of Studies on Alcohol, 51*(5), 389–395.

Miller, E. T. (2000). Preventing alcohol abuse and alcohol-related negative consequences among freshmen college students: Using emerging computer technology to deliver and evaluate the effectiveness of brief intervention efforts. *Dissertation Abstracts International, 61*(8).

Miller, E. T., Roberts, L. J., Neal, D. J., Cressler, S. O., Metrik, J., & Marlatt, G. A. (2000). Test–retest reliability of alcohol measures: Is there a difference between Internet-based assessment and traditional methods? *Psychology of Addictive Behaviors.*

Miller, W. R., & Rollnick, S. (1991). *Motivational interviewing: Preparing people to change addictive behavior.* New York: The Guilford Press.

Mills, K. C., & McCarty, D. (1983). A data based alcohol abuse prevention program in a university setting. *Journal of Alcohol and Drug Education, 28,* 15–27.

Nathan, P. E. (1983). Failures in prevention: Why we can't prevent the devastating effects of alcoholism and drug abuse. *American Psychologist, 38,* 459–467.

National Highway Traffic Safety Administration. (1994). *Traffic safety facts 1993: A compilation of motor vehicle crash data from the fatal accident reporting system and the general estimates system.* Washington, DC: Author.

National Institute on Alcohol Abuse and Alcoholism. (1992). Moderate drinking. *Alcohol Alert, 16,* 1.

Newcomb, M. D., & Bentler, P. M. (1988). *Consequences of adolescent drug use.* Newbury Park, CA: Sage.

Norris, J., Nurius, P. S., & Dimeff, L. A. (1996). Through her eyes: Factors affecting women's perception of and resistance to acquaintance sexual aggression threat. *Psychology of Women Quarterly, 20*(1), 123–145.

O'Malley, P. M., & Wagenaar, A. C. (1991). Effects of minimum drinking age laws on alcohol use, related behaviors and traffic crash involvement among American youth: 1976–1987. *Journal of Studies on Alcohol, 52*(5), 478–491.

Plant, M., Single, E., & Stockwell, T. (Eds.). (1997). *Alcohol: Minimising the harm—what works?* London: Free Association Books.

Pope, H. G., Ionescu, P. M., Aizley, H. G., & Varma, D. K. (1990). Drug use and life style among college undergraduates in 1989: A comparison with 1969 and 1978. *American Journal of Psychiatry, 147*(8), 998–1001.

Presley, C. A., Meilman, P. W., & Lyerla, R. (1994). Development of the Core Alcohol and Drug Survey: Initial findings and future directions. *Journal of American College Health, 42*(6), 248–255.

Prochaska, J. O., & DiClemente, C. C. (1986). Toward a comprehensive model of change. In W. R. Miller & N. Heather (Eds.), *Treating addictive behaviors: Processes of change* (pp. 3–27). New York: Plenum Press.

Prochaska, J. O., DiClemente, C. C., & Norcross, J. C. (1992). In search of how people change: Applications to addictive behaviors. *American Psychologist, 47*(9), 1102–1114.

Reis, J., Riley, W., Lokman, L., & Baer, J. (in press). Interactive multimedia preventive alcohol education: A technology application in higher education. *Journal of Drug Education.*

Roberts, L. J., Neal, D., Kivlahan, D. R., Baer, J. S., & Marlatt, G. A. (2000). Individual drinking changes following a brief intervention among college students: Clinical significance in an indicated preventive context. *Journal of Consulting and Clinical Psychology, 68*(3), 500–505.

Saltz, R., & Elandt, D. (1986). College student drinking studies: 1976–1985. *Contemporary Drug Problems, 13*(1), 117–159.

Samson-Herman, H., Maxwell, C. O., & Doyle, T. F. (1989). The relation of initial alcohol experiences to current alcohol consumption in a college population. *Journal of Studies on Alcohol, 50*(3), 254–260.

Sanchez-Craig, M., Wilkinson, D. A., & Walker, K. (1987). Theory and methods for secondary prevention of alcohol problems: A cognitively based approach. In W. M. Cox (Ed). *Treatment and prevention of alcohol problems: A resource manual* (pp. 287–331). Orlando, FL: Academic Press.

Shedler, J., & Block, J. (1990). Adolescent drug use and psychological health: A longitudinal inquiry. *American Psychologist, 45*(5), 612–630.

Single, E. (1996). Harm reduction as an alcohol-preventive strategy. *Alcohol Health and Research World, 20,* 239–243.

Skinner, H. A. (1988). *Executive summary: Spectrum of drinkers and intervention responses.* Paper presented to the IOM Committee for the Study of Treatment and Rehabilitation Services for Alcoholism and Alcohol Abuse.

Sobell, L. C., Cunningham, J. A., Sobell, M. B., Agrawal, S., Gavin, D. R., Leo, G. I., & Singh, K. N. (1996). Fostering self-change among problem drinkers: A proactive community intervention. *Addictive Behaviors, 21,* 817–833.

Stenmark, D. E., Walfish, S., & Brennan, A. F. (1981). A three course sequence in substance abuse prevention at the baccalaureate level. *Teaching of Psychology, 8*(2), 82–85.

Strunin, L., & Hingson, R. (1992). Alcohol, drugs, and adolescent sexual behavior. *International Journal of the Addictions, 27*(2), 129–146.

Tarter, R. E., & Vanyukov, M. (1994). Alcoholism: A developmental disorder. *Journal of Consulting and Clinical Psychology, 62,* 1096–1107.

Vaillant, G. E. (1996). A long-term follow-up of male alcohol abuse. *Archives of General Psychiatry, 53,* 243–249.

Wagenaar, A. C., & Perry, C. L. (1995). Community strategies for the reduction of youth drinking: Theory and application. In G. M. Boyd, J. Howard, & R. Zucker (Eds.), *Alcohol problems among adolescents: Current directions in prevention research* (pp. 197–223). Hillsdale, NJ: Erlbaum.

Wechsler, H. (1996). Alcohol and the American college campus: A report from the Harvard School of Public Health. *Change, 28*(4), 20–25.

Wechsler, H., Davenport, A., Dowdall, G., Moeykens, B., & Castillo, S. (1994). Health and behavioral consequences of binge drinking in college. *Journal of the American Medical Association, 272*(21), 1672–1677.

Wechsler, H., & Isaac, N. (1992). "Binge" drinkers at Massachusetts colleges. *Journal of the American Medical Association, 267,* 292–293.

Wechsler, H., Moeykens, B., Davenport, A., Castillo, S., & Hansen, J. (1995). The adverse impact of heavy episodic drinkers on other college students. *Journal of Studies on Alcohol, 56,* 628–634.

Weinstein, N. D., & Klein, W. M. (1995). Resistance of personal risk perceptions to debiasing interventions. *Health Psychology, 14*(2), 132–140.

Winerip, M. (1998, January 4). Binge nights: The emergency on campus. *The New York Times,* pp. 29–31, 42.

Zucker, R. A. (1986). The four alcoholisms: A developmental account of the etiologic process. In P. C. Rivers (Ed.), *Nebraska Symposium on Motivation: Vol. 34. Alcohol and addictive behaviors* (pp. 27–83). Lincoln: University of Nebraska Press.

Zucker, R. A., Fitzgerald, H. E., & Moses, H. D. (1995). Emergence of alcohol problems and several alcoholisms: A developmental perspective on etiologic theory and life course trajectory. In D. Cicchetti & D. J. Cohen (Eds.), *Developmental psychopathology* (Vol. 2, pp. 677–711). New York: Wiley.

3

Assessing Adolescent Substance Use Problems and Other Areas of Functioning

State of the Art

KEN C. WINTERS

Adolescent drug involvement is still a major public health concern. American teenagers are showing an increased involvement in substance use since 1992. For example, in a 1997 survey, 22% of 8th graders, 39% of 10th graders, and 42% of 12th graders reported having used an illicit substance in the past year (Johnston, O'Malley & Bachman, 1997). This increased rate of illicit drug use is primarily due to an increase in current marijuana use, which has increased from 1992 to 1997 by more than 16 percentage points among 12th graders (an increase of about 76%) and by more than 10 percentage points among 8th graders (an increase of about 146%). Also, girls are nearly equivalent with boys in substance use rates (Johnston et al., 1997) and may even have surpassed them in some drug categories, such as tobacco (see, e.g., Pascale & Evans, 1993).

Although no large-scale national epidemiological surveys of diagnosable substance use disorder rates in general adolescent populations exist, estimates based on limited community surveys have been recently published. Cohen and colleagues (1993) found in a representative household sample of 676 youths aged 10 to 20 in New York state that alcohol abuse disorders ranged from 3.5% for 14- to 16-year-olds to 14.6% for youth aged 17 to 20. In perhaps the largest investigation of its kind, Harrison and colleagues (Harrison, Fulkerson, & Beebe, 1998) surveyed 74,000 Minnesota high school students and found that for 9th graders, 7% met criteria for substance abuse and 4% for substance dependence and that for 12th graders, 16% met substance abuse criteria and 7% met substance dependence criteria.

From a public health standpoint, adolescent drug abuse has far-reaching social and economic ramifications (Children's Defense Fund, 1991; Johnston, O'Malley, & Bachman, 1992), particularly when its onset is early and when the disorder does not remit. Adverse consequences associated with problematic youth drug abuse include psychiatric comorbidity and suicidality (Kaminer, 1991; Shedler & Block, 1990), mortality from drug-related traffic crashes (Kokotailo, 1995), risky sexual practices (MacKenzie, 1993), and substantial direct health care costs (Drug Abuse Warning Network [DAWN], 1996). Whereas preliminary evidence exists that various treatment approaches can reduce drug use and the related consequences among clinic-referred adolescents (Winters, Latimer & Stinchfield, 1999), little attention has been given to the potential value of brief intervention strategies (see Monti, Barnett, O'Leary, & Colby, Chapter 5, this volume). There is a need for a meaningful effort to identify youth having few but significant substance use problems and to address them efficiently outside the context of specialized treatment. Suitable methods of identification require conceptual agreement as to which assessment variables are relevant and accurate measures of such variables. Because drug involvement and related problems occur along a continuum of severity, and given the potential relevance of diagnostic boundaries in determining referral criteria, both dimensional and categorical measurement strategies are needed in the field.

This chapter begins with a discussion of the problem severity continuum and its heterogeneity, followed by a discussion of the abuse threshold. It considers core variables and domains relevant to adolescent substance abuse assessment and several issues related to the assessment process, including developmental considerations and the validity of self-report. Finally, the chapter provides an overview of prominent screening and comprehensive assessment instruments.

THE PROBLEM SEVERITY CONTINUUM

Given the heterogeneity of adolescent drug involvement, a broad definition of adolescent substance abuse is warranted. Clearly, few teenagers who use drugs, even regularly, are drug dependent. Yet, when problems associated with drug involvement are severe and when frequency of use is habitual and long-standing, a substance dependence disorder may emerge. At the other end of the spectrum is the more common pattern, in which use is infrequent and consequences are minimal and transient. If we take a traditional diagnostic view of drug involvement, "abuse" is defined as use of psychoactive substances that increases risk of harmful and hazardous consequence, and "dependence" is defined as a pattern of compulsive seeking and using substances despite the presence of severe personal and negative consequences. However, these distinctions often do not consider the special case of adolescents (Martin & Winters, 1998). The term "abuse" is often used to refer to any use by adolescents, because on legal grounds alone, any use of substances is illegal, or because some believe that use of any substance contributes to the "abuse" of a developing body and personality. Several other limitations of traditional diagnostic criteria for adolescents have been noted, including that: (1) diagnostic symptoms ignore reasons for drug use; (2) excessive heterogeneity is produced by the one-symptom threshold for a substance abuse diagnosis; (3) abuse symptoms do not always precede the onset of dependence symptoms in youth, which is contrary to expectations about the progression of substance use involvement; and (4) an appreciable percentage of heavy and regular users report one or two dependence symptoms but no abuse symptoms and thus do not meet criteria for any substance use disorder (Kaczynski & Martin, 1995; Martin, Kaczynski, Maisto, & Tarter, 1996; Winters et al., 1999).

Given these considerations, it is useful to take a developmental perspective and consider the following points along a hypothetical drug use problem severity continuum:

1. Abstinence
2. Experimental use. Minimal use, typically associated with recreational activities; often limited to alcohol use
3. Early abuse. More established use, often involving more than one drug; greater frequency; adverse consequences begin to emerge
4. Abuse. Regular and frequent use over an extended period; several adverse consequences emerge
5. Dependence. Continued regular use despite repeated severe consequences; signs of tolerance; adjustment of activities to accommodate drug seeking and drug use
6. Recovery. Return to abstinence; some youths may relapse and cycle through the stages again.

This perspective offers three categories that address level of involvement below the dependence threshold (experimental use, early abuse, and abuse).

Because adolescent users who fall short of meeting dependence criteria are a heterogeneous group (Kaczynski & Martin, 1995), the traditional abuse–dependence distinction may lack verisimiltude for adolescents.

Naturally, any response to an adolescent who is using substances should be consistent with the severity of involvement. Thus treatment interventions should vary along a continuum as well, ranging from brief intervention strategies (e.g., abstinence contract, risk elimination, harm reduction, pattern normalization) to minimal interventions to long-term residential treatment. Although no explicit guidelines exist, the most intensive treatment services should be devoted to youths who show signs of dependency, that is, a history of regular and chronic use, with the presence of multiple personal and social consequences and evidence of an inability to control or stop using substances. Of course, any system that matches client problem severity with an appropriate level of care is irrelevant if such a continuum of treatment does not exist.

TARGETING YOUTHS APPROPRIATE FOR BRIEF INTERVENTIONS

No formal system exists for determining which adolescents would maximally benefit from brief interventions. However, it stands to reason that youths who show abusive-like use are the most likely candidates for brief interventions. Thus it is important to arrive at a working definition of the clinical characteristics and phenomena that define the heterogenous concept of abuse.

The Abuse Threshold

We begin with the issue of whether use equals abuse. The idea that any use of psychoactive substances constitutes abuse is widely accepted at present, at least in part because it is illegal for adolescents to use almost all psychoactive substances, including alcohol and tobacco. Some authorities have therefore asserted that there is no meaningful distinction between use and abuse.

There are problems with the simplest forms of this claim. Because the majority of adolescents experiment with alcohol and many experiment with other substances, to define "abuse" as "use" implies that virtually every adolescent requires some sort of drug abuse intervention. This creates a definition of abuse that is too heterogeneous to be meaningful. Many of those who use alcohol or other drugs when they are young, particularly when their use does not become a regular pattern or lead to serious adverse consequences, do not reveal serious substance abuse problems as they transition into young adulthood (Shedler & Block, 1990). Given the scarcity of treatment services, equating use and abuse seems impractical because it hinders the identification of those who should receive early intervention or more intensive treatment.

One alternative is to conceptualize the abuse threshold and the stages that precede and follow it in terms of a combination of use patterns that place the individual at unacceptable levels of health risk, as well as in terms of negative consequences resulting from such use. This conceptualization further assumes that it is important to identify several stages that precede the far end of the severity continuum, that is, the dependent stage. Thus the single heterogeneous "abuse" category would be replaced by more specific ones. The "early abuse" and "abuse" distinction noted previously is one such example. It is further recommended that the delineation of stages should be sensitive to identifying those users who are most appropriate targets for a given level of treatment (Newcomb & Bentler, 1989). Before we link drug use behaviors to assignment of youth to particular intervention intensities, we need to consider several factors. First, the use of some drugs (e.g., crack cocaine) is sufficiently dangerous that, by itself and in the absence of any other personal consequences or diagnostic symptoms, it is a cause for intervention. Second, making age distinctions is important in that any regular use (apart from other considerations) in a child or very young adolescent (e.g., 12 or 13 years old) may be a warning flag for further drug involvement, so that these individuals should be referred for early intervention. Third, prolonged use of intermediate quantities of drugs or acute ingestion of large quantities of drugs at any age is sufficiently risky that such behavior probably justifies intervention. Fourth, use in particularly inappropriate settings (e.g., prior to driving or during school hours) may be considered "abuse" even in the absence of the overtly negative consequences of such use; it makes no sense to delay intervention until the person advances to more serious consequences, such as getting arrested or involved in an automobile accident. Fifth, in the event that an ambiguous pattern of risky substance use exists, intervention is warranted when the individual has experienced negative social or psychological effects of use. Because the major purpose of any drug abuse intervention is to reverse its negative effects, concern for consequences legitimately preempts concern for specific patterns of use. Sixth, and perhaps the most controversial, is the case in which drug use and consequences are absent but several drug use risk factors are present, such as a family history of drug addiction or alcoholism, drug involvement by older siblings, presence of conduct disorder or ADHD, positive expectancy effects for future drug use, and so forth. Whether targeted intervention strategies for such individuals is effective in reducing future drug abuse still remains an empirical question.

Problems with DSM-IV

The discussion of the abuse threshold would be incomplete without considering the fourth edition of the *Diagnostic and Statistical Manual of Mental Disorders* (DSM-IV; American Psychiatric Association, 1994) criteria for substance use disorders. The applicability of the criteria for adolescents has been called into question (Martin & Winters, 1998). For example, some *DSM-IV* criteria appear to have limited diagnostic utility because they have a very low prevalence, even in clinical samples. This appears to be the case for withdrawal and drug-related medical problems, which likely emerge in most persons only after years of continued drinking or drug use. Relatedly, tolerance appears to have low specificity because the development of tolerance for alcohol in particular is likely a normal developmental phenomenon that happens to most adolescent drinkers. Martin and colleagues (Martin, Kaczynski, Maisto, Bukstein, & Moss, 1995) found that tolerance was highly prevalent among adolescents with and without alcohol dependence even when symptom assignment required an average quantity per drinking occasion of five or more standard drinks. There appear to be other limitations of *DSM-IV* criteria when applied to adolescence. The broad range of problems covered by the *DSM-IV* abuse symptoms, plus the one-symptom threshold (in which endorsing just one abuse symptom results in a diagnosis), produces a great deal of heterogeneity among those with an abuse diagnosis. There is evidence that symptoms of alcohol abuse do not precede symptoms of alcohol dependence, contrary to the notion that abuse should be a prodromal category compared to dependence (Martin et al., 1996).

Furthermore, there is the problem of "diagnostic orphans." This term is used to describe individuals who reveal one or two dependence symptoms but no abuse symptoms and who therefore do not qualify for any diagnosis (Hasin & Paykin, 1998). Several investigations have found that diagnostic orphans are common among adolescents; reported rates range from 10% to 30% (Harrison et al., 1998; Kaczynski & Martin, 1995; Lewinsohn, Rohde, & Seeley, 1996). Kaczynski and Martin (1995) found that diagnostic orphans showed levels of drinking and drug use that were similar to those of adolescents with alcohol abuse and significantly highly than other adolescent regular drinkers without an alcohol diagnosis. These findings suggest either that these individuals have "fallen through the cracks" of the *DSM-IV* system or that, as a result of the too-liberal one-symptom threshold for *DSM-IV* abuse criteria, these individuals are actually diagnostic "imposters" (Martin & Winters, 1998). Although research is needed to further understand the meaning of diagnostic orphans, this group may be appropriate for early intervention strategies.

Normative Considerations

An important factor in the assessment of drug involvement among adolescents is the need to separate the normative and developmental roles played by drug use in this age group. It is difficult to determine when adolescent drug use has negative long-term implications and when it has short-term effects and social payoff. In a strict sense, a "normal" trajectory for adolescents is to experiment with the use of psychoactive substances. As described in the seminal work by Kandel and colleagues (Kandel, 1975; Yagamuchi & Kandel, 1984), adolescents' experiences with substance use most often take place first in a social context and involve the use of "gateway" substances, such as alcohol and cigarettes, which are legal for adults and readily available to minors. Almost all adolescents experiment with gateway drugs, yet relatively few advance to later and more serious levels of substance use, such as the regular use of marijuana and other illicit drugs (Kandel, 1975). Moreover, the presence of some abuse symptoms is not all that rare among adolescents who use substances, even for those who do not use at heavy levels. For example, the Minnesota student survey (Harrison et al., 1998) found that among youths who reported *any* recent substance use, 14% of 9th graders and 23% of 12th graders reported at least one abuse symptom. Also, it has been observed that youths who drink regularly (i.e., at least once a month for at least 6 months) but who do not meet *DSM-IV* criteria for an alcohol use disorder reveal relatively high rates of personal consequences associated with such use (Kaczynski & Martin, 1995).

CORE CONSTRUCTS FOR ASSESSMENT

Any meaningful assessment of adolescent substance abuse requires attention to a wide range of variables. I consider two major sets of assessment variables here. One set has been traditionally included in standardized screening and comprehensive assessment tools and is viewed as essential to the identification, referral and treatment of problems associated with adolescent drug involvement. A list of these key variables is provided in Table 3.1. These variables serve to assist the clinician in determining the extent of the problem, what factors may underlie it, and what intervention response is the most appropriate.

The second set of variables represents cognitive variables that traditionally are not included in existing adolescent substance abuse assessment instruments. Nevertheless, these variables not only have a role in helping to determine level of treatment, particularly brief intervention strategies, but they also may mediate and moderate change behaviors and thus are relevant to outcome research. These cognitive variables are discussed in the following section.

TABLE 3.1. Traditional Content Domains for Determining Level and Nature of Intervention

Drug abuse problem severity

- Onset of initial drug use; onset of regular (e.g., weekly or more frequent) use of drugs.
- Frequency, quantity, and duration for specific drugs, with an emphasis on the preferred drug; both recent (e.g., the previous 6 months) and lifetime use should be covered.
- Review of signs and symptoms of abuse (i.e., hazardous and harmful use) and dependence (deemphasis on withdrawal symptoms).
- Reasons for use (e.g., social, coping, psychological).
- Personal consequences due to drug use, including social, emotional, family, legal, school, HIV/AIDS risk behaviors, and physical.

Risk and protective factors

- Personal adjustment (e.g., self-image, conventionality of values, delinquency proneness, psychological status, school affiliation, learning abilities).
- Peer environment (e.g., peer drug use, peer norms, abstinent role models).
- Home environment (e.g., family togetherness, parenting practices, parental drug use behaviors and attitudes, sexual/physical abuse, sibling drug use behaviors, family norms and expectations about drug use).
- Community and neighborhood characteristics (e.g., population density, level of crime, socioeconomic status).

Cognitive Domains: Possible Mediators and Moderators of Change

A growing body of research highlights the development of substance-related beliefs or schemas and their role in mediating and moderating early substance use (Christensen & Goldman, 1983; Christensen, Smith, Roehling, & Goldman, 1989; Zucker, Kincaid, Fitzgerald, & Bingham, 1995). Research on the cognitive precursors of drug use behaviors has been directed at demonstrating either that groups with different behaviors, such as alcohol consumption patterns, possess different cognitions (Johnson & Gurin, 1994) or, conversely, that groups with different cognitions show more likelihood of future drug use behaviors (Christensen et al., 1989).

Naturally, developmental considerations are important with respect to assessing cognitive factors in adolescents. Cognitive capacities for abstract thinking begin to take a more prominent role during early adolescence, yet older adolescents are better equipped to consider the future consequences of their actions (Keating & Clark, 1980). Another consideration is that environmental and personal adjustment variables interact with cognitive variables to influence and promote behavioral change. For example, social support from peers and family members will likely affect self-efficacy.

Four cognitive variables related to behavioral change that have been prominently discussed in the substance abuse literature include: reasons for drug use, expectancies about behavioral outcomes (and the related construct of risk perception), readiness to change, and confidence in general ability to accomplish personal goals (or self-efficacy).

Reasons for Drug Use

Research suggests that drug use by adolescents may be associated with several motivations, including recreational benefits (e.g., to have fun), social conformity, mood enhancement, and coping with stress (Petraitis, Flay, & Miller, 1995). There is some evidence that youths with a substance-use-dependence disorder ascribe greater benefits to the social conformity and mood enhancement effects of drug involvement compared with non-dependent adolescents (Henly & Winters, 1988).

Expectancies

For adolescents, it is relevant to measure drug-related expectancies pertaining to negative physical effects, negative psychosocial effects, future health concerns, positive social effects, and reduction of negative affect (Christiansen, Goldman, & Brown, 1985). Similar concepts discussed in the literature are risk perception or perceived cost versus benefit of the behavior. Individuals who have knowledge about the hazards and risks of a given health behavior show a consistent tendency to deny that they personally are at risk. This denial can lead to two cognitive processes: (1) belief perseverance, in which individuals selectively attend to messages that support their beliefs (Festinger, 1957) and exhibit counterarguments when faced with disconfirming evidence (Nisbit & Ross, 1980) and (2) optimistic bias or erroneous beliefs that personal risk is less than the risk faced by others (Janis & Mann, 1977). Some variables relevant for measurement of expectancies and risk perception include perceived vulnerability to and knowledge about the health risks of drug use, perceived personal vulnerability to drug-related consequences, and the person's belief that quitting drug use will reduce his or her personal risk for such consequences. Also, there may be merit in measuring what has been referred to as "optimistic bias" for personal risk. Participants can be asked to rate their chances of developing certain consequences of drug use behaviors (e.g., much lower than average, lower than average, above average, etc.) and their responses can be compared with estimates of actual consequences obtained from national data (Weinstein, 1984). (See Smith & Anderson, Chapter 4, this volume, for more discussion on the relationship of substance use and expectancy effects.)

Readiness for Behavior Change

This domain involves problem recognition, readiness for action, treatment suitability (availability and accessibility), and influences that lead to coercive pressure to seek treatment. These motivational factors may affect adolescents' attitudes toward subsequent treatment, including their inclination to adhere to treatment plans (Prochaska, DiClemente, & Norcross, 1992). We know very little about the determinants of motivational variables that promote positive change in adolescents. It stands to reason, however, that adolescents are subject to many of the same underlying motivational forces that influence change in adults suffering from addictions. For example, drug involvement often creates an awareness within the individual that the drug use offers personal benefits, despite the recognition that such use leads to a destructive behavior pattern. The result is that efforts to change these behaviors often fail. As a double-edged sword, drug use produces ambivalence for the person who is thinking about change, a simultaneous sense of both wanting and not wanting to change (Prochaska, DiClemente, & Norcross, 1992; Shaffer, 1997). The effects of ambivalence can manifest in the following way (Shaffer, 1997): At the outset, the person ignores the obvious destructive power of drug involvement and thus is inclined to cling to the part of this experience that produces positive consequences, such as relief from painful emotions; however, as negative consequences mount, the drug user becomes aware of their ambivalence and begins to express a wish to quit; the individual identifies the addictive behavior as the source of the many problems he or she is experiencing; however, until the individual begins to realize that the costs of the addictive behavior exceed the benefits, he or she is unlikely to want to stop. For developmental reasons, young people may have more trouble than adults projecting the consequences of their use into the future (Erikson, 1968). Their drug involvement has not yet occurred over an extended period of time, and thus multiple and chronic negative consequences have not yet accumulated and the possible long-term consequences of risky behaviors are minimized. To further aggravate the change process, the adolescent may have experienced coercive pressure to seek and continue treatment. There are no empirical studies that provide reliable estimates of the extent and type of coercion that occurs in the process of youths seeking and receiving drug treatment, but conventional wisdom suggests that many adolescents have explicitly or implicitly been coerced into attending treatment. Coercive influences can take several forms, such as exclusion from the decision-making process about seeking treatment, use of force and deceit to impose treatment on the individual, and use of restraint to retain the person in treatment (Monahan et al., 1995). Consequently, at the outset of treatment, counselors must be

sensitive to motivational barriers that may be linked to circumstances surrounding the youth's contact with the service.

Self-Efficacy

Self-efficacy, or the confidence in personal ability, has a central role in
many conceptionalizations about behavioral control and change (see, e.g.,
Bandura, 1977). Self-efficacy has been shown to predict a variety of health
behavior outcomes (Grembowski et al., 1993; O'Leary, 1985), including alcohol treatment outcome (Miller & Rollnick, 1991). Self-efficacy affects
not only one's choice of activities, such as behavior change goals, but also
how much effort is expended in such activities and how long one will persist in the face of adversity. Because levels of self-efficacy have predicted
goal achievement (Borrelli & Mermelstein, 1994), it may be that self-
efficacy influences outcome by affecting the attention one pays to achieving
goals. Thus self-efficacy measures should be accompanied by measures of
goal setting and achievement, as well as other constructs believed to underlie self-efficacy, such as the client's perceptions of his or her own ability to
overcome barriers to change (Miller, 1983).

CRITICAL MEASUREMENT ISSUES

Developmental Considerations

The measurement process is affected by developmental factors. Substance-
abusing youths have been characterized as developmentally delayed in
terms of their cognitive, social, and emotional functioning (Noam &
Houlihan, 1990). These delays may affect perception of and willingness to
report problems, as well as receptivity to treatment. It stands to reason that
admitting to a serious drug problem requires a modicum of self-insight.
Many youths may not be emotionally prepared to take an open view of
their behavior and to recognize the negative effects that continued drug use
may elicit. Stage of change theory suggests that a lack of problem recognition impedes engagement in treatment (Prochaska et al., 1992).

There are other developmental considerations as well. It has been observed that some youths compromise their self-reports by overstating problems, as evidenced by admitting on a questionnaire that they took a fake
drug (e.g., "cadrines"; Winters, Stinchfield, Henly, & Schwartz, 1991). Although there may be several reasons for this type of tendency to "fake
bad," it may be influenced by social immaturity factors often seen during
adolescence, such as self-aggrandizement. Also, the selection of assessment
questionnaires and interviews requires that the assessor consider the devel-

opmental appropriateness of the instrument. Some tools have been primarily normed and validated on older adolescents, and also the reading and comprehension levels required may be inappropriate for younger adolescents. To determine the suitability of an instrument, one should review its manual.

Validity of Self-Report

The use of diagnostic assessment measures assumes that self-reports are valid, although the validity of self-report of drug use behavior has been the subject of considerable debate (Babor, Stephens, & Marlatt, 1987; Watson, Tilleskjor, Hoodecheck-Show, Pucel, & Jacobs, 1984). In addition to purposely distorting the truth, clients' responses can be distorted due to lack of insight, inattentiveness, or misunderstanding of a question. The clinical literature is relatively sparse in terms of the extent to which compromised self-report occurs and what factors contribute to it. However, an examination of the instrumentation literature provides some support for the validity of self-report: (1) admissions of illicit drug use by a large proportion of respondents in clinic-referred settings; (2) low rates of endorsements of items indicative of "faking bad"; (3) higher rates of drug use and accompanying psychosocial problems in clinical samples compared with community or school samples; (4) a pattern of convergence when self-report is compared with reports of other informants (e.g., parents and teachers) and archival records; and (5) a general consistency of disclosures across time (see, e.g., Brown et al., 1998; Maisto, Connors, & Allen, 1995; Shaffer et al., 1993; Winters et al., 1991).

Inconsistent self-reports, nevertheless, have been noted in the literature. When adolescents are asked about past drug use that was sporadic or infrequent (Single, Kandel, & Johnson, 1975) and when queried over a 1-year period about the reported age of first use of alcohol and marijuana (Bailey, Flewelling, & Rachal, 1992), significant inconsistencies have been observed. Relatedly, there have been discrepancies noted when intake data are compared with similar data collected at treatment completion. This issue was investigated by Stinchfield (1997) and speaks to the potential problem, often noted from clinical experience, that drug abusers tend to minimize the extent or level of their drug use. Stinchfield compared self-reports of drug use problems obtained from adolescents at two points in time: at drug assessment intake and at completion of treatment 1 month later. In both instances, participants were instructed to base their self-reports on the same historical time frame, namely, 1 year prior to treatment. When test scores were compared, the scores at discharge were significantly higher than the scores at intake. The lower intake scores may have been the result of a self-report dampening effect caused by denial and the general reluctance of individuals to fully self-disclose under difficult situations. Test effects can affect relative levels of self-reported drug use. Does the study suggest that self-report data are useless? Even given the lower levels of reported drug use at intake, the clinic-referred adolescents indicated levels of drug use much higher than those of a nonclinical, community comparison sample. Thus the impact of the so-called "intake–discharge" effect, whatever its causes, does not appear to disregard self-report data.

However, this effect is relevant to brief interventions, especially those that focus on the use of motivational interviewing techniques. These approaches rely heavily on self-report as part of personalized feedback and for the decisional balance exercise. Clearly, as the therapist builds rapport with the client, the dampening effect is lessened. Also, the use of both standardized questionnaires and structured interviews serves as a vehicle for improving the validity of self-report. Standardized instruments have several advantages, including minimized rate or bias, tendency for clients to feel less threatened by this testing process, and inclusion of scales designed to assess response bias. Interviews can promote validity of self-report in three ways. First, the interviewer has an opportunity to express concern about the client's situation. When a client feels intimidated by the assessment or is resistant to questioning, expressions of empathy may improve his or her willingness to self-disclose. Second, general information may be gained by observing nonverbal clues, such as emotional and physical characteristics. Third, follow-up questioning may elicit information that would have been difficult to obtain through the forced-choice format of a questionnaire.

Parents' Report

An issue related to the validity of adolescent self-report is the value of parents' reports. Diagnoses of childhood disorders have historically depended on the report of the parent (primarily the mother), although the adolescent psychopathology literature suggests that parents' and adolescents' reports are fairly congruent with each other for some problem areas, particularly externalizing behaviors, but not for internalized behaviors and symptoms (Ivens & Rehm, 1988). Clinical experience has long suggested that parents cannot always provide meaningful details about their child's possible alcohol and other drug use behaviors. Empirically, the limited data that do exist on this topic provide a mixed picture. Diagnostic agreement between mothers' and children's reports of substance use disorders have shown a considerable range. Edelbrock and colleagues (Edelbrock, Costello, Dulcan, & Kalas, 1986) reported an average mother–child agreement of 63% for substance use disorder symptoms, whereas Weissman's research team reported an average agreement between mothers' and sons' reports of only 17%

(Weissman et al., 1987). A recent agreement study examined reports of adolescents in drug clinics and their mothers on a wide range of drug use behaviors and consequences (Winters, Anderson, Bengston, Stinchfield, & Latimer, 2000). They found that mothers concurred at a 78% level with their child in terms of reporting the highest level of recent substance use. However, when mothers were asked about more specific details about the child's substance involvement, concordance with child data was only moderate.

Assessment Practices

Appropriate use of assessment instruments in clinical settings, including those in which brief intervention approaches are practiced, requires a sensitivity to sound assessment practices. Provided here are four testing practices that can serve as a guide for appropriate use of questionnaires and interviews (Eyde, Moreland, Robertson, Primoff, & Most, 1988). The relevance of these guidelines for brief interventions is noted.

1. *Proper test understanding and use.* Responsible and competent use of a test includes making sure the test actually measures what it is supposed to be measuring. The test's manual should describe the traits and characteristics that the test is intended to measure and the types of patients for whom and settings in which the use of the test is appropriate. Relatedly, test users need to have knowledge about the test's reliability and validity. The psychometric data should be relevant for the intended use of the test. Test results must be interpreted with caution if its use does not match the conditions under which the test was psychometrically evaluated. If scales are to be used as part of a pre–post comparison, it is especially important to consider their standard error of measurement. Because candidates for brief interventions should be administered tests that can adequately measure mild to moderate levels of drug involvement severity, the test's psychometric evidence should address this issue.

2. *Appropriate use of norms and criterion data.* For norm-based tests, the norms associated with the test must be appropriate for the given sample being tested. It would be unwise to use a test in a clinical setting that did not have clinical norms. For criterion-based tests (e.g., diagnostic interviews), it is important to make sure that all criterion measures that were established in the development of the test are appropriate for the patients being tested. It also is important to ensure that the condition and setting under which the norms and criterion data were collected are similar to those of the present application of the test. This consideration is quite relevant, given that testing an individual during a relatively brief clinic stay may produce different demand characteristics and other sources of report-

ing variance compared with longer term situations, such as a residential treatment program.

3. *Scoring accuracy.* The test administrator must take responsibility for checking scoring accuracy when the test is hand scored. Computerized score reports that provide narrative summaries and recommendations for treatment should be interpreted cautiously because they are based on generalities.

4. *Interpretative feedback.* The user must have the skills to give interpretation and provide appropriate feedback to the individual being tested. Successful brief interventions, particularly when they are based on motivational interviewing strategies, depend in large part on the therapist imparting clear feedback to the client about the client's behavior, feelings, and options for change. Test scores are a vital tool for the therapist as he or she helps the client recognize the negative consequences of drug-using behaviors and how others who have produced similar test scores have been referred for intervention or treatment.

Use of Structured and Semistructured Diagnostic Interviews

It is relevant to consider the special case of structured and semistructured diagnostic interviews. This is the optimal method when attempting to determine the presence or absence of a substance use disorder. Given that determining the appropriateness for brief intervention approaches likely requires ruling out a dependence diagnosis, such interviews provide an efficient means to begin the client–treatment matching process.

The structured and semistructured formats differ in the degree of clinical judgment that the interviewer must employ when assigning symptoms, ratings, and diagnoses. Highly structured interviews direct the interviewer to read each question exactly as it is written and then decide whether the described symptom is absent or present (or, in some cases, absent, subclinical, or present). These interviews can be administered with acceptable reliability by a well-trained layperson because the client answers objective questions with fixed-response categories. With the advent of definable criteria for alcohol use disorders, such as in *DSM-IV*, it is possible with structured interviews to more precisely identify the information needed to make a diagnosis. In contrast, semistructured interviews require more clinical judgment by the assessor, who elicits the client's initial response and then determines through further probing whether a symptom is present or not. Users of these interviews usually require advanced training in assessment and psychopathology. Such interviews grant the interviewer considerable latitude in adapting questions to suit the respondent, and they allow the interviewer to probe further depending on the response. This exploration lies somewhere between client self-report and clinician rating.

Naturally, it is vital to match the skill level of the assessor with the training requirements of these two interview formats. The clinical skill level of the assessor is more crucial when administering semistructured interviews; obtaining a diagnosis from such interviews may require a considerable degree of expertise. On the other hand, the very highly structured interviews that contain strictly fixed formats for responses and for which little judgment is required (i.e., record a "yes" or "no" based on the participant's response) can be reliably administered by well-trained laypersons. This is not to say that all structured interviews are judgment free. It is common for the more recent structured interviews (e.g., Adolescent Diagnostic Interview Schedule [ADI], Winters & Henly, 1993; Diagnostic Interview for Children and Adolescents [DICA], Herjanic & Campbell, 1977; Structured Clinical Interview for the DSM-III-R [SCID], Spitzer, Williams, & Gibbon, 1987) to require that the rater make fairly sophisticated decisions between the presence and possible presence (subclinical) of symptoms.

REVIEW OF ASSESSMENT INSTRUMENTS

It is quite cost effective to take advantage of the assessment work of others, given the considerable amount of technical expertise, time, and resources that are required to develop sound instruments. Although there are several instruments available to researchers and clinicians, locating and reviewing appropriate tools can be challenging. Sorting through them to determine their accuracy and utility, particularly with respect to brief intervention approaches, can also be a time-consuming task. Fortunately, many of the more recent instruments have been well studied and have favorable psychometric properties, and the process of reviewing them is simplified because several handbooks and review articles can serve as reference guides (Allen & Columbus, 1995; Center for Substance Abuse Treatment, 1999; Farrow, Smith, & Hurst, 1993; Leccese & Waldron, 1994).

Table 3.2 provides brief summaries of the more prominent screening and comprehensive tools (interview and paper-and-pencil formats) reported in the literature. The relatively shorter screening instruments may be most relevant for use with brief interventions. These tools are useful because they can succinctly estimate a youth's position along the problem severity continuum. Screening measures typically yield conservative scoring decisions (e.g., "probable substance abuser" or "needs a comprehensive assessment") in an effort to guard against the mistake of claiming that there is no substance use problem when in fact one exists (i.e., a false negative). A screening tool's full value is appreciated when it is used to determine the

TABLE 3.2. Screening and Comprehensive Instruments for Assessing Adolescent Drug Involvement

Instrument name	Author	Type	Length	Content	Source for psychometrics
		Screening instruments			
Adolescent Alcohol Involvement Scale (AAIS)	Mayer & Filstead (1979)	Self-report	14-item	Drug involvement	Mayer & Filstead (1979); Moberg (1983)
Adolescent Drinking Index (ADI)	Harrell & Wirtz (1989)	Self-report	24-item	Drug involvement and psychosocial factors	Harrell & Wirtz (1989)
Adolescent Drug Involvement Scale (ADIS)	Moberg & Hahn (1991)	Self-report	13-item	Drug involvement	Moberg & Hahn (1991)
Client Substance Index (CSI)	Moore (1983)	Self-report	113-item	Drug involvement	Moore (1983)
Client Substance Index—Short (CSI-S)	Thomas (1990)	Self-report	15-item	Drug involvement	Thomas (1990)
Drug and Alcohol Problem (DAP) Quick Screen	Schwartz & Wirtz (1990)	Self-report	30-item	Drug involvement	Schwartz & Wirtz (1990)
Drug Use Screening Inventory—Revised (DUSI-R)	Tarter et al. (1992)	Self-report	159-item	Drug involvement, psychiatric comorbidity, and psychosocial factors	Kirisci et al. (1995); Tarter et al. (1992)
Personal Experience Screening Questionnaire (PESQ)	Winters (1992)	Self-report	40-item	Drug involvement, psychosocial factors, and response distortion	Winters (1992)
Problem Oriented Screening Questionnaire (POSIT)	Rahdert (1991)	Self-report	139-item	Drug involvement and psychosocial factors	Dembo et al. (1997); Latimer et al. (1997); McLaney et al. (1994); Rahdert (1991)

Instrument	Reference	Type	Items	Content	Citations
Rutgers Alcohol Problem Index (RAPI)	White & Labouvie (1989)	Self-report	23-item	Drug involvement and psychosocial factors	White & Labouvie (1989)
Substance Abuse Subtle Screening Inventory (SASSI)	Miller (1990)	Self-report	81-item	Drug involvement	Miller (1990); Risberg, Stevens, & Graybill (1995)
Comprehensive instruments					
Adolescent Diagnostic Interview (ADI)	Winters & Henly (1993)	Interview	Varies[a]	Drug involvement, psychosocial factors ans response distortion	Winters & Henly (1993); Winters, Stinchfield, Fulkerson, & Henly (1993)
Adolescent Drug Abuse Diagnoses (ADAD)	Friedman & Utada (1989)	Interview	150-item	Drug involvement and psychosocial factors	Friedman & Utada (1989)
Adolescent Problem Severity Index (APSI)	Metzger et al. (1991)	Interview	Varies[a]	Drug involvement and psychosocial factors	Metzger et al. (1991)
Comprehensive Addiction Severity Index for Adolescents (CASI-A)	Meyers (1991)	Interview	Varies[a]	Drug involvement and psychosocial factors	Meyers (1991)
Customary Drinking and Drug Use Record (CDDR)	Brown et al. (1998)	Interview	Varies[a]	Drug involvement	Brown et al. (1998)
Diagnostic Interview for Children and Adolescents (DICA)	Reich et al. (1982, 1992)	Interview	Varies[a]	Drug involvement, psychiatric comorbidity, and psychosocial factors	Psychometric evidence specific to SUD not yet published
Diagnostic Interview Schedule for Children (DISC)	Costello et al. (1985); Shaffer et al. (1996)	Interview	Varies[a]	Drug involvement, psychiatric comorbidity, and psychosocial factors	Costello et al. (1985); Fisher et al. (1993); Roberts et al. (1996); Shaffer et al. (1996)

(continued)

TABLE 3.2. (continued)

Instrument name	Author	Type	Length	Content	Source for psychometrics
Comprehensive instruments (continued)					
Kiddie SADS (K-SADS)	Endicott & Spitzer (1978)	Interview	Varies[a]	Drug involvement and psychiatric comorbidity	Endicott & Spitzer (1978); Orvaschel (1985, 1995); Puig-Antich & Ryan (1986)
Prevention Management Evaluation System (PMES)	Simpson (1991)	Interview	Varies[a]	Drug involvement and psychosocial factors	Barrett et al. (1988); Simpson (1991)
Structured Clinical Interview for the DSM (SCID)	Spitzer et al. (1992)	Interview	Varies[a]	Drug involvement and psychiatric comorbidity	Martin et al. (1995); Spitzer et al. (1987, 1992)
Teen Severity Index (T-ASI)	Kaminer et al. (1991)	Interview	Varies[a]	Drug involvement, psychiatric comorbidity, and psychosocial factors	Kaminer et al. (1991)
Adolescent Chemical Health Inventory (ACHI)	Renovex (1988)	Self-report (computer-adapted)	Varies[a]	Drug involvement and psychosocial factors	Renovex (1988)
Adolescent Self-Assessment Profile (ASAP)	Wanberg (1992)	Self-report	225-item	Drug involvement	Wanberg (1992)
Chemical Dependency Assessment Profile (CDAP)	Harrell et al. (1991)	Self-report	235-item	Drug involvement	Harrell et al. (1991)
Hilson Adolescent Profile (HAP)	Inwald et al. (1986)	Self-report	310-item	Drug involvement and psychiatric comorbidity	Inwald et al. (1986)

Instrument	Reference	Format	No. of items	Construct	Reference(s)
Juvenile Automated Substance Abuse Evaluation (JASAE)	ADE (1987)	Self-report (computer-adapted)	108-item	Drug involvement	ADE (1987)
Personal Experience Inventory (PEI)	Winters & Henly (1989)	Self-report	276-item	Drug involvement, psychiatric comorbidity, and psychosocial factors	Winters & Henly (1989); Winters et al. (1993)
Other measures					
Alcohol Expectancies Questionnaire—Adolescent Version (AEQ-A)	Brown et al. (1987)	Self-report	90-item	Alcohol expectancies	Brown et al. (1987); Christiansen et al. (1989)
Decisional Balance Scale	Migneault et al. (1997)	Self-report	16-item	Pros and cons of drinking	Migneault et al. (1997)
Perceived-Benefit-of-Drinking and Drug Use Scales	Petchers & Singer (1987)	Self-report	10-item	Beliefs about the personal benefits of drug use	Petchers & Singer (1987, 1990)
Problem Recognition Questionnaire (PRQ)	Cady et al. (1996)	Self-report	24-item	Readiness for change	Cady et al. (1996)
Circumstances, Motivation, Readiness and Suitability Scales (CMRS)	Jainchill et al. (1995)	Self-report	25-item	Readiness for change and suitability for treatment	Jainchill et al. (1995)
Drug Avoidance Self-Efficacy Scale (DASES)	Martin et al. (1995)	Self-report	—	Self-efficacy for abstinence	Martin et al. (1995)

[a]Number of items and administration time varies widely, based on adolescent's level of drug involvement.

appropriateness of a more complete assessment and for determination of treatment needs.

In contrast to screening measures, comprehensive, multidimensional tools are aimed at verifying the presence of a substance abuse problem and determining the level of treatment and what individual treatment goals are relevant in the event treatment is warranted. Generally, comprehensive interviews in this field are organized around diagnostic criteria, such as *DSM-III-R* and *DSM-IV*, whereas multiscale instruments provide norm-based scale scores. Our review includes prominent child and adolescent psychiatric interviews that contain modules for substance use disorders, substance use disorder interviews, and paper-and-pencil questionnaires. Finally, we summarize other measures that may be particularly relevant for brief interventions, including expectancy, readiness for change, and self-efficacy measures.

SUMMARY AND SUGGESTED RESEARCH DIRECTIONS

The recent proliferation of adolescent substance abuse assessment instruments is a double-edged sword. Professionals and researchers have a number of different screening and comprehensive tools from which to choose. On the other hand, selecting the right one for a given individual for a particular situation can be a difficult task. There are numerous screening tools, and there is redundancy in that several interviews are closely modeled after the adult-based Addiction Severity Index (McLellan, Luborsky, Woody, & O'Brien, 1980). An empirical comparison of the instruments has not been conducted, and so little is known about how these various measures perform differentially in different clinical situations and with varying subgroups of youth. In Leccese and Waldron's (1994) critical review of the adolescent substance abuse assessment area, they concluded that some of the existing instruments have promising psychometric properties and "that recent progress in this field is encouraging" (p. 561).

In terms of content coverage, the existing instruments provide adequate attention to drug use problem severity and related psychosocial risk and protective factors. Nevertheless, future research should expand into domains that have been promoted by the adult treatment literature, such as readiness for change, and should consider variables likely to be important to matching adolescent substance abusers to brief intervention strategies, including self-efficacy, risk perception, and coercion. Also, we know little about the role of assessment in enhancing behavior change among drug-using youth. The personal feedback obtained from the assessment process can be persuasive input for convincing clients to change (Miller, Sovereign, & Krege, 1988).

Other brief intervention assessment challenges merit further research attention. First are issues related to the validity of self-report. Most tools have reported validity data on severe-end cases. Thus we have relatively less confidence in existing scales with respect to their accuracy in assessing drug use severity at the lower end of the continuum. Measurement error may be greater for moderate cases. For example, it has been shown that reports of prior drug use are more unreliable when such use is infrequent (Single et al., 1975), and a similar problem of unreliability may occur when measuring infrequent and less severe negative consequences associated with infrequent use. Also, it stands to reason that minimization by the adolescent may be greater when use is moderate and severe consequences have not yet occurred; and it is unlikely that parents, traditionally poor corroborators of their child's drug involvement, can be relied on to provide highly useful data.

There is also a need for more research as to the value of response distortion scales to detect dishonesty among drug-abusing youths. Many existing adolescent defensiveness measures are based on adult scales and thus may not be developmentally appropriate for adolescents. It is difficult to judge whether the scales are measuring true denial or simply reflecting natural impression management tendencies of young people to see oneself in a favorable light. Finally, we know little about how assessment mode affects disclosure of drug use. There is some literature on the comparability of computer versus paper-and-pencil administration, yet the differential effect on self-report of paper-and-pencil format compared with face-to-face and telephone interviews is an understudied area (Aquilino, 1994). This is an important research area given that brief intervention approaches depend on adequate self-disclosure by the client within time constraints.

The potential of brief interventions for adolescents with mild to moderate problems associated with use of alcohol and other drugs will likely become clearer as research in this area expands. It will be important for the assessment literature to address the administration and measurement validity challenges posed by brief interventions. These challenges include how to maximize a blend between brief and comprehensive assessment, measuring motivational variables, and use of assessment results as a feedback tool to bring clients to the action phase.

REFERENCES

A.D.F. (1987). *Juvenile Automated Substance Abuse Evaluations (JASAE)*. Clarkston, MI: Author.

Allen, J. P., & Columbus, M. (Eds.). (1995). *Assessing alcohol problems: A guide for clinicians and researchers* (NIAAA Treatment Handbook Series 4). Bethesda, MD: National Institute on Alcohol Abuse and Alcoholism.

American Psychiatric Association. (1994). *Diagnostic and statistical manual of mental disorders* (4th ed.). Washington, DC: Author.

Aquilino, W. S. (1994). Interview mode effects in surveys of drug and alcohol use. *Public Opinion Quarterly, 58*, 210–240.

Babor, T. F., Stephens, R. S., & Marlatt, G. A. (1987). Verbal report methods in clinical research on alcoholism: Response bias and its minimization. *Journal of Studies on Alcohol, 48*, 410–424.

Bailey, S. L., Flewelling, R. L., & Rachal, J. V. (1992). The characteristics of inconsistencies in self-reports of alcohol and marijuana use in longitudinal study of adolescents. *Journal of Studies on Alcohol, 53*, 636–647.

Bandura, A. (1977). *Social learning theory.* Englewood Cliffs, NJ: Prentice-Hall.

Barrett, M. E., Simpson, D. D., & Lehman, W. E. (1988). Behavioral changes among adolescents in drug abuse intervention programs. *Journal of Clinical Psychology, 44*, 461–473.

Borrelli, B., & Mermelstein, R. (1994). Goal setting and behavior change in a smoking cessation program. *Cognitive Therapy and Research, 18*, 68–83.

Brown, S. A., Christiansen, B. A., & Goldman, M. S. (1987). The Alcohol Expectancies Questionnaire: An instrument for the assessment of adolescent and adult alcohol expectancies. *Journal of Studies on Alcohol, 48*, 483–491.

Brown, S. A., Creamer, V. A., & Stetson, B. A. (1987). Adolescent alcohol expectancies in relation to personal and parental drinking patterns. *Journal of Abnormal Psychology, 96*, 117–121.

Brown, S. A., Myers, M. G., Lippke, L., Tapert, S. F., Stewart, D. G., & Vik, P. W. (1998). Psychometric evaluation of the Customary Drinking and Drug Use Record (CDDR): A measure of adolescent alcohol and drug involvement. *Journal of Studies on Alcohol, 59*, 427–438.

Cady, M., Winters, K. C., Jordan, D., & Solheim, K. (1996). Motivation to change as a predictor of treatment outcome for adolescent substance abusers. *Journal of Child and Adolescent Substance Abuse, 5*, 73–91.

Center for Substance Abuse Treatment. (1999). *Screening and assessing adolescents for substance use disorders* (Treatment Improvement Protocol [TIP] Series 31). Rockville, MD: Substance Abuse Mental Health Services Administration.

Children's Defense Fund. (1991). *The adolescent and young adult fact book.* Washington, DC: Author.

Christiansen, B. A., & Goldman, M. S. (1983). Alcohol-related expectancies versus demographic background variables in the prediction of adolescent drinking. *Journal of Consulting and Clinical Psychology, 51*, 249–257.

Christiansen, B. A., Goldman, M. S., & Brown, S. A. (1985). The differential development of adolescent alcohol expectancies may predict adult alcoholism. *Addictive Behaviors, 10*, 299–306.

Christiansen, B. A., Smith, G. T., Roehling, P. V., & Goldman M. S. (1989). Using alcohol expectancies to predict adolescent drinking behavior after one year. *Journal of Consulting and Clinical Psychology, 57*, 93–99.

Cohen, P., Cohen, J., Kasen, S., Velez, C. M., Hartmark, C., Johnson, J., Rojas, M., Brook, J., & Streuning, E. L. (1993). An epidemiological study of disorder in late childhood and adolescence: 1. Age- and gender-specific prevalence. *Journal of Child Psychology and Psychiatry, 34*, 851–867.

Costello, E. J., Edelbroch, C., & Costello, A. J. (1985). Validity of the NIMH Diagnostic Interview Schedule for Children: A comparison between psychiatric and pediatric referrals. *Journal of Abnormal Child Psychology, 13,* 570–595.

Dembo, R., Schmeidler, J., Borden, P., Chin Sue, C., & Manning, D. (1997). Use of the POSIT among arrested youths entering a juvenile assessment center: A replication and update. *Journal of Child and Adolescent Substance Abuse, 6,* 19–42.

Drug Abuse Warning Network. (1996). *1996 DAWN report.* Washington, DC: Substance Abuse and Mental Health Service Administration.

Edelbrook, C., Costello, A. J., Dulcan, M. K., & Kalas, R. (1986). Parent–child agreement on child psychiatric symptoms assessed via structured interview. *Journal of Child Psychology and Psychiatry, 27,* 181–190.

Endicott, J., & Spitzer, R. L. (1978). A diagnostic interview: The Schedule for Affective Disorder and Schizophrenia. *Archives of General Psychiatry, 35,* 837–844.

Erikson, E. H. (1968). *Identity, youth and crisis.* New York: Norton.

Eyde, L. D., Moreland, K. L., Robertson, G. J., Primoff, E. S., & Most, R. B. (1998). *Test user qualifications: A data-based approach to promoting good test use* [Executive summary]. Joint Committee on Testing Practices, Test User Qualifications Working Group. Washington, DC: American Psychological Association.

Farrow, F. A., Smith, W. R., & Hurst, M. D. (1993). *Adolescent drug and alcohol assessment instruments in current use: A critical comparison.* Seattle: University of Washington.

Festinger, L. (1957). *A theory of cognitive dissonance.* Stanford, CA: Stanford University Press.

Fisher, P., Shaffer, D., Piacentini, J. C., Lapkin, J., Kafantaris, V., Leonard, H., & Herzog, D. B. (1993). Sensitivity of the Diagnostic Interview Schedule for Children—2nd Edition (DISC-2.1) for specific diagnoses of children and adolescents. *Journal of the American Academy of Child and Adolescent Psychiatry, 32,* 666–673.

Friedman, A. S., & Utada, A. (1989). A method for diagnosing and planning the treatment of adolescent drug abusers: Adolescent Drug Abuse Diagnosis instrument. *Journal of Drug Education, 19,* 285–312.

Grembowski, D., Patrick, D., Diehr, P., Durham, M., Beresford, S., Kay, E., & Hecht, J. (1993). Self efficacy and health behavior among older adults. *Journal of Health and Social Behavior, 34,* 89–104.

Harrell, T. H., Honaker, L. M., & Davis, E. (1991). Cognitive and behavioral dimensions of dysfunction in alcohol and polydrug abusers. *Journal of Substance Abuse, 3,* 415–426.

Harrell, A., & Wirtz, P. M. (1989). Screening for adolescent problem drinking: Validation of a multidimensional instrument for case identification. *Psychological Assessment, 1,* 61–63.

Harrison, P. A., Fulkerson, J. A., & Beebe, T. J. (1998). DSM-IV substance use disorder criteria for adolescents: A critical examination based on a statewide school survey. *American Journal of Psychiatry, 155,* 486–492.

Hasin, D., & Paykin, A. (1998). Dependence symptoms but no diagnosis: Diagnostic orphans in a "community" sample. *Drug and Alcohol Dependence, 50,* 19–26.

Henly, G. A., & Winters, K. C. (1988). Development of problem severity scales for the assessment of adolescent alcohol and drug abuse. *International Journal of the Addictions, 23*, 65–85.

Herjanic, B., & Campbell, W. (1977). Differentiating psychiatrically disturbed children on the basis of a structured interview. *Journal of Abnormal Child Psychology, 5*, 127–134.

Inwald, R. E., Brobst, M. A., & Morissey, R. F. (1986). Identifying and predicting adolescent behavioral problems by using a new profile. *Juvenile Justice Digest, 14*, 1–9.

Ivens, C., & Rehm, L. P. (1988). Assessment of childhood depression: Correspondence between reports by child, mother, and father. *Journal of the American Academy of Child and Adolescent Psychiatry, 6*, 738–741.

Jainchill, N., Bhattacharya, G., & Yagelka, J. (1995). Therapeutic communities for adolescents. In E. Rahdert & D. Czechowicz (Eds.), *Adolescent drug abuse: Clinical assessment and therapeutic interventions* (Research Monograph No. 156, pp. 190–217). Rockville, MD: National Institute on Drug Abuse.

Janis, I. L., & Mann, L. (1977). *Decision making: A psychological analysis of conflict, choice and commitment*. New York: The Free Press.

Johnson, P. B., & Gurin, G. (1994). Negative affect, alcohol expectancies, and alcohol-related problems. *Addiction, 89*, 581–586.

Johnston, L., O'Malley, P., & Bachman, J. (1997). *National survey results on drug use from the Monitoring the Future study, 1997*. Rockville, MD: National Institute on Drug Abuse.

Johnston, L. D., O'Malley, P. M., & Bachman, J. G. (1992). *National survey results on drug use from the monitoring the future study, 1975–1992: Vol. 1: Secondary school students*. Rockville, MD: National Institute on Drug Abuse.

Kaczynski, N. A., & Martin, C. S. (1995, June). *Diagnostic orphans: Adolescents with clinical alcohol symptomatology who do not qualify for DSM-IV abuse or dependence diagnosis*. Paper presented at the annual meeting of the Research Society on Alcoholism, Steamboat Springs, CO.

Kaminer, Y. (1991). Adolescent substance abuse. In R. J. Frances & S. I. Miller (Eds.), *Clinical textbook of addictive disorders* (pp. 320–346). New York: Guilford Press.

Kaminer, Y., Bukstein, O., & Tarter, R. E. (1991). The Teen-Addiction Severity Index: Rationale and reliability. *International Journal of the Addictions, 26*, 219–226.

Kandel, D. B. (1975). Stages in adolescent involvement in drug use. *Science, 90*, 912–914.

Keating, D. P., & Clark, C. L. (1980). Development of physical and social reasoning in adolescence. *Developmental Psychology, 16*, 23–30.

Kirisci, L., Mezzich, A., & Tarter, R. (1995). Norms and sensitivity of the adolescent version of the Drug Use Screening Inventory. *Addictive Behaviors, 20*, 149–157.

Kokotailo, P. (1995). Physical health problems associated with adolescent substance abuse. In E. Rahdert & D. Czechowicz (Eds.), *Adolescent drug abuse: Clinical assessment and therapeutic interventions* (NIDA Research Monograph No. 156, NIH Publication No. 95–3908, pp. 112–129). Rockville, MD: National Institute on Drug Abuse.

Latimer, W. W., Winters, K. C., & Stinchfield, R. D. (1997). Screening for drug abuse among adolescents in clinical and correctional settings using the Problem Oriented Screening Instrument for Teenagers. *American Journal of Drug and Alcohol Abuse, 23,* 79–98.

Leccese, M., & Waldron, H. B. (1994). Assessing adolescent substance use: A critique of current measurement instruments. *Journal of Substance Abuse Treatment, 11,* 553–563.

Lewinsohn, P. M., Rohde, P., & Seeley, J. R. (1996). Alcohol consumption in high school adolescents: Frequency of use and dimensional structure of associated problems. *Addiction, 91,* 375–390.

MacKenzie, R. G. (1993). Influence of drug use on adolescent sexual activity. *Adolescent Medicine: State of the Art Reviews, 4,* 112–115.

Maisto, S. A., Connors, G. J., & Allen, J. P. (1995). Contrasting self-report screens for alcohol problems: A review. *Alcoholism: Clinical and Experimental Research, 19,* 1510–1516.

Martin, C. S., Kaczynski, N. A., Maisto, S. A., Bukstein, O. M., & Moss, H. B. (1995). Patterns of *DSM-IV* alcohol abuse and dependence symptoms in adolescent drinkers. *Journal of Studies on Alcohol, 56,* 672–680.

Martin, C. S., Kaczynski, N. A., Maisto, S. A., & Tarter, R. E. (1996). Polydrug use in adolescent drinkers with and without *DSM-IV* alcohol abuse and dependence. *Alcoholism: Clinical and Experimental Research, 20,* 1099–1108.

Martin, C. S., & Winters, K. C. (1998). Diagnosis and assessment of alcohol use disorders among adolescents. *Alcohol Health and Research World, 22,* 95–106.

Martin, G. N., Wilkinson, D. A., & Paulos, C. X. (1995). The drug avoidance self-efficacy scale. *Journal of Substance Abuse, 7,* 151–163.

Mayer, J., & Filstead, W. J. (1979). The Adolescent Alcohol Involvement Scale: An instrument for measuring adolescent use and misuse of alcohol. *Journal of Studies on Alcohol, 40,* 291–300.

McLaney, M. A., Del-Boca, F., & Babor, T. (1994). A validation study of the Problem Oriented Screening Instrument for Teenagers (POSIT). *Journal of Mental Health-United Kingdom, 3,* 363–376.

McLellan, A. T., Luborsky, L., Woody, G. E., & O'Brien, C. P. (1980). An improved diagnostic evaluation instrument for substance abuse patients: The Addiction Severity Index. *Journal of Nervous and Mental Disease, 186,* 26–33.

Metzger, D., Kushner, H., & McLellan, A. T. (1991). *Adolescent Problem Severity Index.* Philadelphia: University of Pennsylvania.

Meyers, K. (1991). *Comprehensive Addiction Severity Index for Adolescents.* Philadelphia: University of Pennsylvania.

Migneault, J. P., Pallonen, U. E., & Velicer, W. F. (1997). Decisional balance and stage of change for adolescent drinking. *Addictive Behaviors, 22,* 339–351.

Miller, G. (1990). *The Substance Abuse Subtle Screening Inventory–Adolescent Version.* Bloomington, IN: Substance Abuse Subtle Screening Inventory Institute.

Miller, W. R. (1983). Motivational interviewing with problem drinkers. *Behavioural Psychotherapy, 1,* 147–172.

Miller, W. R., & Rollnick, S. (1991). *Motivational interviewing: Preparing people to change addictive behavior.* New York: Guilford Press.

Miller, W. R., Sovereign, R. G., & Krege, B. (1988). Motivational interviewing with problem drinkers: II. The Drinker's Check-up as a preventive intervention. *Behavioural Psychotherapy, 16*, 251–268.

Moberg, D. P. (1983). Identifying adolescents with alcohol problems: A field test of the Adolescent Alcohol Involvement Scale. *Journal of Studies on Alcohol, 44*, 701–721.

Moberg, D. P., & Hahn, L. (1991). The adolescent drug involvement scale. *Journal of Adolescent Chemical Dependency, 2*, 75–88.

Monahan, J., Hoge, S. K., Lidz, C., Roth, L. H., Bennett, N., Gardner, W., & Mulvey, E. (1995). Coercion and commitment: Understanding involuntary mental hospital admission. *International Journal of Law and Psychiatry, 18*, 249–263.

Moore, D. (1983). *Client Substance Index*. Olympia, WA: Olympic Counseling Services.

Newcomb, M. D., & Bentler, P. M. (1989). Substance use and abuse among children and teenagers. *American Psychologist, 44*, 242–248.

Nisbit, R. E., & Ross, L. (1980). *Human inference: Strategies and shortcomings of social judgement*. Englewood Cliffs, NJ: Prentice-Hall.

Noam, G. G., & Houlihan, J. (1990). Developmental dimensions of *DSM-III* diagnoses in adolescent psychiatric patients. *American Journal of Orthopsychiatry, 60*, 371–378.

O'Leary, A. (1985). Self-efficacy and health. *Behavior Research and Therapy, 23*, 437–451.

Orvaschel, H. (1985). Psychiatric interviews suitable for use in research with children and adolescents. *Psychopharmacology Bulletin, 21*, 737–745.

Orvaschel, H. (1995). *Schedule for Affective Disorders and Schizophrenia for School-Age Children—Epidemiologic Version—5 (K-SADS-E-5)*. Fort Lauderdale, FL: Nova Southeast University.

Pascale, P. J., & Evans, W. J. (1993). Gender differences and similarities in patterns of drug use and attitudes of high school students. *Journal of Drug Education, 23*, 105–116.

Petchers, M., & Singer, M. (1987). Perceived-Benefit-of-Drinking Scale: Approach to screening for adolescent alcohol abuse. *Journal of Pediatrics, 110*, 977–981.

Petchers, M., & Singer, M. (1990). Clinical applicability of a substance abuse screening instrument. *Journal of Adolescent Chemical Dependency, 1*, 47–56.

Petraitis, J., Flay, B. R., & Miller, T. Q. (1995). Reviewing theories of adolescent substance use: Organizing pieces of the puzzle. *Psychological Bulletin, 117*, 67–86.

Prochaska, J. O., DiClemente, C. C., & Norcross, J. C. (1992). In search of how people change: Applications to addictive behaviors. *American Psychologist, 47*(9), 1102–1114.

Puig-Antich, J., & Ryan, N. (1986). *Schedule for Affective Disorders and Schizophrenia for School-Age Children (6–19 Years)—Kiddie-SADS-Present Episode (K-SADS-P) (4th Working Draft)*. Pittsburgh, PA: University of Pittsburgh School of Medicine, Western Psychiatric Institute and Clinic.

Rahdert, E. (Ed.). (1991). *The Adolescent Assessment/Referral System Manual* (DHHS Publication No. ADM 91-1735). Rockville, MD: National Institute on Drug Abuse.

Reich, W., Herjanic, B., Welner, Z., & Gandhy, P. R. (1982). Development of a structured psychiatric interview for children: Agreement on diagnosis comparing child and parent interviews. *Journal of Abnormal Child Psychology, 10*, 325–336.

Reich, W., Shayla, J. J., & Taibelson, C. (1992). *The Diagnostic Interview for Children and Adolescents—Revised (DICA-R).* St. Louis, MO: Washington University.

Renovex. (1988). *Adolescent Chemical Health Inventory.* Minneapolis, MN: Author.

Risberg, R. A., Stevens, M. J., & Graybill, D. F. (1995). Validating the adolescent form of the Substance Abuse Subtle Screening Inventory. *Journal of Child and Adolescent Substance Abuse, 4*, 25–41.

Roberts, R. E., Solovitz, B. L., Chen, Y. W., & Casat, C. (1996). Retest stability of *DSM-III-R* diagnoses among adolescents using the Diagnostic Interview Schedule for Children (DISC-2.1C). *Journal of Abnormal Child Psychology, 24*, 349–362.

Schwartz, R. H., & Wirtz, P. W. (1990). Potential substance abuse: Detection among adolescent patients using the Drug and Alcohol Problem (DAP) Quick Screen, a 30-item questionnaire. *Clinical Pediatrics, 29*, 38–43.

Shaffer, H. J. (1997). The psychology of stage change. In J. H. Lowinson, P. Ruiz, R. B. Millman, & J. G. Langrod (Eds.), *Substance abuse: A comprehensive textbook* (pp. 100–106). Baltimore, MD: Williams & Wilkins.

Shaffer, D., Fisher, P., & Dulcan, M. (1996). The NIMH Diagnostic Interview Schedule for Children (DISC 2. 3): Description, acceptability, prevalences, and performance in the MECA study. *Journal of the American Academy of Child and Adolescent Psychiatry, 35*, 865–877.

Shedler, J., & Block, J. (1990). Adolescent drug use and psychological health: A longitudinal inquiry. *American Psychologist, 45*(5), 612–630.

Simpson, D. D. (1991). *The TCU Prevention Intervention Management and Evaluation System (PMES).* Fort Worth, TX: Texas Christian University, Institute of Behavioral Research.

Single, E., Kandel, D., & Johnson, B. D. (1975). The reliability and validity of drug use responses in a large scale longitudinal survey. *Journal of Drug Issues, 5*, 426–443.

Spitzer, R., Williams, J., & Gibbon, B. (1987). *Instruction Manual for the Structured Clinical Interview for the DSM-III-R.* New York: New York State Psychiatric Institute.

Spitzer, R. L., Williams, J. B., Gibbon, M., & First, M. B. (1992). The Structured Clinical Interview for *DSM-III-R* (SCID): 1. History, rationale and description. *Archives of General Psychiatry, 49*, 624–629.

Stinchfield, R. D. (1997). Reliability of adolescent self-reported pretreatment alcohol and other drug use. *Substance Use and Misuse, 32*, 63–76.

Tarter, R. E., Laird, S. B., Bukstein, O., & Kaminer, Y. (1992). Validation of the Adolescent Drug Use Screening Inventory: Preliminary findings. *Psychology of Addictive Behaviors, 6*, 322–236.

Thomas, D. W. (1990). *Substance Abuse Screening Protocol for the Juvenile Courts.* Pittsburgh, PA: National Center for Juvenile Justice.

Wanberg, K. W. (1992). *Adolescent Self Assessment Profile.* Arvada, CO: Center for Alcohol/Drug Abuse Research and Evaluation.

Watson, C., Tilleskjor, C., Hoodecheck-Show, E., Pucel, J., & Jacobs, L. (1984). Do alcoholics give valid self-reports? *Journal of Studies on Alcohol, 45,* 344–348.

Weinstein, N. D. (1984). Why it won't happen to me: Perceptions of risk factors and illness susceptibility. *Health Psychology, 3,* 431–457.

Weissman, M. M., Wickramaratne, P., Warner, V., John, K., Prusoff, B. A., Merikangas, K. R., & Gammon, G. D. (1987). Assessing psychiatric disorders in children: Discrepancies between mothers' and children's reports. *Archives of General Psychiatry, 44,* 747–753.

White, H. R., & Labouvie, E. W. (1989). Towards the assessment of adolescent problem drinking. *Journal of Studies on Alcohol, 50,* 30–37.

Winters, K. C. (1992). Development of an adolescent alcohol and other drug abuse screening scale: Personal Experience Screening Questionnaire. *Addictive Behaviors, 17,* 479–490.

Winters, K. C., Anderson, N., Bengston, P., Stinchfield, R. D., & Latimer, W. W. (2000). Development of a parent questionnaire for use in assessing adolescent drug abuse. *Journal of Psychoactive Drugs, 32,* 3–13.

Winters, K. C., & Henly, G. A. (1989). *Personal Experience Inventory and Manual.* Los Angeles: Western Psychological Services.

Winters, K. C., & Henly, G. A. (1993). *Adolescent Diagnostic Interview Schedule and Manual.* Los Angeles: Western Psychological Services.

Winters, K. C., Latimer, W. W., & Stinchfield, R. D. (1999). *DSM-IV* criteria for adolescent alcohol and cannabis use disorders. *Journal of Studies on Alcohol, 60,* 337–344.

Winters, K. C., Stinchfield, R. D., Fulkerson, J., & Henly, G. A. (1993). Measuring alcohol and cannabis use disorders in an adolescent clinical sample. *Psychology of Addictive Disorders, 7,* 185–196.

Winters, K. C., Stinchfield, R. D., Henly, G. A., & Schwartz, R. H. (1991). Validity of adolescent self-report of alcohol and other drug involvement. *International Journal of Addictions, 25,* 1379–1395.

Yagamuchi, K., & Kandel, D. B. (1984). Patterns of drug use from adolescence to young adulthood: 3. Patterns of progression. *American Journal of Public Health, 74,* 673–681.

Zucker, R. A., Kincaid, S. B., Fitzgerald, H. E., & Bingham, C. R. (1995). Alcohol schema acquisition in preschoolers: Differences between children of alcoholics and children of nonalcoholics. *Alcoholism: Clinical and Experimental Research, 19,* 1011–1017.

4

Personality and Learning Factors Combine to Create Risk for Adolescent Problem Drinking

A Model and Suggestions for Intervention

GREGORY T. SMITH and KRISTEN G. ANDERSON

This chapter sets forth a model that describes how some adolescents may be prone to drink problematically. The model combines what are traditionally considered to be personality trait factors, which are thought to have a substantial genetic loading, with what are traditionally considered to be learning factors, which are thought to be based on environmental experience. We do this in the following steps. First, we present a general discussion of adolescence and drinking, relying on broad developmental stage theories. Second, we describe key trait and learning factors and how they combine in this risk model. Third, we discuss general treatment issues for the adolescent population, as well as specific treatment implications of the model we propose. Fourth and finally, we place the discussion in a sociocultural context by describing similarities and differences in the risk process as a function of race.

ADOLESCENT STAGE THEORY AND DRINKING

Broadband developmental stage or developmental task theories, such as that of Erikson (1950), provide a vantage point from which to understand adolescent behavior in general and adolescent drinking behavior specifically. A number of theorists conceptualize adolescence as a time of transition and experimentation during which adolescents experiment with or sample from a variety of potential adult roles (cf. Erikson, 1950; Havighurst, 1972). Adolescents are thought to face the task of differentiating themselves from parents and family: The experimental adoption of a number of different values, beliefs, and behaviors is considered an adaptive part of performing this developmental task. This experimentation can take on the form of challenging social prohibitions, testing limits and personal boundaries, and general risk taking. Such behaviors may be important contributors to the tasks of achieving autonomy and of identity formation (Schulenberg, Maggs, & Hurrelmann, 1997).

Thus, as adolescents broaden their range of experiences while becoming less subject to parental protection or control, one challenge they face is learning how to gauge the likely consequences, both positive and negative, of new and potentially risky behaviors and, relatedly, learning how to control urges and impulses when both positive and negative behavioral outcomes are likely. Havighurst (1972) has argued that these efforts are also part of the process of developing internal controls over one's behavior. The development of internal controls over impulses (Havighurst, 1972) makes possible the pursuit of long-term goals over immediate gratifications, an important aspect of a stable, adult identity. A second important developmental challenge is managing one's social and relational experiences (cf. Ganiere & Enright, 1989; Sullivan, 1947). The social experience of the adolescent and his or her acquisition of social and interpersonal skills is also crucial to successful developmental adaptation. Often, these two challenges are interrelated. Adolescents may take risks or try out unfamiliar behaviors precisely in an effort to manage or improve their social or relational experience.

A number of investigators have provided evidence indicating that teenage drinking can be conceptualized as part of this normal developmental process: Teenage drinkers are asserting autonomy from parents, they are taking risks, they are indulging impulses, and they are typically pursuing social facilitation (Chassin, Presson, & Sherman, 1989; Donovan & Jessor, 1978; Jessor, 1987; Shedler & Block, 1990; Smith, Goldman, Greenbaum, & Christiansen, 1995). An important clinical issue then becomes to determine when and how this normal developmental process goes awry. What factors contribute to problem drinking during adolescence, and what kinds of interventions are helpful?

The model we propose emphasizes individual differences in disinhibition, such that individuals who are highly disinhibited will have more difficulty managing risk taking in a healthy way, and it emphasizes individual differences in expectations for social benefits from drinking. There are a number of hints in the existing literature that some versions of these factors are likely important for early-onset problem drinking. First, researchers have studied a range of constructs called disinhibition, impulsivity, or behavioral undercontrol (Sher & Trull, 1994; Sher, Walitzer, Wood, & Brent, 1991; Windle, 1990). Evidence suggests that this cluster of constructs represents a rather stable personality trait, detectable early in life (Kagan, Reznick, & Snidman, 1987), that has a substantial genetic loading (cf. Jang, McCrae, Angleitner, Riemann, & Livesley, 1998, and Finkel & McGue, 1997, for the heritability of the broadly opposite construct of harm avoidance). This broad trait correlates with, and apparently predicts, early-onset alcohol use (Sher et al., 1991; Windle, 1990; for substance use, see Shedler & Block, 1990). Disinhibited individuals are likely to drink more and to have more problems from their drinking than are others. Our model also emphasizes learned expectations about alcohol's effects. Alcohol expectancy research has shown that adolescents who, prior to beginning drinking, expect more strongly than others that alcohol will enhance their social lives, drink earlier and are more likely to be problem drinkers (Christiansen, Smith, Roehling, & Goldman, 1989; Smith, McCarthy, & Goldman, 1995). Thus some combination of trait risk and psychosocial learning risk might help to explain how, for some adolescents, normal developmental experimentation results in a problem drinking outcome. We now offer a theoretical model that combines these categories of risk factors.

TOWARD INTEGRATING PERSONALITY AND LEARNING MODELS OF RISK: ACQUIRED PREPAREDNESS FOR ALCOHOLISM

Although trait-based personality theories and learning theories are described as proceeding from entirely different paradigms (Peterson, 1992), in some respects this distinction is artificial. It certainly seems necessary to draw on both kinds of theories to explain any complex behavior such as alcohol use. We propose the following broad model of problem drinking risk, based on an integration of selected literature from both fields. Trait disinhibition, typically described as a personality risk factor, should be considered a nonspecific risk factor for acting out behavior in general. Learning-based risk factors are alcohol-specific risk factors for drinking that develop both through direct and vicarious experience: Family history influences, peer influences, and general social influences shape individuals' beliefs and assumptions about alcohol. These two sets of factors combine to create what we will call an *acquired preparedness* for alcohol-related problems. As we describe subsequently, there is reason to believe that personality traits influence what individuals learn about alcohol: Certain traits may make it more likely that individuals will learn to expect more reinforcement than punishment from alcohol. High-risk status for problem drinking, then, represents a readiness or preparedness to drink more heavily—and to drink in hazardous situations—that is acquired or developed, typically as a joint product of certain broad personality traits and specific learning about alcohol and its putative effects. This form of high-risk status may be especially important for adolescent problem drinking, because adolescents are faced with risk-taking and impulse-control challenges, as well as with the goal of finding behaviors likely to facilitate social experience. The next sections present a selective review of both the personality-risk and learning-risk literatures, followed by our integration of the two.

Individual Differences in Personality and Alcoholism Risk

Although a variety of personality-based risk models exist, investigators have typically focused on three constructs (or sets of constructs): *neuroticism/emotionality* (Patterson & Newman, 1993; Sher & Trull, 1994; Tarter & Vanyukov, 1994); *extraversion* or *sociability* (Sher & Trull, 1994; Tarter & Vanyukov, 1994); and *impulsivity* or *disinhibition*, sometimes referred to by the umbrella term *behavioral undercontrol* (Sher & Trull, 1994; Sher et al., 1991; Windle, 1990). Other researchers have reviewed the relationship of these constructs to alcohol abuse (cf. Sher & Trull, 1994). We offer a very brief overview of those findings, discuss problems with these concepts, and then review a recent integrative model of disinhibition that pertains to each of these constructs (Patterson & Newman, 1993).

Neuroticism/Emotionality

This construct refers to high levels of emotional reactivity to events, as well as high levels of worry or anxiety. Although individuals with alcohol problems score higher on such measures than controls (Barnes, 1983; Cox, 1985) and although anxiety disorders co-occur with alcoholism (Kushner, Sher, & Beitman, 1990), it remains unclear whether neuroticism presages later alcohol problems (Sher & Trull, 1994). Some prospective studies do not support this inference (cf. Jones, 1968; Robins, Bates, & O'Neal, 1962), and others suggest that neurotic symptoms increase as a function of alcoholism (Kammeier, Hoffman, & Loper, 1973). On the other hand, still others have found that high-risk individuals are more neurotic than low-risk individuals (Finn & Pihl, 1987; Sher et al., 1991). A few prospective studies do suggest that neurotic traits predict alcoholism (Sieber, 1981), perhaps especially for women (Jones, 1971).

The heterogeneity of these findings may well be a function of different types of alcohol problems represented in different studies. Zucker (1987) identified one type of person with alcohol problems for whom negative affectivity was primary, and personality-based cluster analysis studies often identify a single alcoholic subtype characterized by anxiety and subjective distress (Sheppard, Smith, & Rosenbaum, 1988). If neuroticism is a risk factor, it probably applies only to a subset of problem-drinking individuals. Obviously, it will pertain only to those adolescents who are high on that trait.

Extraversion/Sociability

Here, too, whether extraversion predicts alcohol problems is difficult to determine. Some studies do not find reliable associations between extraversion and alcoholism (Barnes, 1983; Cox, 1985), and sociability appears not to be closely related to a family history of alcoholism (Sher, 1991). One study even found lower levels of extraversion to be related to serious alcohol dependence (Rankin, Stockwell, & Hodgson, 1982). However, prospective studies suggest the opposite: that individuals who subsequently developed alcohol problems were rated as more expressive, gregarious, and sociable than controls (Jones, 1968; Sieber, 1981). Because social introversion may increase as a function of alcoholism (Kammeier et al., 1973), it may be that high sociability predicts the onset of drinking problems, with clinical alcoholism masking this trait (Sher & Trull, 1994). Others have argued that what appears to be sociability may really be disinhibition (Tarter & Vanyukov, 1994). In sum, the role of sociability as a main effect predictor of alcoholism remains unclear.

Impulsivity/Disinhibition/Behavioral Undercontrol

Numerous studies have identified some variable in this domain as a significant predictor of alcohol problems, typically for men but sometimes for women as well (cf. Brook, Gordon, Whiteman, & Cohen, 1986; Hawkins, Catalano, & Miller, 1992; Jackson & Matthews, 1988; McCarthy & Smith, 1995; Sher et al., 1991; Smith, 1994; West, Drummond, & Eames, 1990; Wood, Nagoshi, & Dennis, 1992; Zucker & Gomberg, 1986). By using questionnaires with titles such as "Behavioral Undercontrol" or "Disinhibition," most of these researchers have made the assumption that they have measured some underlying personality construct common to a variety of acting out behaviors. This notion is, of course, intuitively appealing and etiologically significant.

We believe that this assumption is not warranted. When measuring these constructs, one typically does so by inquiring into other forms of acting out behavior. Items measuring behavioral undercontrol reflect reports of various forms of delinquency, problem behavior, and antisocial acts: physical fights, lying, cruelty, lawbreaking, failure to honor financial obligations, recklessness, abuse of other drugs, and so on. To say, then, that high scores on scales of this kind predict alcohol problems is to say only that acting out in several areas predicts acting out in another area (increased drinking or hazardous drinking). From our point of view, there is little etiological gain by noting that various forms of acting out behavior predict each other. As essential as it is to remember that the emergence of some form of acting out behavior in adolescence (or before) predicts a range of other acting out behaviors in the future, this observation does not highlight some core personality risk process. By itself, it does little to illuminate the psychological process of risk for alcohol abuse. Of course, these findings do suggest a direction in which such work could go; there may well be some basic psychological process underlying impulsivity or disinhibition.

In sum, the existing literature on personality risk identifies two constructs of uncertain relation to alcohol abuse (neuroticism and extraversion) and a set of behaviors solidly related to alcohol abuse suggestive of some core process involved in disinhibition. We now turn to one model that integrates these three risk variables and that illustrates the kind of role personality variables are likely to play in the etiology of alcohol abuse.

Patterson and Newman's Model of Disinhibition

Based on a wide range of experimental findings, Patterson and Newman (1993) propose the following model. First, individuals differ in how readily they form approach-for-reward response sets and how intensely those sets are maintained. Thus some individuals are more highly focused on the pursuit of reward, and others are more highly focused on the avoidance of punishment. The difference between these two groups becomes especially important when considering behaviors that might bring both reward and punishment. In such a situation, approach-for-reward individuals will have a greater focus on seeking reward and so, the model maintains, will be less likely to stop and modulate a response given punishment cues. In particular, extraverts appear more forcefully motivated for reward and, as a result, are less likely to learn from punishment trials when focused on the possibility of reward. Thus extraversion is associated with a greater likelihood to maintain an optimistic expectation that reward is likely. Second, individuals differ in their reactions when they expect reward and instead experience punishment. Individuals high on neuroticism or emotional reactivity are thought to experience a greater boost in arousal than others. As noted previously, neuroticism here refers to a heightened emotional reactivity to events. Persons high on this trait react more intensely and with more arousal to unexpected events than do others. Their boost in arousal, when combined with extraversion (tendency for active responding), competes with the tendency to stop and reflect on the punishment cues. As a result, it increases the likelihood of *response facilitation*: neurotic extraverts continue to act based on the original, reward-based motivational set. In sum, neurotic extraverts appear likely to respond to punishment with an increased likelihood to continue to seek the reward. Again, this tendency makes them less likely to stop, pause and reflect, and learn to inhibit their behavior because of the new threat of punishment. Because such individuals are more likely to continue a behavior that has been punished in the past, they are referred to as disinhibited. Experimental evidence shows that, when learning which of a set of responses is reinforced and which is punished, neurotic extraverts make more errors of commission than others (they keep seeking reward, having failed to learn that punishment is the anticipated outcome), and they have shorter response latencies after a punishing outcome—implying less processing of the punishment result (Patterson & Newman, 1993).

This model integrates the three personality traits most often identified as risk factors for problem drinking: neuroticism, extraversion, and disinhibition. It describes a general, broad- based personality risk for disinhibited behavior. Neurotic or emotionally reactive extraverts are more likely to pursue reward than to avoid punishment when both outcomes are possible. Perhaps more important, because they tend not to stop, pause, and reflect after a punishing event (as indicated by their short response latencies), they are less likely to form associations involving cues that predict punishment. They are more apt to form associations predictive of reward, given their reward-based response set. As a result, their responding is more likely to be swayed by expectations of reward than by cautionary thoughts (see Patterson & Newman, 1993). The model is an important advance in a number of ways. First, it is based on extensive experimental evidence that Patterson and Newman (1993) summarize rather than on questionnaires that may include multiple constructs related to acting out behavior. Second, it describes a psychological process for disinhibition, in contrast to approaches that, without identifying a disinhibitory process, simply measure a set of behaviors that are thought to point to some unarticulated process. Third, it is a broad model that describes a bias toward active, disinhibited responding generally; it therefore could underlie a number of different disinhibition syndromes. Fourth, the model describes how individuals learn stronger expectations of reward than of punishment, thereby suggesting how a trait-like response could shape future learning.

The importance of this model is twofold: Having an active, reward-based personality style makes one more likely to engage in behaviors, such as heavy alcohol use, that are perceived as both rewarding and potentially punishing. Second, once active reward-seeking individuals engage in heavy drinking, they are more likely to focus on and remember the rewarding aspects of the experience. They should attend to and recall less of the negative, punishing side of the event. Patterson and Newman's (1993) model describes individuals who have a higher probability of engaging in heavy alcohol use and of encoding the experience as rewarding.

To return to our consideration of adolescence, although most studies in this area have been done on either adults or late adolescents (ages 17–19), there is good evidence that the relevant personality traits are highly heritable (Finkel & McGue, 1997; Jang et al., 1998), stable, and detectable early in life (Kagan et al., 1987). The few studies conducted on adolescents support the presence of these broad traits (cf. Merikangas, Swendsen, Preisig, & Chazan, 1998). In addition to this empirical evidence, clinicians frequently provide anecdotal reports that appear to describe disinhibited adolescents. Typically, these adolescents take more risks with their drinking, evidently in the pursuit of greater rewards, and end up experiencing greater punishment, either in injury or arrest. They appear to be differentiated from their peers, including some drinking peers, by a failure to assess adequately the risks of their behaviors. Thus there is good reason to believe that trait disinhibition is manifest in some adolescents. Because adolescents are beginning to try out new, more mature behaviors and are therefore taking risks with an absence of supervision, those adolescents with trait disinhibition are more likely to experience negative outcomes from their actions due to their bias to pursue, and their bias even to notice, rewards but not punishments.

Of course, this model of disinhibition is not sufficient to explain problem alcohol use in particular; rather, it describes a process that makes an array of behaviors more likely, by some factor, in certain individuals. It does not describe a process by which the consumption of alcohol is automatically commandeered because of personality style. Of course, it is hard to imagine any personality theory that would or could point to an inevitable result of drinking alcohol: This is a given limitation of personality models. A certain personality style can make some complex behaviors more likely, but it cannot explain the actual acquisition of a given behavior.

From Personality to Specific Behavioral Expression: The Importance of Learning

How does disinhibition ultimately find some specific behavioral expression? It is important here to briefly consider the fundamental connection between personality and learning perspectives. From a learning perspective, the disinhibition model really describes a general learning bias: Disinhibited individuals are more likely to learn the reinforcing consequences of events and less likely to learn the punishing consequences. Trait disinhibition indicates a general tendency to learn the rewards more strongly than the punishments for a given behavior. The behavior of disinhibited individuals reflects this learning bias. Thus traits can be thought of as indicating a top-down preparedness for certain kinds of learning. Ultimately, the specific preparedness to perceive that, for example, drinking is rewarding, is acquired: The general preparedness for disinhibition must meet up with specific alcohol-related learning to become a risk factor for problem drinking. Thus one's alcohol-related psychosocial learning history mediates the influence of disinhibition on problem-drinking risk.

Classic learning theories of expectancy development and their application to alcohol abuse address this step in the risk process. We offer a brief review of expectancy theory and then turn to its application to alcohol abuse.

Alcohol Expectancies and Problem Drinking

Psychological expectancy theory is a basic learning theory, that is, a theory of how new behaviors are acquired. Its aim is to identify the mechanism by which early learning experiences come to influence later behavioral choices. It can be traced to James (1890); it was explicitly formulated by Tolman (1932) and further developed by MacCorquodale and Meehl (1953), Rotter (1954), Bolles (1972), and others. It represents one specific version of a number of related theories, each of which is concerned with the cognitive mechanisms by which early learning experiences come to influence later behavioral choices (see, for example, Bagozzi, 1992). Expectancy theory, then, is a theory of how any new behavior is acquired: It emphasizes cognition and memory. Briefly, the repeated perception of an association between a given behavior and certain outcomes will lead to the storage of these associations in memory in the form of expectancies of if–then relations between the behavior and its consequences. These stored associations then influence decisions made at future choice points; expectations of valued reinforcers from a given behavior will increase the likelihood of that behavior. In this manner, early learning experiences can serve as early or distal influences on later behavior. The influence of learning experiences is transmitted forward in time by stored information concerning the behavior (i.e., expectancies), which function as the proximal influence that mediates the influence of distal factors on current behavior (Goldman, Brown, Christiansen, & Smith, 1991; Goldman & Rather, 1993; Henderson, Goldman, Coovert, & Carnevalla, 1994; Sher et al., 1991; Smith, 1989, 1994; Stacy, Newcomb, & Bentler, 1991). In recent years, expectancy formulations have been usefully applied to a wide range of topics in psychology, including classical and operant conditioning (Anderson, 1983; Bolles,

1972; Rescorla, 1988), psychopathology (Alloy & Tabachnik, 1984), hypnosis (Kirsch, 1985), interpersonal processes (Jones, 1986; Miller & Turnbull, 1986), and even affect (cf. Carver & Scheier, 1990).

As applied to alcohol use, then, expectancy theory proposes a mechanism by which early learning experiences come to exert an influence on drinking choices later in time (Goldman et al., 1991; Goldman & Rather, 1993; Smith, 1989). Information from learning experiences relating alcohol consumption to anticipated reinforcement or punishment is stored in memory; it then influences the decision to drink at later drinking choice points. Expectancy is a summary label for this stored information.

Of course, the learning experiences could be direct experiences with alcohol, such as the experience of a jovial time with friends or the negative experience of feeling sick. It is important to note, though, that the acquisition of alcohol expectancies need not involve direct experience with alcohol. Modern social learning formulations (cf. Abrams & Niaura, 1987; Bandura, 1986) emphasize the role of vicarious learning or modeling, and numerous studies indicate that young children without appreciable drinking experience are forming clear views of both the appropriateness (Casswell, Gilmore, Silva, & Brasch, 1988; Spiegler, 1983) and the effects (Bauman & Bryan, 1980; Kraus, Smith, & Ratner, 1994; Miller, Smith, & Goldman, 1990) of drinking alcohol. This is an important feature of the model, because it suggests that children form expectancies *before* they begin to drink.

More specifically, alcohol expectancy theory includes the following predictions. First, one should be able to measure individuals' alcohol expectancies reliably and comprehensively. Second, because expectancies are thought to be a cause of drinking based on earlier learning, expectancy scores should (1) correlate with drinking behavior, (2) predict the subsequent onset of drinking, and (3) mediate the influence of markers of early learning on later drinking; also, expectancy manipulations should influence subsequent drinking. Expectancies should have a further influence on the shaping of drinking behavior: For individuals who are beginning to drink (who, based on the model, presumably already have more expectancies for reinforcement than nondrinkers) early use should lead to *increased* expectancies for reinforcement in the future, for three reasons. First, predrinking expectancies, which are vicariously learned relations between a behavior and its consequences, may accurately predict drinking sequelae. Drinking experience would then provide another learning event to reinforce (strengthen) the expectancy. Second, expectancy for drinking consequences, such as social confidence and comfort, may help produce those very consequences, and drinking experience would again reinforce initial expectancy. Third, expectancies may influence attention so that expectancy-consistent outcomes are selectively registered: The expectancy-consistent perception would also constitute a reinforcing event (Smith, Goldman, et al., 1995). It follows that one should see a positive feedback or reciprocal influence process: Individuals with initially more positive expectancies drink first and drink more, and their drinking experience in turn leads them to expect even more reinforcement in the future, leading to increased drinking (Smith, Goldman, et al., 1995).

We briefly review evidence for these hypotheses before considering the integration of expectancy theory with Patterson and Newman's (1993) model.

Empirical Evidence for Alcohol Expectancy Theory

We describe a series of studies undertaken in our laboratories, as well as findings from a recent meta-analysis, to investigate expectancy's hypothesized role. Although a great deal of research in this burgeoning field has come from other laboratories as well, the scope and space limitations of this chapter constrain extensive review of this material. Interested readers are advised to consult any of a number of recent reviews (cf. Connors & Maisto, 1988; Connors, Maisto, & Dermen, 1992; Goldman et al., 1991; Goldman & Rather, 1993).

Step 1: Measurement of Alcohol Expectancies

A number of authors have developed expectancy scales (Brown, Goldman, Inn, & Anderson, 1980; Christiansen, Goldman, & Inn, 1982; Connors, O'Farrell, Cutter, & Thompson, 1986; Leigh, 1987; Leigh & Stacy, 1993; Miller, Smith, & Goldman, 1990; Southwick, Steele, Marlatt, & Lindell, 1981; Stout & Fromme, 1989; Young & Knight, 1989). In general, the scales measure individuals' currently held expectancies, which are presumably formed on the basis of numerous prior learning experiences. Thus what we measure is thought to be the sum product of the influence of earlier learning: We are, therefore, measuring a very immediate, proximal influence on drinking—expectancies as currently stored in memory. A recent meta-analysis concluded that the expectancy measures with the strongest effect sizes were those that were highly reliable and that had a broad range of content coverage (McCarthy & Smith, 1996; see Smith & McCarthy, 1995, for the importance of breadth of coverage to validity).

Although there has been some controversy concerning alcohol expectancy measurement (see Goldman et al., 1991; Leigh, 1989; Smith & Goldman, 1994), there is general consistency in the expectancy content reflected in subscales. The most commonly used scales are the Alcohol

Expectancy Questionnaire (AEQ; Brown et al., 1980) and the Alcohol Expectancy Questionnaire–Adolescent Version (AEQ-A; Christiansen et al., 1982). The subscale names of the AEQ are based on the beliefs that alcohol leads to (1) global positive changes, (2) sexual enhancement, (3) social and physical pleasure, (4) social assertiveness, (5) relaxation, and (6) arousal/ aggression. All six of these scales are thought to reflect perceived reinforcement from drinking. The AEQ-A has five scales that reflect reinforcement expectancies, one bipolar scale, and one negative expectancy scale. The reinforcement expectancy scales are: (1) global positive changes, (2) improved cognitive and motor functioning, (3) sexual enhancement, (4) increased arousal, (5) relaxation. The bipolar scale reflects an expectation for either social enhancement or social impairment. The purely negative scale reflects an expectation for deteriorated cognitive and motor functioning.

Other authors have expanded the coverage of negative expectancies. For example, Leigh and Stacy (1993) have subscales that reflect negative social effects, negative emotional effects, negative physical effects, and negative cognitive and performance effects. Fromme, Stroot, and Kaplan (1993) also expanded coverage by developing a measure that assesses positive expectancies, negative expectancies, and the subjective evaluation of those effects.

Step 2: Expectancies Correlate with Drinking

To date, numerous studies have documented the relationship between expectancies and the drinking behavior of *adults*, from low-level social drinkers to alcoholics (cf. Brown, 1985a, 1985b; Brown, Goldman, & Christiansen, 1985; Connors et al., 1986; Cooper, Russell, Skinner, Fromme, & Mudar, 1992; Mann, Chassin, & Sher, 1987), and of *adolescents* (Brown, Creamer, & Stetson, 1987; Christiansen & Goldman, 1983; Christiansen et al., 1989; Smith & Goldman, 1990; Stacy et al., 1991), leaving little doubt that alcohol expectancy correlates highly with drinking behavior across a wide range of age and drinking groups. In their meta-analysis, McCarthy and Smith (1996) reported the following effect sizes. Reinforcement expectations had an average effect size when predicting drinking of $r = .35$; when the drinking criteria were both quantity and frequency and alcohol-related problems, the average effect size was .44. The average negative (punishment) effect size was lower: .22, although the largest effect sizes were observed when positive and negative expectancies were combined (.47). (Of course, the measurement considerations noted previously suggest that these are underestimates of the true expectancy–drinking relationship because the average effect sizes include estimates from studies with too few expectancy items and lower reliability.)

Step 3: Expectancies Predict Future Onset of Teen Drinking

To help address the hypothesis that alcohol expectancies cause drinking behavior, researchers have employed longitudinal designs in which the putative cause (expectancy) naturally preceded the effect (problem drinking behavior); this approach makes it possible to assess the influence of expectancy measured prior to onset of problem drinking on individuals' subsequent engagement in problem drinking. In the first such study, Christiansen and colleagues (1989) studied young adolescents, many of whom were engaging in their first drinking experiences. Five of seven expectancy scales as assessed in seventh and eighth graders successfully discriminated between non-problem drinkers and those teens who subsequently became problem drinkers over the ensuing 1-year period. Smith (1994) isolated a subsample of 353 nondrinking adolescents and studied their drinking behavior 1 year later: expectancies held at Year 1, when they were nondrinkers, accounted for 22% of the variance in their Year 2 drinking behavior.

A different approach from this "natural experiment" design is to control statistically for early use levels when evaluating expectancy predictions of later use. Using this method, Stacy and colleagues (1991) found that adolescent expectancies predicted adult drug use 9 years later, controlling for adolescent drug use. Thus, over short- and long-term longitudinal periods, whether using a "natural experiment" by studying teens making the transition to problem drinking behavior or using statistical means to control for prior use and whether measuring alcohol consumption alone or other drugs as well, expectancy appears to predate and predict subsequent use. McCarthy and Smith (1996) found that the average effect size of expectancy in predicting later drinking levels was $r = .32$. Indirect support also comes from Miller, Smith, and Goldman (1990) and Kraus, Smith, and Ratner (1994), who reported evidence that alcohol expectancies apparently form as early as the third grade.

Step 4: Expectancies Mediate Learning Influences on Teen Drinking

There is no obvious way to assess early alcohol-related learning experiences. If there were, there would be no reason to assess expectancies; we would measure learning directly instead. However, we can assess markers that reflect the probability of positive learning about alcohol and relate the markers to expectancy and consumption. Smith and Goldman (1990) compiled a composite index of family drinking variables to represent the likely influence of such variables on adolescent consumption using a sample of high school juniors and seniors. The index included: (1) history of alcoholism in first-, second-, and third-degree relatives; (2) history of problems associated with drinking in the same relatives; (3) parents' experience of a set of life problems associated with drinking, including hangovers, blackouts, family problems, work problems, legal difficulties, fighting, early-morning drinking, and drinking alone; (4) frequency of both father's and mother's drinking; and (5) each parent's attitude toward adult drinking. The mediation hypothesis was tested following Baron and Kenny (1986), who described the conditions necessary for demonstration of mediation: (1) the bivariate correlations among the predictor (family drinking), the putative mediator (expectancy), and the criterion (adolescent drinking) are found to be significant; and (2) the indirect path from the predictor (family drinking) to the criterion (teen drinking) through the mediator (expectancy) is significant as well. This set of relationships results in a significant drop in the predictor–criterion correlation when the mediator is introduced.

Smith and Goldman (1990), in fact, found just such a set of relationships: All three variables were significantly related, and the drop in the relationship between family variables and teen drinking when expectancy was introduced was statistically significant. Interestingly, expectancy accounted for over 10 times more of the variance in teen drinking than did the family influence composite by itself (nearly 40% vs. 3.6%). Expectancies likely mediate other early causes as well.

Expectancy's mediational influence was only partial; with expectancies included, the family variables' independent influence on teen drinking, though smaller (accounting for 1% of the variance), remained statistically significant. Another recent study (Sher et al., 1991) also supported the partial mediating influence of expectancies.

Step 5: Experimental Manipulation of Expectancy Reduces Alcohol Consumption

All correlational designs are, at best, quasi-experimental in nature, and experimental manipulations that isolate the proposed cause provide more compelling evidence for causal inference. One recent study used a true experimental design to test whether expectancies could be manipulated with a consequent change in drinking levels. Darkes and Goldman (1993) told a sample of heavy-drinking college students (some of whom were drinking at problem levels) that they and others might or might not receive alcohol in a masked beverage and that they would participate in a party. Participants were challenged to identify those among them who had actually received alcohol. Afterward, these participants were asked to monitor environmental cues for expectancies, for example, advertising, media influences, other drinkers, and so forth. Later, the same participants returned to the lab and participated in a second party, again with the goal of identifying who among them had received alcohol. Participants learned that they could not identify the true drinkers at better than chance levels. Two control groups were used: students in a "traditional" college program for teaching responsible drinking and a no-treatment group. In addition, expectancies were assessed using an instrument (Levine & Goldman, 1989) sensitive to situational and short-term changes in expectancies. Results showed that only the expectancy manipulation reduced drinking over the 2 weeks following the experimental manipulation and that drinking decreases paralleled decreases in measured expectancies. It was noteworthy that the expectancy challenge showed the most striking impact on the heaviest drinkers, suggesting that these procedures might be influencing a central drinking mechanism. These findings, of course, have implications for the development of future prevention and intervention programs, but further studies using more extensive challenges and follow-ups of a considerably longer period are certainly necessary to establish the utility of these practical applications.

Step 6: The Positive Feedback Loop or Reciprocal Influence between Expectancies and Early Drinking

Smith and colleagues (1995) used a 2-year, three-wave longitudinal design with adolescents—most of whom had not begun to drink at the outset of the study—to test this hypothesis. They found that expectancy significantly predicted drinking behavior 1 year later, over and above the relation between prior and subsequent drinking; and that drinking experience predicted expectancy endorsement 1 year later, over and above the relation between prior and subsequent expectancy scores. This finding supports the notion of a reciprocal influence between expectancy and drinking among adolescents who are first beginning to drink. It is important to note that the influence was of a positive feedback variety: Expectancy for reinforcement predicted increases in future drinking, and increased drinking predicted increases in subsequent reinforcement expectancies. There was no sign of a "corrective" feedback process, in which drinking experience might have caused a tempering of reinforcement expectancy. Apparently, before adolescents first drink, there are already individual differences in the consequences they expect from consumption that predict who will drink early in life; further, the individual differences in expectancy are only strengthened by those early drinking experiences.

In sum, alcohol expectancy theory has received powerful support. Expectancies, even those held prior to drinking experience, predict future drinking. Perhaps more important, an expectancy manipulation has proved successful in reducing drinking. There is, then, considerable evidence for this learning theory-based model of risk. It appears that specific learning about alcohol's expected consequences plays an important role in shaping subsequent drinking behavior.

Acquired Preparedness: An Integration of Personality and Learning Risk Factors

We propose that the two risk factors reviewed here—trait disinhibition and concrete learning about alcohol's effects—combine to create an acquired preparedness to develop alcohol abuse problems. We use the term "acquired preparedness" to indicate the following. The genetically influenced trait of disinhibition implies that one is prone to learn the reinforcing, rather than the punishing, consequences of behaviors; in other words, the disinhibited person is prone to form positive expectancies about behaviors. Thus disinhibition implies that the probability of acting out behaviors in general is increased. Ultimately, the development of alcohol problems in particular is acquired, when the trait, that is, the learning bias, combines with specific alcohol-related learning. We propose that disinhibited teens are more likely, from a given learning event, to learn that drinking will bring a range of reinforcers than are other teens. We use the term "preparedness" to note that even with both risk factors in place, alcohol abuse is far from an automatic outcome. Preparedness implies a readiness to manifest alcohol problems: It denotes an increased probability of a problem drinking outcome. We use the term "acquired" to indicate that the general preparedness of disinhibition becomes a risk factor for alcohol abuse only when the disinhibited teen is exposed to alcohol-related learning.

One implication of this model is that disinhibited individuals' drinking should have a positive feedback quality. After each drinking event, there will be a tendency for the individual to remember or encode its reinforcing aspects more than its punishing aspects, leading to the probability of increased future drinking. This deduction dovetails nicely with Smith, Goldman, and colleagues' (1995) finding that drinking experience led to more positive expectancies and increased risk for future drinking.

In its pure form, the model we have proposed is illustrated in Figure 4.1. This figure includes one further distinction we have yet to discuss: the distinction between drinking levels and alcohol-related problems (life difficulties that stem from drinking). Studies have shown that these are two distinct, although related, factors (Smith, McCarthy, & Goldman, 1995). The model proposes that although disinhibition will have a significant bivariate correlation with both drinking and problems, once expectancy is added into the model, disinhibition's direct influence on drinking will go to zero. In other words, disinhibition's influence on drinking will be indirect—fully mediated by expectancy. However, we hypothesize that disinhibition will maintain a direct influence on alcohol-related problems, even with expectancy included in the model: The notion is that a disinhibited person is more likely to get into trouble than a nondisinhibited person when both have consumed the same amount of alcohol. The model is constructed to reflect presumed time lags in the causal chain: Disinhibition helps shape expectancy, which influences drinking, and both disinhibition and expectancy influence alcohol-related problems.

We have recently conducted two tests of the model. Full reports of those tests can be found in dissertations by Kroll (1998) and McCarthy (1998), and an initial report of their work was included in Smith, McCarthy, Kroll, and Miller (1998). Because Patterson and Newman's (1993) experimental demonstrations of disinhibition by neurotic extraverts were conducted with men, Kroll (1998) first tested the acquired preparedness model in a sample of 17- to 20-year-old men. He used a pool of more than 400 participants and defined disinhibition dichotomously: Neurotic extraverts were identified as disinhibited, and stable introverts (the opposite quadrant in a two-dimensional space defined by neuroticism–stability and extraversion–introversion) were classified as inhibited. He then used structural equation analysis to test, in a cross-sectional sample of 170, an approximation of the model depicted in Figure 4.1. Kroll (1998) found the following: the bivariate correlations of disinhibition with drinking and alcohol-related problems were, respectively, .26 and .33; both were significant. Disinhibition also correlated significantly, .32, with expectancy. When this set of variables was entered into a structural equation model with paths as depicted in Figure 4.1, the influence of disinhibition on expectancy dropped from .26 to .07 (nonsignificant); the drop itself is statistically significant. This finding is consistent with the hypothesis that the influence of disinhibition on drinking is fully mediated by its influence on expectancy:

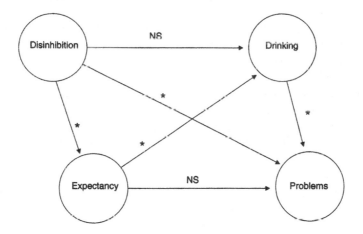

FIGURE 4.1. Schematic representation of the acquired preparedness model. *denotes significant influences; NS denotes nonsignificant paths.

The indirect effect of disinhibition on drinking level through expectancy was significant. Also as hypothesized, disinhibition's influence on alcohol-related problems was not mediated by expectancy: It did not drop significantly when expectancy was included (Smith et al., 1998).

McCarthy (1998) expanded on this work in two ways. First, he included a sample of 17- to 20-year-old women to test whether the model generalizes across sex. Second, he also conducted the laboratory test of disinhibition cited by Patterson and Newman (1993). On the combined male–female sample, McCarthy (1998) replicated Kroll's (1998) findings: Expectancy appeared to mediate disinhibition's influence on drinking but not its influence on alcohol-related problems. When analyzed separately by sex, the indirect (mediated) effect was significant for men (p .01) and marginally significant for women (p .10). Interestingly, results supported McCarthy's (1998) additional hypothesis that disinhibition would be more strongly related to drinking for women than for men. The notion is that drinking is more normative for adolescent men but requires more disinhibition for women. Thus, although there is some support for the key mediational hypothesis in women, there may be additional factors that alter the predictive process for women that require further investigation (Smith et al., 1998).

McCarthy (1998) also tested whether male and female neurotic extraverts showed the same disinhibition on the laboratory task measuring disinhibited errors. Both male and female neurotic extraverts made more errors of commission (responding in the hope of reward in a punishment condition). Interestingly, male neurotic extraverts showed the shorter response latency after punishment, but for female neurotic extraverts, that effect was not quite significant. Here again, further exploration of the utility of this model for female drinkers is warranted.

Both Kroll (1998) and McCarthy (1998) tested one other hypothesis of the model: Disinhibition should correlate significantly more strongly with positive alcohol expectancies than with negative alcohol expectancies, if the reward-based bias is present. Both studies confirmed that hypothesis.

Although these studies provide promising initial evidence for the acquired preparedness model, there are two important limitations to these data. The most important limitation is that these studies were conducted on older adolescent participants. It is crucial to show that this process also operates in early adolescence, when teens are first beginning to drink. The second limitation is that these studies were cross-sectional. Clearly, longitudinal tests of this process are necessary. On the other hand, considerable evidence in the literature supports the temporal ordering of these variables. Disinhibition appears to be a rather stable trait that is detectable early in life (Kagan et al., 1987; Lynam, 1996; Shaw & Winslow, 1997). Alcohol expectancies appear to emerge around the third grade (Kraus, Smith, & Ratner, 1994; Miller et al., 1990). Drinking onset typically occurs during early to mid-adolescence, and longitudinal work has shown that both disinhibition and alcohol expectancy predict subsequent drinking behavior (Sher & Trull, 1994; Smith, 1994; Smith, Goldman, et al., 1995). As we also noted previously, further exploration of this model and of the general role of disinhibition on adolescent girls' drinking is indicated. Alterations in the model as a function of gender may prove valuable.

Acquired Preparedness and Types of Alcoholics

Any etiological proposal such as this one must account for the finding that there are different types of alcoholics with both different personality styles and different drinking patterns. Although an extensive review of alcoholic subtyping is beyond our scope, our model does relate to some of the key typing distinctions in the literature.

One type of person with alcohol problems that has been identified repeatedly (cf. Sheppard et al., 1988; Zucker, 1987) is the person who experiences high subjective distress and who is often described as drinking to self-medicate. This group tends to have high reactivity to stress and some acting out tendencies (cf. Sheppard et al., 1988; Sher & Trull, 1994) that make them more likely to respond to their distress by drinking. Neurotic extraverts may be well represented among this group of alcoholics.

Similar logic may apply to the adolescent risk process. If a general developmental task of adolescence involves risk taking with new behaviors, evaluating the likely positive and negative outcomes of new, prospective behaviors, and impulse control (Smith & Miller, 1992), then disinhibited adolescents probably reflect a personality type likely to have particular difficulty with this developmental task. There are likely to be other avenues of risk as well: This model is meant to describe one possible pathway of difficulty for adolescents.

What is less clear from our discussion so far is how this model might account for the less anxious, more purely psychopathic type of alcoholic described by most subtypers (Babor et al., 1992; Cloninger, 1987; Sheppard et al., 1988; Zucker, 1987). There is another aspect to Patterson and Newman's work that addresses this point. They describe a series of studies that show similarities and differences between psychopaths and neurotic extraverts with respect to disinhibition. Neurotic extraverts experience heightened arousal after punishment, which makes them less able to modulate their responses, which leads them to rely on their dominant, active response mode—hence the lack of reflection on punishment cues. Psychopaths respond somewhat differently: They do not show signs of greater activation and exaggerated responding as neurotic extraverts do. Instead, they seem to have a kind of attentional difficulty: They have difficulty switching their attention from a reward to a new punisher. Patterson and

Newman (1993) describe this as an automatic processing deficit. With a lifelong learning history deficient in this attentional switch, psychopaths are less likely to develop a range of responses to punishment cues (Patterson & Newman, 1993). This basic processing deficit and the lifelong diminished learning about punishment associated with it may help to explain the psychopathic type of problem drinker, who generally is experiencing less subjective distress than the neurotic extravert.

Treatment Implications: General

First, we briefly mention one aspect of adolescent alcohol-related treatment that, we believe, must be integrated into any treatment approach. Frequently, adolescents are somewhat pressured or coerced into treatment for alcohol abuse, that is, they enter treatment because their behavior has alarmed parents or other caretaking authorities rather than because of a personally recognized need to change. A related concern is that in most settings, adolescents cannot enter treatment without parental informed consent. For these reasons, they may tend to enter treatment with a lower level of motivation than many adults, and it has been speculated that what motivation they do possess may be more driven by the desire to receive rewards and privileges while avoiding punishment than by a readiness to change their behavior (Morehouse, 1989). Research has suggested that the adolescent problem drinker typically has not experienced serious ongoing problems as a consequence of alcohol use (or does not perceive drinking as the cause of negative experiences) and thus does not view his or her drinking as a problem (Morehouse, 1989). Many of the more serious consequences of alcohol abuse that might serve as long-term motivations (e.g., avoiding cirrhosis of the liver) are not perceived by adolescents as personally relevant. Consequently, the typical adolescent abuser is thought to be harder to motivate for treatment than the typical adult abuser. In a recent study applying the stages of change perspective (Prochaska & DiClemente, 1983), Migneault, Pallonen, and Velicer (1997) found that 49% of a sample of 10th- and 11th-grade drinkers were in the precontemplation stage.

For these reasons, we argue that a stages of change perspective tailored toward adolescents, along with application of appropriate motivational interviewing strategies, should routinely be part of any form of adolescent treatment (Miller, 1996). Monti, Barnett, O'Leary, and Colby (Chapter 5, this volume) suggest that brief interventions, using motivational interviewing, may be effectively modified to meet the therapeutic needs of adolescents. As well as presenting a structured approach for this type of treatment, they provide information to assist in tailoring the intervention to different settings, different ages, and cultural groups.

Expectancy Challenge Treatment

The acquired preparedness model emphasizes the importance of the alcohol-related expectancies individuals ultimately form. One recent study suggests some promise in an intervention aimed at reducing positive alcohol expectancies. Darkes and Goldman (1993) challenged college students' positive alcohol expectancies in two ways. First, heavy drinking students participated in a drinking party, with the understanding that some of the students were given alcohol and others were given a placebo and that they, too, received either alcohol or placebo. Their task was to identify which students actually had received alcohol. Students could not identify drinkers at any better than chance rates, and they were given feedback about this failure. The students were then taught about expectancies and instructed to monitor expectancy-relevant information they were exposed to in the media. They later returned to the lab and participated in another party, again learning that they could not identify the drinkers reliably. They were taught that many social messages encourage various positive expectancies about drinking, but they also learned that they could not pick out those who had consumed alcohol from those who had consumed a placebo with any reliability. All this information presumably implied that many of the positive effects they had attributed to alcohol were not a result of the pharmacology of the drug but resulted instead from social expectations. Outcome findings were that students in the expectancy-treatment group had significantly greater reductions in drinking than did students in either a traditional alcohol-reduction program or a no-treatment control group. Also, expectancy-reduction participants reduced their positive alcohol expectancies, but the other two groups did not. Finally, the impact of this intervention appeared strongest on the heaviest drinkers.

This intervention appears promising. However, it would require some changes for implementation with adolescents: Adolescents cannot be given alcohol to consume, nor can they be led to believe they had consumed alcohol. It may be possible to have them observe parties of legal drinkers without participating. Such an intervention has not yet been tested on an adolescent population. Some optimism for this approach can be gleaned from Kraus and colleagues (1994), who modified alcohol expectancies in a sample of 9- to 11-year-olds. Kraus and colleagues (1994) found that a video in which puppets expressed positive beliefs about alcohol's effects and then experienced negative consequences from drinking reduced children's positive expectancies at 4-week follow-up. They also found that a video in which adults drank and behaved boorishly *increased* children's positive expectancies, perhaps because any drinking by adults is perceived as desirable, as children are learning how to become adults. Thus great care needs to be exercised in developing interventions of this kind.

Speculations on Treatment Implications of the Acquired Preparedness Model

The model holds that the subset of adolescents high on trait disinhibition have a bias toward learning the positive or reinforcing aspects of events and against learning the negative or punishing aspects. The failure to learn the punishing aspects of drinking could happen in a few different ways:

1. Disinhibited individuals may simply fail to attend to the punishing aspects. This possibility is implied in the finding that, for men at least, disinhibited individuals spend less time processing a punishing event than they do a reinforcing event. Recent memory research also emphasizes the possible failure to attend to uncomfortable information (Isbell, Smith, & Wyer, 1998).

2. Wyer and Srull's (1986) memory model proposes that information is stored and retrieved according to one's particular goals: Disinhibited individuals may be more likely to store drinking information in reward-based "bins" or categories, such as "fun with friends," diminishing the probability of recalling the negative aspects of consumption. This possibility presupposes that negative consequences were attended to but were stored in "bins" that are less likely to be accessed.

3. Another model suggests a slightly different possibility. Lazarus (1982) proposed that a person's detailed encoding of an event is preceded by a more undifferentiated evaluation of the event, perhaps as either potentially positive or potentially negative. Which aspects of the event are subsequently encoded may well be influenced by this general affect-based evaluation (see Isbell et al., 1998). Here again, a reward-biased disinhibited adolescent may tend to store reward-relevant information more fully than less relevant, punishment-related data.

Each of these three possibilities involves a kind of "top-down" memory process, suggesting that both what is recalled and the form in which it is recalled are subject to motivational or biasing influences. All three models are broadly consistent with the hypothesis that disinhibited individuals have a bias toward learning rewarding outcomes over punishing outcomes. It seems possible that strategies aimed to alter one's attention allocation or to alter the form of one's memory structures may prove beneficial. Again, such strategies are only likely to be successful once readiness to change has been considered and addressed.

Our first treatment speculation concerns attentional processes. A motivated adolescent might well benefit from an intervention tailored after self-instruction training, which has been employed with ADHD children (Barkley, 1989; Meichenbaum & Goodman, 1971). Perhaps one could train a disinhibited adolescent to review mentally both the good and the bad consequences of a given drinking event, with a special emphasis on balancing the good consequences with aversive consequences. One could also encourage such a client to brainstorm about the wider range of potential consequences the drinking experience might have led to, again encouraging a wide range of both positive and negative outcomes. One could go on to have the client imagine future drinking episodes and imagine both the positive and negative outcomes of those episodes. The aim of this intervention would be to broaden the disinhibited adolescent's attentional focus, so that both rewarding and punishing outcomes of drinking can enter into awareness and thus into memory. Although self-instruction has had mixed success with ADHD children (Barkley, 1989), it merits consideration with a target disinhibited adolescent population.

The second and third possibilities, based on memory models, may require a kind of metamemory intervention (Lucanegli, Galderisi, & Cornoldi, 1995, describe transfer effects following metamemory training). If an adolescent is more prone to think about "fun with friends" than "risks to myself," he or she may tend to access memories about drinking episodes that are primarily positive (even if the negative outcomes were stored in memory). The intervention challenge in such a case can be thought of as altering the memory structure. Perhaps a willing adolescent can learn, through rehearsal, to broaden the "memory bin" from "fun with friends" to "fun with friends that won't get me in trouble" or at least "fun with friends that won't get me grounded, thus limiting my fun with friends." Here again, the intervention would have a strong cognitive component, as the clinician encourages the adolescent to both recall and consider punitive or, at a minimum, risky consequences, perhaps finding a way to illustrate the value of a broader "memory bin" that can allow for more accurate predictions of life consequences from drinking.

A similar intervention ought to be considered following Lazarus's (1982) model. Willing adolescents might learn the benefits of encoding memories of events, such as drinking, in both positive and negative terms, again so as to enhance prediction of life outcomes. One could certainly illustrate that such memory changes are likely to help the adolescent meet long-term goals more effectively, even if those long-term goals are social in nature. In this way, adolescents could develop positive affect for more complex memories that include both reward and punishment.

Developmental researchers have shown that adult-mediated metacognitive experiences can lead to metacognitive growth in children, that is, growth in the ability to think about one's own reasoning (Fry, 1992). This finding augurs well for metamemory efforts of the kind we are suggesting. Perhaps an increased ability to appreciate the biases in one's memory structure could lead to improved recall and hence more informed decision making and a reduction in harm to oneself and others (see Miller, Turner, & Marlatt, Chapter 2, this volume).

Prevention Implications

Some adaptation of the interventions we have described could certainly be applied in a prevention format. Certainly the acquired preparedness model (Smith, McCarthy, & Kroll, in press) and alcohol expectancy theory (Smith & Goldman, 1994) each suggest ways of identifying one group of high-risk adolescents. Adolescents high on disinhibition, who already hold strong positive alcohol expectancies, might benefit most from both expectancy interventions (Darkes & Goldman, 1993; Kraus et al., 1994) and attentional and memory interventions as described previously. At a broad level, the approach we have described involves identifying a group of adolescents likely to have trouble with the risk-taking aspects of adolescent development (Havighurst, 1972) and teaching cognitive skills that may help them to negotiate the developmental challenge.

Sociocultural Considerations

One limitation of most of the research in this field is that it has been conducted primarily on white men. Its generalizability to women and ethnic minorities is, therefore, unclear. We have described one study on disinhibition in women, and clearly more needs to be done with respect to gender. There is some research on similarities and differences in drinking patterns between whites and blacks, and we have conducted one study on acquired preparedness as a function of race.

Different racial and ethnic groups apparently exhibit different characteristic rates and patterns of alcohol use and related consequences (Lex, 1985, 1987; Spiegler, Tate, Aitken, & Christian, 1989), suggesting that risk processes may not be the same across groups. Researchers have found that blacks start to drink at later ages and in smaller proportions than whites and that adolescent blacks tend to have fewer alcohol-related problems than do adolescent whites (Barnes & Welte, 1986; Catalano et al., 1992; Johnston, O'Malley, & Bachman, 1987; Singer & Petchers, 1987). With respect to the risk processes central to acquired preparedness, studies have disagreed as to whether black and white samples differ in mean expectancy endorsement (Connors, Maisto, & Wilson, 1988; Dermen & Cooper, 1994; Kline, 1990; Reese & Friend, 1994) and as to whether the relationship between expectancy and drinking differs in black and white samples

(Kline, 1990; Reese & Friend, 1994). Although there is some evidence that blacks and whites may differ in sensation seeking (Carrol & Zuckerman, 1977; Kurtz & Zuckerman, 1978; Sutker, Archer, & Allain, 1978), they may not differ in disinhibition in particular (Carrol & Zuckerman, 1977; Karoly, 1975; Kurtz & Zuckerman, 1978; Sutker, Archer, & Allain, 1978). Many researchers have failed to control for potential group differences in socioeconomic status, which may account in part for the equivocal nature of these findings.

McCarthy, Miller, Smith, and Smith (1998) conducted a cross-sectional test of the acquired preparedness model on a sample of 279 whites and 200 blacks. Using structural equation modeling, they found that the structural–correlational model supported acquired preparedness in both samples and that the model parameters were not significantly different between groups. Although the predictive patterns were the same for both races, blacks drank significantly less and experienced significantly fewer alcohol-related problems. Thus the risk process appeared similar even though group mean levels of use were quite different. More studies of this kind are necessary.

Regarding treatment, there is an extensive theoretical literature on the kinds of approaches that may work best with different ethnic groups and on the kinds of special issues that may arise (see Sue & Sue, 1990, for a review of this literature). At this point, there is a very clear need for more systematic empirical investigation of these issues. The development of treatment samples that are representative of more than one ethnic group is an important first step (see Waldron, Brody, & Slesnick, Chapter 7, this volume, for one such study). There may well be important differences in the approaches one must take as a function of the ethnic and cultural background of one's client. Against this background, it is interesting that the acquired preparedness risk process appears to be common to both black and white samples.

SUMMARY

We have described a model of adolescent risk for problem drinking that integrates personality and learning risk factors. The model seems relevant for some adolescents as they negotiate classic adolescent developmental tasks. The acquired preparedness model holds that disinhibited adolescents are prepared to learn the reinforcing aspects of risky behaviors more strongly than the punishing aspects. When this preparedness interacts with specific alcohol-related learning, disinhibition leads to the biased formation of positive alcohol expectancies over negative alcohol expectancies. Alcohol expectancies, in turn, predict the onset of drinking and the onset of alcohol-related problems. Thus alcohol expectancies mediate disinhibition's influence on drinking. We have summarized initial support for this model, and we have described the kinds of studies yet to be done that will test the model further.

We have discussed issues in intervention with adolescent problem drinkers. Empirical support exists for our advocacy of motivational interviewing and expectancy challenge procedures. From the theoretical perspective of the model, we have gone on to speculate on the kinds of interventions likely to be useful for this type of high-risk adolescent. We have suggested interventions aimed at improving attention to the punishing aspects of drinking, as well as interventions aimed at altering memory structures to make negative consequences of drinking more accessible. Before any such interventions are warranted, considerably more research is needed to identify the specific locus of difficulty (i.e., attention or memory). We believe the acquired preparedness model is a start toward identifying one subgroup of high-risk adolescents, and we hope that interventions based on the model will add to the arsenal clinicians bring to adolescent treatment.

REFERENCES

Abrams, D. B., & Niaura, R. S. (1987). Social learning theory. In H. T. Blane & K. E. Leonard (Eds.), *Psychological theories of drinking and alcoholism* (pp. 131–178). New York: Guilford Press.

Alloy, L. B., & Tabachnik, N. (1984). Assessment of covariation by humans and animals: The joint influence of prior expectations and current situational information. *Psychological Review, 91,* 112–149.

Anderson, J. R. (1983). A spreading activation theory of memory. *Journal of Verbal Learning and Verbal Behavior, 22,* 261–295.

Babor, T. F., Hoffman, M., DelBoca, F. K., Hesselbrock, V., Meyer, R. E., Dolinsky, Z. S., & Rounsaville, B. (1992). Types of alcoholics: 1. Evidence for an empirically derived typology based on indicators of vulnerability and severity. *Archives of General Psychiatry, 49,* 599–608.

Bagozzi, R. P. (1992). The self-regulation of attitudes, intentions, and behavior. *Social Psychology Quarterly, 55,* 178–204.

Bandura, A. (1986). *Social foundations of thought and action.* Englewood Cliffs, NJ: Prentice-Hall.

Barkley, R. A. (1989). Attention-deficit hyperactivity disorder. In E. J. Mash & R. A. Barkley (Eds.), *Treatment of childhood disorders* (pp. 39–72). New York: Guilford Press.

Barnes, G. (1983). Clinical and prealcoholic personality characteristics. In B. Kissin & H. Begleiter (Eds.), *The pathogenesis of alcoholism* (Vol. 6, pp. 113–195). New York: Plenum Press.

Barnes, G. M., & Welte, J. W. (1986). Adolescent alcohol abuse: Subgroup differences and relationships to other problem behaviors. *Journal of Adolescent Research,* 1, 79–94.

Baron, R. M., & Kenny, D. A. (1986). The moderator–mediator variable distinction in social psychological research: Conceptual, strategic, and statistical considerations. *Journal of Personality and Social Psychology,* 51, 1173–1182.

Bauman, K. E., & Bryan, E. S. (1980). Subjective expected utility and children's drinking. *Journal of Studies on Alcohol,* 41, 952–958.

Bolles, R. C. (1972). Reinforcement, expectancy, and learning. *Psychological Review,* 79, 394–409.

Brook, J. S., Gordon, A. S., Whiteman, M., & Cohen, P. (1986). Dynamics of childhood and adolescent personality traits and adolescent drug use. *Developmental Psychology,* 22, 403–414.

Brown, S. A. (1985a). Expectancies versus background in the prediction of college drinking patterns. *Journal of Consulting and Clinical Psychology,* 53, 123–130.

Brown, S. A. (1985b). Reinforcement expectancies and alcoholism treatment outcome after a one-year follow-up. *Journal of Studies on Alcohol,* 46, 304–308.

Brown, S. A., Creamer, V. A., & Stetson, B. A. (1987). Adolescent alcohol expectancies in relation to personal and parental drinking practices. *Journal of Abnormal Psychology,* 96, 117–121.

Brown, S. A., Goldman, M. S., & Christiansen, B. A. (1985). Do alcohol expectancies mediate drinking patterns of adults? *Journal of Consulting and Clinical Psychology,* 53, 512–519.

Brown, S. A., Goldman, M. S., Inn, A. M., & Anderson, L. (1980). Expectancies of reinforcement from alcohol: Their domain and relation to drinking patterns. *Journal of Consulting and Clinical Psychology,* 48, 419–426.

Carrol, E. N., & Zuckerman, M. (1977). Psychopathology and sensation seeking in "downers," "speeders," and "trippers": A study of the relationship between personality and drug choice. *International Journal of the Addictions,* 12, 591–601.

Carver, C. S., & Scheier, M. F. (1990). Origins and functions of positive and negative affect: A control process view. *Psychological Review,* 97, 19–35.

Casswell, S., Gilmore, L. L., Silva, P., & Brasch, P. (1988). What children know about alcohol and how they know it. *British Journal of Addictions,* 83, 223–227.

Catalano, R. F., Morrison, D. M., Wells, E. A., Gillmore, M. R., Iritani, B. M., & Hawkins, J. D. (1992). Ethnic differences in family factors related to early drug initiation. *Journal of Studies on Alcohol,* 53, 208–217.

Chassin, L., Presson, C. C., & Sherman, S. J. (1989). "Constructive" vs. "destructive" deviance in adolescent health-related behaviors. *Journal of Youth and Adolescence,* 18, 245–262.

Christiansen, B. A., & Goldman, M. S. (1983). Alcohol-related expectancies versus demographic background variables in the prediction of adolescent drinking. *Journal of Consulting and Clinical Psychology,* 51, 249–258.

Christiansen, B. A., Goldman, M. S., & Inn, A. M. (1982). Development of alcohol-related expectancies in adolescents: Separating pharmacological from social learning influences. *Journal of Consulting and Clinical Psychology,* 50, 336–344.

Christiansen, B. A., Smith, G. T., Roehling, P. V., & Goldman, M. S. (1989). Using alcohol expectancies to predict adolescent drinking behavior after one year. *Journal of Consulting and Clinical Psychology, 57,* 93–99.

Cloninger, C. R. (1987). Neurogenetic adaptive mechanisms in alcoholism. *Science, 236,* 410–416.

Connors, G. J., & Maisto, S. A. (1988). The alcohol expectancy construct: Overview and clinical applications. *Cognitive Therapy and Research, 12,* 487–504.

Connors, G. J., Maisto, S. A., & Dermen, K. H. (1992). Alcohol-related expectancies and their applications to treatment. In R. R. Watson (Ed.), *Drug and alcohol abuse reviews: Vol. 3. Alcohol abuse treatment* (pp. 203–231). Totowa, NJ: Humana Press.

Connors, G. J., Maisto, S. A., & Wilson, D. W. (1988). Racial factors influencing college students' ratings of alcohol's usefulness. *Drug and Alcohol Dependence, 21,* 247–252.

Connors, G. J., O'Farrell, T. J., Cutter, H. S. G., & Thompson, D. C. (1986). Alcohol expectancies among male alcoholics, problem drinkers and nonproblem drinkers. *Alcoholism: Clinical and Experimental Research, 10,* 667–671.

Cooper, M. L., Russell, M., Skinner, J. B., Fromme, M. R., & Mudar, P. (1992). Stress and alcohol use: Moderating effects of gender, coping, and alcohol expectancies. *Journal of Abnormal Psychology, 101,* 139–152.

Cox, W. M. (1985). Personality correlates of substance abuse. In M. Galizio & S. A. Maisto (Eds.), *Determinants of substance abuse* (pp. 209–246). New York: Plenum Press.

Darkes, J., & Goldman, M. S. (1993). Expectancy challenge and drinking reduction: Experimental evidence for a mediational process. *Journal of Consulting and Clinical Psychology, 61,* 344–353.

Dermen, K. H., & Cooper, M. L. (1994). Sex-related alcohol expectancies among adolescents: Scale development. *Psychology of Addictive Behaviors, 8,* 152–160.

Donovan, J. E., & Jessor, R (1978). Adolescent problem drinking: Psychosocial correlates in a national sample study. *Journal of Studies on Alcohol, 39*(9), 1506–1524.

Erikson, E. H. (1950). *Childhood and society.* New York: Norton.

Finkel, D., & McGue, M. (1997). Sex differences and nonadditivity in heritability of the multidimensional personality questionnaire scales. *Journal of Personality and Social Psychology, 72,* 929–938.

Finn, P. R., & Pihl, R. O. (1987). Men at high risk for alcoholism: The effect of alcohol on cardiovascular response to unavoidable shock. *Journal of Abnormal Psychology, 96,* 230–236.

Fromme, K., Stroot, E. A., & Kaplan, D. (1993). Comprehensive effects of alcohol: Development and psychometric assessment of a new expectancy questionnaire. *Psychological Assessment, 5*(1), 19–26.

Fry, P. S. (1992). *Fostering children's cognitive competence through mediated learning experiences.* Springfield, IL: Thomas.

Ganiere, D. M., & Enright, R. D. (1989). Exploring three approaches to identity development. *Journal of Youth and Adolescence, 18*(3), 283–295.

Goldman, M. S., Brown, S. A., Christiansen, B. A., & Smith, G. T. (1991). Alcoholism and memory: Broadening the scope of alcohol-expectancy research. *Psychological Bulletin, 110,* 137–146.

Goldman, M. S., & Rather, B. C. (1993). Substance use disorders: Cognitive models and architecture. In N. P. Kendall & K. S. Dobson (Eds.), *Psychopathology and cognition* (pp. 245–292). Orlando, FL: Academic Press.

Havighurst, R. J. (1972). *Developmental tasks and education* (3rd ed.). New York: McKay.

Hawkins, J. D., Catalano, R. F., & Miller, J. (1992). Risk and protective factors for alcohol and other drug problems in adolescence and early adulthood: Implications for substance abuse prevention. *Psychological Bulletin, 112,* 64–105.

Henderson, M. J., Goldman, M. S., Coovert, M. D., & Carnevalla, N. (1994). Covariance structure models of expectancy. *Journal of Studies on Alcohol, 55,* 315–326.

Isbell, L. M., Smith, H. L., & Wyer, R. S. (1998). Consequences of attempts to disregard social information. In J. M. Golding & C. M. MacLeod (Eds.), *Intentional forgetting: Interdisciplinary approaches* (pp. 289–320). Mahwah, NJ: Erlbaum.

Jackson, C. P., & Matthews, G. (1988). The prediction of habitual alcohol use from alcohol related expectancies and personality. *Alcohol and Alcoholism, 23,* 305–314.

James, W. (1890). *The principles of psychology* (Vol. 1). New York: Holt.

Jang, K. L., McCrae, R. R., Angleitner, A., Riemann, R., & Livesley, W. J. (1998). Heritability of facet-level traits in a cross-cultural twin sample: Support for a hierarchical model of personality. *Journal of Personality and Social Psychology, 74,* 1556–1565.

Jessor, J. (1987). Problem-behavior theory, psychosocial development, and adolescent problem drinking. *British Journal of Addiction, 82,* 331–342.

Johnston, L. D., O'Malley, P. M., & Bachman, J. G. (1987). *National trends in drug use and related factors among American high school students and young adults 1975–1986* (NIDA Research Monograph, DHHS Publication No. ADM 87–1535). Washington, DC: U.S. Government Printing Office.

Jones, E. E. (1986). Interpreting interpersonal behavior: The effects of expectancies. *Science, 234,* 41–46.

Jones, M. C. (1968). Personality antecedents and correlates of drinking patterns in adult males. *Journal of Consulting and Clinical Psychology, 32,* 2–12.

Jones, M. C. (1971). Personality antecedents and correlates of drinking patterns in women. *Journal of Consulting and Clinical Psychology, 36,* 61–69.

Kagan, J., Reznick, S. R., & Snidman, N. (1987). The physiology of behavioral inhibition in children. *Child Development, 58,* 1459–1473.

Kammeier, M. L., Hoffman, H., & Loper, R. G. (1973). Personality characteristics of alcoholics as college freshman and at time of treatment. *Quarterly Journal of Studies on Alcohol, 34,* 390–399.

Karoly, P. (1975). Comparison of psychological values in delinquent and nondelinquent females. *Psychological Reports, 36,* 567–570.

Kirsch, I. (1985). Response expectancy as a determinant of experience and behavior. *American Psychologist, 40,* 1189–1202.

Kline, R. B. (1990). The relation of alcohol expectancies to drinking patterns among alcoholics: Generalization across gender and race. *Journal of Studies on Alcohol, 51,* 175–182.

Kraus, D., Smith, G. T., & Ratner, H. H. (1994). Modifying alcohol-related expectancies in grade-school children. *Journal of Studies on Alcohol, 55,* 535–542.

Kroll, L. S. (1998). *An integration of learning based factors and personality risk factors in the prediction of drinking problems.* Unpublished doctoral dissertation, University of Kentucky.

Kurtz, J. P., & Zuckerman, M. (1978). Race and sex differences on the Sensation Seeking Scales. *Psychological Reports, 43,* 529–530.

Kushner, M., Sher, K. J., & Beitman, B. (1990). The relation between alcohol problems and the anxiety disorders. *American Journal of Psychiatry, 147,* 685–695.

Lazarus, R. S. (1982). Thoughts on the relation between emotion and cognition. *American Psychologist, 37,* 1019–1024.

Leigh, B. C. (1987). Beliefs about the effects of alcohol in self and others. *Journal of Studies on Alcohol, 48,* 467–475.

Leigh, B. C. (1989). In search of the seven dwarves: Issues of measurement and meaning in alcohol expectancy research. *Psychological Bulletin, 105,* 361–373.

Leigh, B. C., & Stacy, A. W. (1993). Alcohol outcome expectancies: Scale construction and predictive utility in higher order confirmatory models. *Psychological Assessment, 5,* 216–229.

Levine, B., & Goldman, M. S. (1989, August). *Situational variations in expectancies.* Paper presented at the annual convention of the American Psychological Association, New Orleans, LA.

Lex, B. W. (1985). Alcohol problems in special populations. In J. H. Mendelson & N. K. Mello (Eds.), *The diagnosis and treatment of alcoholism* (pp. 89–187). New York: McGraw-Hill.

Lex, B. W. (1987). Review of alcohol problems in ethnic minority groups. *Journal of Consulting and Clinical Psychology, 55,* 293–300.

Lucanegli, E., Galderisi, D., & Cornoldi, C. (1995). Specific and general transfer effects following metamemory learning. *Learning Disabilities Research and Practice, 10,* 11–21.

Lynam, D. R. (1996). Early identification of chronic offenders: Who is the fledgling psychopath? *Psychological Bulletin, 120,* 209–234.

MacCorquodale, K., & Meehl, P. E. (1953). Preliminary suggestions as to a formalization of expectancy theory. *Psychological Review, 60,* 55–63.

Mann, L. M., Chassin, L., & Sher, K. J. (1987). Alcohol expectancies and the risk for alcoholism. *Journal of Consulting and Clinical Psychology, 55,* 411–417.

McCarthy, D. M. (1998). *Towards an integrative model of disinhibition and learning risk for alcohol abuse.* Unpublished doctoral dissertation, University of Kentucky.

McCarthy, D. M., Miller, T. L., Smith, G. T., & Smith, J. R. (1998, July). *General and specific risk for substance use.* Paper presented at the annual meeting of the Research Society on Alcoholism, Hilton Head, SC.

McCarthy, D. M., & Smith, G. T. (1995, August). *Issues in the measurement of risk for substance abuse.* Paper presented at the 103rd annual convention of the American Psychological Association, New York, NY.

McCarthy, D. M., & Smith, G. T. (1996, June). *Meta-analysis of alcohol expectancy.* Paper presented at the annual meeting of the Research Society on Alcoholism, Washington, DC.

Meichenbaum, D., & Goodman, J. (1971). Training impulsive children to talk to themselves: A means of developing self-control. *Journal of Abnormal Psychology, 77,* 115–126.

Merikangas, K. R., Swendsen, J. D., Preisig, M. A., & Chazan, R. Z. (1998). Psychopathology and temperament in parents and offspring: Results of a family study. *Journal of Affective Disorders, 51,* 63–74.

Migneault, J. P., Pallonen, U. E., & Velicer, W. F. (1997). Decisional balance and stage of change for adolescent drinking. *Addictive Behaviors, 22,* 339–351.

Miller, D. T., & Turnbull, W. (1986). Expectancies and interpersonal processes. *Annual Review of Psychology, 37,* 233–256.

Miller, P. M., Smith, G. T., & Goldman, M. S. (1990). Emergence of alcohol expectancies in childhood: A possible critical period. *Journal of Studies on Alcohol, 51,* 343–349.

Miller, W. R. (1996). Motivational interviewing: Research, practice, and puzzles. *Addictive Behaviors, 21,* 835–842.

Morehouse, E. R. (1989). Treating adolescent alcohol abusers. *Social Casework: The Journal of Contemporary Social Work, 70,* 355–363.

Patterson, C. M., & Newman J. P. (1993). Reflectivity and learning from aversive events: Toward a psychological mechanism for syndromes of disinhibition. *Psychological Review, 100,* 716–736.

Peterson, C. (1992). *Personality* (2nd ed.). Fort Worth, TX: Harcourt Brace Jovanovich.

Prochaska, J. O., & DiClemente, C. C. (1983). Stages and processes of self-change of smoking: Toward an integrative model of change. *Journal of Consulting and Clinical Psychology, 51,* 390–395.

Rankin, H., Stockwell, T., & Hodgson, R. (1982). Personality and alcohol dependence. *Personality and Individual Differences, 3,* 145–151.

Reese, F. L., & Friend, R. (1994). Alcohol expectancies and drinking practices among Black and White undergraduate males. *Journal of College Student Development, 35,* 319–325.

Rescorla, R. A. (1988). Pavlovian conditioning. *American Psychologist, 43,* 151–160.

Robins, L. N., Bates, W., & O'Neal, P. (1962). Adult drinking patterns of former problem children. In D. Pittman & C. R. Snyder (Eds.), *Society, culture, and drinking patterns* (pp. 395–412). New York: Wiley.

Rotter, J. B. (1954). *Social learning and clinical psychology.* Englewood Cliffs, NJ: Prentice-Hall.

Schulenberg, J., Maggs, J. L., & Hurrelmann, K. (1997). Negotiating developmental transitions during adolescence and young adulthood: Health risks and opportunities. In J. Schulenberg, J. L. Maggs, & K. Hurrelmann (Eds.), *Health risks and developmental transitions during adolescence* (pp. 1–19). New York: Cambridge University Press.

Sieber, M. F. (1981). Personality scores and licit and illicit substance use. *Personality and Individual Differences, 2,* 235–241.

Shaw, D. S., & Winslow, E. B. (1977). Precursors and correlates of antisocial behavior from a learning perspective. In D. M. Stoff, J. Breiling, & J. D. Maser (Eds.), *Handbook of antisocial behavior* (pp. 148–158). New York: Wiley.

Shedler, J., & Block, J. (1990). Adolescent drug use and psychological health: A longitudinal inquiry. *American Psychologist, 45*(5), 612–630.

Sheppard, D., Smith, G. T., & Rosenbaum, G. (1988). Use of MMPI subtypes in predicting completion of a residential alcoholism treatment program. *Journal of Consulting and Clinical Psychology, 56,* 590–596.

Sher, K. J. (1991). *Children of alcoholics: A critical appraisal of theory and research.* Chicago: University of Chicago Press.

Sher, K. J., & Trull, T. J. (1994). Personality and disinhibitory psychopathology: Alcoholism and antisocial personality disorder. *Journal of Abnormal Psychology, 103,* 92–102.

Sher, K. J., Walitzer, K. S., Wood, P. K., & Brent, E. E. (1991). Characteristics of children of alcoholics: Putative risk factors, substance use and abuse, and psychopathology. *Journal of Abnormal Psychology, 100,* 427–448.

Singer, M. I., & Petchers, M. K. (1987). A biracial comparison of adolescent alcohol use. *American Journal of Drug and Alcohol Abuse, 13,* 461–474.

Smith, G. T. (1989). Expectancy theory and alcohol: The situation insensitivity hypothesis. *Psychology of Addictive Behaviors, 2,* 108–115.

Smith, G. T. (1994). Psychological expectancy as mediator of vulnerability to alcoholism. *Annals of the New York Academy of Sciences, 708,* 165–171.

Smith, G. T., & Goldman, M. S. (1990, August). *Toward a mediational model of alcohol expectancy.* Paper presented at the annual convention of the American Psychological Association, Boston, MA.

Smith, G. T., & Goldman, M. S. (1994). Alcohol expectancy theory and the identification of high-risk adolescents. *Journal of Research on Adolescence, 4,* 229–247.

Smith, G. T., Goldman, M. S., Greenbaum, P. E., & Christiansen, B. A. (1995). The divergent paths of high-expectancy and low-expectancy adolescents. *Journal of Abnormal Psychology, 104,* 32–40.

Smith, G. T., & McCarthy, D. M. (1995). Methodological considerations in the refinement of clinical assessment instruments. *Psychological Assessment, 7,* 300–308.

Smith, G. T., McCarthy, D. M., & Goldman, M. S. (1995). Self-reported drinking and alcohol-related problems among adolescents: Dimensionality and validity over 24 months. *Journal of Studies on Alcohol, 56,* 383–394.

Smith, G. T., McCarthy, D. M., & Kroll, L. (in press). Toward integrating personality and learning models of alcoholism: Acquired preparedness for alcoholism. In R. Vrasti & L. Towle (Eds.), *Alcoholism: New research perspectives.* London: Wiley.

Smith, G. T., McCarthy, D. A., Kroll, L., & Miller, T. L. (1998, August). Combining personality and learning risk factors: The acquired preparedness model. In M. Kilbey (Chair), *Expectancies: A cognitive science approach to alcohol and drug abuse.* Symposium conducted at the annual meeting of the American Psychological Association, San Francisco.

Smith, G. T., & Miller, T. L. (1992). Toward a developmental framework for the treatment of adolescent alcohol abuse: Current findings and future directions. In R. R. Watson (Ed.), *Alcohol and drug abuse reviews: Vol. 3. Alcohol abuse treatment* (pp. 87–113). Totowa, NJ: Humana Press.

Southwick, L., Steele, C., Marlatt, A., & Lindell, M. (1981). Alcohol-related expectancies: Defined by phase of intoxication and drinking experience. *Journal of Consulting and Clinical Psychology, 49,* 713–721.

Spiegler, D. L., Tate, D. A., Aitken, S. S., & Christian, C. M. (Eds.). (1989). *Alcohol use among U.S. ethnic minorities* (NIAAA Research Monograph No. ADM 89-1435). Washington, DC: U.S. Government Printing Office.

Spiegler, D. L. (1983). Children's attitudes toward alcohol. *Journal of Studies on Alcohol, 44,* 545–552.

Stacy, A. W., Newcomb, M. D., & Bentler, P. M. (1991). Cognitive motivation and drug use: A 9-year longitudinal study. *Journal of Abnormal Psychology, 100,* 502–515.

Stroot, E. A., & Fromme, K. (1989, November). *Comprehensive effects of alcohol: Development of a new expectancy questionnaire.* Paper presented at the annual meeting of the Association for Advancement of Behavior Therapy, Washington, DC.

Sue, D. W., & Sue, D. (1990). *Counseling the culturally different: Theory and practice.* New York: Wiley Interscience.

Sullivan, H. S. (1947). *Conceptions of modern psychiatry.* Washington, DC: William Alanson White Psychiatric Foundation.

Sutker, P. B., Archer, R. P., & Allain, A. N. (1978). Drug abuse patterns, personality characteristics, and relationships with sex, race and sensation seeking. *Journal of Consulting and Clinical Psychology, 46,* 1374–1378.

Tarter, R. E., & Vanyukov, M. (1994). Alcoholism: A developmental disorder. *Journal of Consulting and Clinical Psychology, 62,* 1096–1107.

Tolman, E. C. (1932). *Purposive behavior in animals and man.* New York: Century.

West, R., Drummond, D., & Eames, K. (1990). Alcohol consumption, problem drinking and anti-social behavior in a sample of college students. *British Journal of Addictions, 85,* 479–486.

Windle, M. (1990). Temperament and personality attributes of children of alcoholics. In M. Windle & J. S. Searles (Eds.), *Children of alcoholics: Critical perspectives* (pp. 129–167). New York: Guilford Press.

Wood, M. D., Nagoshi, C. T., & Dennis, D. A. (1992). Alcohol norms and expectancies as predictors of alcohol use and problems in a college student sample. *American Journal of Alcohol Abuse, 18,* 461–476.

Wyer, R. S., & Srull, T. K. (1986). Human cognition in its social context. *Psychological Review, 93,* 322–359.

Young, R., & Knight, R. C. (1989). The Drinking Expectancy Questionnaire: A revised measure of alcohol-related beliefs. *Journal of Psychopathology and Behavior Assessment, 11,* 99–112.

Zucker, R. A. (1987). The four alcoholisms: A developmental account of the etiologic process. In P. C. Rivers (Ed.), *Nebraska Symposium on Motivation: Vol. 34. Alcohol and addictive behaviors* (pp. 27–83). Lincoln: University of Nebraska Press.

Zucker, R. A., & Gomberg, E. S. L. (1986). Etiology of alcoholism reconsidered: The case for a biopsychosocial process. *American Psychologist, 41,* 783–793.

II

Empirical Illustrations Linked to Part I/Clinical Applications of Brief Interventions

5

Motivational Enhancement for Alcohol-Involved Adolescents

PETER M. MONTI, NANCY P. BARNETT,
TRACY A. O'LEARY, and SUZANNE M. COLBY

Adolescent substance use and abuse is a significant public health concern due to its prevalence and associated negative consequences (see Winters, Chapter 3; Brown & Lourie, Chapter 8; Myers, Brown, Tate, Abrantes, & Tomlinson, Chapter 9, this volume). According to the 1998 Monitoring the Future survey (Johnston, O'Malley, & Bachman, 1999), nearly one fourth of 8th graders (23%) and over one half of 12th graders (52%) reported some alcohol consumption in the last month. Estimates of the prevalence of alcohol use disorders among teenagers range from 3%–4%, according to a sample of 14- to 16-year olds (Cohen et al., 1993), to almost one third of a cohort of high school seniors (32%; Reinhertz, Giaconia, Lefkowitz, Pakiz, & Frost, 1993).

Adolescent drinking has been associated with injuries, motor vehicle crashes, assaults, and suicide attempts (Gould et al., 1998; Hicks, Morris, Bass, Holcomb, & Neblett, 1990; Maio, Portnoy, Blow, & Hill, 1994). Indeed, alcohol-related injuries and crashes are the leading causes of death for young adults (Institute of Medicine, 1990). Whereas adult levels of alcohol consumption have remained relatively steady over the past 25 years in the United States, teenagers are initiating drinking and using drugs at younger ages than ever before.

Because adolescents typically do not identify themselves as problem drinkers, an optimal approach is to develop proactive screening, assessment, and treatment procedures that target settings in which adolescents with substance-related problems are likely to present. Urgent care settings, primary care clinics, and the courts are potentially good intervention sites. Our group has recently focused on detecting alcohol use in teens in an emergency room (Barnett et al., 1998; Colby et al., 1999), on comparing characteristics of alcohol-positive versus alcohol-negative adolescents in this setting (Monti, 1997), and on developing a brief alcohol screen for adolescent problem drinking (Chung et al., 2000).

Although better identification of adolescent alcohol use problems is necessary, it is obviously not sufficient. In contrast to the adult alcohol-treatment literature (see, e.g., Hester & Miller, 1995; Monti, Abrams, Kadden, & Cooney, 1989), relatively little empirical effort has been directed toward developing effective treatment for adolescents. School-based primary prevention programs have met with some success (see, e.g., Botvin, Schinke, Epstein, Diaz, & Botvin, 1995), but they tend not to address cessation and reduction issues for adolescents who are already drinking; they cannot target school dropouts; and they rarely address motivational issues related to use and abuse. (See Miller, Turner, & Marlatt, Chapter 2, this volume, for an overview of the need to address motivational issues in substance use intervention.)

One approach that has been developed by Alan Marlatt and colleagues (see Miller et al., Chapter 2, this volume) addresses the first two of these issues by employing motivational enhancement with heavy-drinking college students. Although the results are very encouraging, to date the approach has been limited to use with college students. It does not address a large segment of the teenage population who are younger and/or may not be attending school. Furthermore, given the increased alcohol and drug-related risks associated with school dropout (Cook & Moore, 1993; Winters, Chapter 3, this volume), it seems important to develop a program in a nonschool environment that could include a wider segment of the population.

Medical settings provide an opportunity to reach adolescents who need intervention but who are not served by other services (Glynn, Anderson, & Schwartz, 1991). Indeed, the efficacy of brief interventions for adult problem drinkers in clinics or medical settings has been well established (Babor & Grant, 1992; Fleming, Barry, Manwell, Johnson, & London, 1997; Miller & Rollnick, 1991; see also Wilk, Jensen, & Havighurst, 1997, for a review). Recently, the World Health Organization (1996) reported results of a multinational trial of brief interventions in primary care settings that showed a significant decrease in daily alcohol consumption following a 5- to 15-minute intervention with a health care provider.

Yet another compelling reason to conduct a brief alcohol intervention in a medical setting is to capitalize on what might be construed a "teachable moment" or a "window of opportunity," especially if the setting is an emergency room (ER). Indeed, adolescents treated in an ER for an alcohol-related event are likely to be especially receptive to an alcohol intervention due to the salience of the event and their negative emotional reaction to it. Furthermore, if they are frightened and upset when they arrive, it is likely that the confusion and often long wait in a busy ER will increase their discomfort. Practitioners can capitalize on such factors to elicit ambivalence from teens about their alcohol use and promote interest in reducing dangerous drinking.

In this chapter we present a motivational intervention (MI) approach that is particularly well suited for use in an ER in that it combines a nonjudgmental and empathic therapeutic style (Miller & Rollnick, 1991) with personal feedback regarding drinking patterns and effects. This approach has proven effective in reducing problem drinking among adults (Miller, 1995). Indeed, Brown and Miller (1993) found enduring changes in the alcohol use of adult heavy drinkers following a single MI session. The brevity of an MI makes it particularly suitable for use in an ER or other opportunistic settings.

This chapter outlines clinical research that has been conducted with adolescents who range from 13 through 19 years of age. All teens were treated individually with the same treatment approach, except that the parents of 13- to 17-year-old-patients were approached for informed consent and possible involvement in the treatment. Although our work has involved adolescents who volunteer to participate in our studies, we feel that our approach may have wide applicability to treatment programs, to programs for adjudicated youths, and to a variety of prevention efforts. Replication research with these populations is warranted.

In the following section, we present detailed step-by-step coverage of our MI approach, illustrated with relevant clinical examples. Next, we present several topics that require special attention, including counselor training, other populations of interest and treatment modality issues, and dealing with other substances of abuse. Finally, we briefly present empirical results for our approach, conclusions, and some future directions for this line of research.

MOTIVATIONAL INTERVENTION SESSION

The MI protocol we have developed for our research program focuses on alcohol consumption and risky behavior, with an emphasis on heavy drinking and driving after drinking. As is consistent with an MI approach, the intervention should be modified, as appropriate, to be meaningful for each teen and his or her level of interest in changing. The session description that follows is typically conducted in 30–45 minutes. Because we are intervening with teens who have been treated in an ER for alcohol-related reasons (e.g., motor vehicle crash, assault, intoxication), we wait for their alcohol levels to decrease and administer a mini-mental status exam to ensure that they are able to understand and provide informed consent to participate in the intervention.

Introduction and Engagement

The introduction can be made prior to the assessment (which may promote more honest responding) or prior to the MI. The purpose of the introduction is to provide the teen with an idea of the content, style, and limitations of the time that will be spent with the counselor. We introduce the session as an opportunity for teens to talk about their thoughts and feelings about the event that brought them to the ER, to get some information about their pattern of drinking and the effects of alcohol, and to spend some time, if they are interested, talking about ways to avoid similar things happening in the future. In our ER setting counselors emphasize that they will not tell the teen what to do; rather it is up to the teen to make decisions and choices about drinking and about things he or she does when drinking. (Of course, this statement about the counselor's orientation should be made only if it is consistent with the program that the teen is attending.) The circumstances that precipitated the ER visit are then reviewed, including how much the teen had been drinking, whom he or she was with, and any injuries sustained or consequences suffered. The use of open-ended questions in this part of the interview enhances rapport and helps the counselor rapidly develop an understanding of the teen's recent drinking patterns and associations. An open-ended question is a question that cannot be answered with one word or very brief responses. For example, asking "How was alcohol a part of what happened?" is open-ended, whereas "What did you drink?" is not.

For sessions that are preventive in nature (i.e., not following an indentifiable concern about a teen, such as a recent alcohol violation or similar event), the purpose of the session can be articulated as an opportunity to talk about experiences with alcohol and to address any concerns or questions the teen might have. Whether or not there is a precipitating event, the counselor should state his or her interest in getting the teen's perspective overtly at the outset and demonstrate that interest throughout the session.

The introduction provides an opportunity to establish rapport and minimize defensiveness. The counselor should present an empathic, concerned, nonauthoritarian, and nonjudgmental style (see, e.g., Miller, 1995). It is important for teens to believe that the counselor respects their ideas, is interested in hearing about their experiences, and will not scold them or make disapproving statements about their behavior. This introduction is straightforward and can be used regardless of the nature of the referral (i.e., voluntary or involuntary). See Table 5.1 for elements to include in the introduction.

The following introductory statements illustrate the manner in which we describe the MI session to teens. We discuss the structure, content, and aim of the session, with repeated emphasis on the teen's personal responsibility and choice regarding changing alcohol use. Notice the collaborative tenor of the introduction, in that the counselor is establishing that the two will work together to generate strategies to avoid similar situations in the future.

"What I'd like to do now is explore with you your alcohol use. We're concerned about risky drinking and other risky behaviors that tend to go along with drinking, like driving. I can't tell you what to do; only you can decide what you'll do. Rather, I'd like to find out what you think about drinking after this experience and maybe see if together we can come up with some ways to avoid these kinds of situations in the future. You're the one who will decide what happens with your drinking. If you choose, you can make changes in your drinking, but that's really up to you. How does that sound? Can we try this out?"

Many teens express concerns about divulging information about their alcohol use. The following illustrates how we broach the sensitive topic of confidentiality with teens in the ER. Brittany, a 17-year-old white female who arrived by ambulance at the ER after being involved in a motor vehicle

---

TABLE 5.1. Elements of the Introduction

Purpose and content: What will be discussed. This may include an overview of the session or sessions.

Counselor's orientation: What the counselor will and won't do. For example, we make it clear that the counselor is "not going to tell [the teen] what to do."

Limitations of confidentiality: With any type of client it is important to provide a definition of confidentiality and an explanation of the circumstances under which confidentiality would be broken. We remind teens of this at every session. Because our intervention for young teens (those not yet 18) requires parental consent and includes parent assessment and intervention, we also make it clear to teens and to their parents that we will not share what one tells us with the other.

Program-specific elements: Special program characteristics, such as attendance requirements or counselor reports to other entities, should be discussed early in the session. For example, in the ER we acknowledge that there may be interruptions to our session (e.g., for medical procedures) and that if that happens the counselor will stay close by but that the discussion would stop until the interruption has ended.

accident in which she was the driver, shares her concerns with the counselor.

COUNSELOR: First, before we begin, I'd like to talk to you about the project and what we'll be doing. I'll be asking you a number of questions about your alcohol use and other substance use, ask you about the events that led up to the car accident tonight, provide you with some information from the questionnaires you completed earlier if you're interested, and talk about some ways you may be able to avoid this kind of thing happening again. How does that sound?

BRITTANY: Well, I don't know. . . . I don't know how much I want to talk about what happened. I don't want this going on my permanent record. I really don't want anyone to know what happened, and besides, I was in a car accident. I probably shouldn't say anything at all.

COUNSELOR: I can understand how you might feel that way. Let me tell you about confidentiality and its limits. Everything you tell us is kept strictly confidential—that means that I will not share the information you give me nor anything you say during our discussion with anyone, including your parents or the staff here at the ER. The only times when I'm required by law to report information to the authorities are as follows: when a person says that they are going to hurt themselves or hurt others or when there's suspicion of child abuse or neglect or elder abuse or neglect. Aside from those instances, everything you tell me is confidential. We don't even put your name or any other potentially identifying material on any project material, except our follow-up forms, which are kept in a separate place in a locked file. What other concerns do you have about participating?

BRITTANY: Um, I don't want the police to know what I say.

COUNSELOR: We also protect your confidentiality outside of the ER setting. So if the police, your school, or anyone else called and wanted information, we couldn't release anything to them. We also don't acknowledge that you even participated in the project. The only way they would know if you participated in this project would be if you decided to tell them.

BRITTANY: Oh, I see. Well, I guess that sounds okay. What if I decide that I don't want to do this anymore? Will you tell anyone then?

COUNSELOR: No. If you decided not to continue in the project, we wouldn't tell anyone about any of the information you gave us. We keep all of the information teenagers give us in a locked filing cabinet, and the only people who have access to it are those directly involved in the research project. Your name is not on any of the questionnaires you answer.

BRITTANY: Okay, I feel a little better about it. You can go ahead with your questions.

COUNSELOR: Great. Let's get started.

Participant Assessment

In our program, assessment instruments serve a dual purpose. They are used as a measure of target behaviors at the initial session and at later assessments to detect any changes over time, and they also are used to provide personalized feedback to teens within the MI session. Assessments are administered after the basic structure of the program has been described. In our ER setting, measures are interviewer administered, but other facilities may prefer to have teens self-administer the questionnaires. Paper-and-pencil versions may be used, or measures can be computerized for ease of administration, data collection, and development of feedback. The structure of the program and the resources available will determine the nature of the assessment. An important distinction when choosing assessments is to decide whether it is an objective of the program to provide teens with a perspective of how they compare with other teens of the same gender and age. In order to provide such "normative information," it is necessary to use measures that have age and gender norms available.

Babor and his colleagues (1994) identified key variables to measure when assessments of outcome are desired, including alcohol consumption, alcohol problems, and quality-of-life variables that are associated with changes in drinking behavior, such as general psychosocial functioning or academic functioning. In an ER setting, our goal is to construct an assessment that is sufficiently comprehensive to obtain an accurate baseline evaluation, as well as feedback for the MI, yet brief enough to keep intervention in the ER feasible. (See Table 5.2 for a listing of the domains we measure.) In other settings, more extensive assessment sessions at baseline may be desirable. (See National Institute on Alcohol Abuse and Alcoholism [NIAAA], 1995; Lecchese & Waldron, 1994; and Winters, Chapter 3, this volume, for information on instruments that are appropriate for use with adolescents.)

Exploration of Motivation

Once the assessment is complete and teens have been oriented to the MI session, they are asked what they like and do not like about drinking. Open-ended questions are used to encourage teens to generate all their likes and dislikes about drinking and to talk about the effects that matter most to them. In our program teens are also asked why they might drive after

TABLE 5.2. Elements of Personalized Feedback

Measure	Assessment feedback sheet
	ALCOHOL USE
Quantity/frequency measure[a]	Your answers to our questions about how much you've drunk in the past 3 months show three things:
	1. You drink more often than _____ out of 10 males/ females your age.
	2. When you drink, you typically drink more than _____ out of 10 males/females your age.
	3. You get drunk more often than _____ out of 10 males/ females your age.
	PHYSICAL DEPENDENCE ON ALCOHOL
Adolescent Drinking Index (Harrell & Wirtz, 1985)[a]	Do you know how to tell that your body is physically dependent on alcohol? There are signs that alcohol has begun to do something to your body. These changes can be an early warning sign of serious problems with alcohol. You showed:
Item #5	(×) Tolerance: You need more alcohol to get the same effect.
Item #25 or #27	(×) Withdrawal: You got sick or had a hangover when you stopped drinking.
Item #9 or #26	(×) Severe intoxication: You drank until you passed out, got sick, or had a blackout.
	EMOTIONAL DEPENDENCE ON ALCOHOL
Adolescent Drinking Index Self-Medication subscale[a]	What do you know about the ways people get emotionally dependent on alcohol?
	Your answers on some of our questions show that you use alcohol to cope with unpleasant feelings more often than _____ out of 10 males/females your age.
	CONSEQUENCES OF ALCOHOL USE
Adolescent Drinking Index Total score[a]	Your answers to questions about unpleasant things that happened to you because of drinking show that you had more problems with family, friends, and school than _____ out of 10 males/females your age.
Adolescent Drinking Index Rebelliousness subscale[a]	Your answers to questions about unpleasant things that happened to you because of drinking show that you had more problems with fighting and getting into trouble than _____ out of 10 males/females your age.

(continued)

TABLE 5.2. *(continued)*

Measure	Assessment feedback sheet
	RISK TAKING AND ALCOHOL
Adolescent Injury Checklist (modified) Total Alcohol Scale score (Jelalian et al., 1997)	You said that ____ times in the past year you were drinking or using drugs when you got injured. To what extent do you think alcohol contributed to your getting hurt?
Reckless Behavior Questionnaire (Shaw, Wagner, Arnett, & Aber, 1992) (modified) Total score and with alcohol	We asked you about a number of risky or dangerous behaviors you have done in the past year. You said that you had done ____% of the ones we asked about. Of the ones you had done, you said alcohol was ____ involved when you did these risky things.
	AVOIDING DRINKING AND DRIVING
Safe Strategies Questionnaire (Farrow, 1989)	So far you have used ____ different methods to avoid driving after drinking or riding with a driver who has been drinking. Using even one strategy decreases your risk of accidents due to drinking and driving.

[a]Measures have available norms.

drinking and what they do not like about driving after drinking (including the worst thing they could imagine happening). They are asked to elaborate on their parents' and friends' attitudes toward drinking and toward drinking and driving and on how those attitudes might affect their own drinking behaviors.

This section of the MI session has several goals (see Table 5.3). The counselor is able to gain an understanding of the teen's decisional balance with regard to drinking. By establishing the list of the teen's pros and cons of drinking, the counselor and teen can develop a shared understanding of what aspects serve as positive reinforcers for drinking and what elements (i.e., consequences of drinking) might serve as reasons for reducing alcohol use. The counselor can then tailor the MI to these personalized pros and cons, while keeping in mind the teen's stage of readiness for changing drinking behavior. This discussion also assists the counselor in identifying influences on the teen's behaviors in the form of peer and parental behavior and attitudes and the importance of these influences, according to the teen.

Jose, a 19-year-old Hispanic male working full time after recently graduating from high school, was seen in the ER after suffering lacerations

TABLE 5.3. Promoting Exploration within the MI Session

Goals of exploration	Strategies
Promote respectful interchange	Use open-ended questions, reflective listening statements.
Identify reinforcers	Ask: "What do you like about drinking?" "What else?"
Identify motivators	"What do you dislike about drinking?" "What's the most important thing?" "What's the worst thing?"
Develop discrepancy and ambivalence	Use double-sided reflection: "So although drinking beer helps you relax and enjoy yourself, it also can make you do things you wish you hadn't."

and contusions following a fight in a local nightclub. The lack of perceived cons of drinking on Jose's part, coupled with his statements regarding his alcohol use, indicate that he is in the precontemplation stage of change: He does not perceive himself to have any alcohol-related problems and has expressed no intentions to change his drinking in the near future.

COUNSELOR: What do you like about your drinking?

JOSE: Hmm . . . I like how I feel when I drink.

COUNSELOR: In what ways?

JOSE: Uh, well, drinking relaxes me.

COUNSELOR: I see. What else?

JOSE: It's a social thing, a way to hang out with my boys and have a good time.

COUNSELOR: You enjoy the socializing you do by drinking and how it makes you feel. What else?

JOSE: I can forget about work. It's a way to celebrate the end of the week for me. I work 60 hours a week doing construction, man. It's hard work.

COUNSELOR: Okay. What else?

JOSE: That's about it.

COUNSELOR: So, let me see if I understand. You like drinking because it makes you feel relaxed and social. It's a means for getting together with friends, enjoying yourself, forgetting about work, and rewarding yourself on the weekends. Is that about right?

JOSE: Yeah, and I like the way it tastes, especially when I've been working outside.

COUNSELOR: How about the things you don't like as much about your drinking? What are they?

JOSE: Well, there's really nothing I don't like about it. I don't have any problems with my drinking. Just because I'm here because I got into a fight at the club doesn't mean I have an alcohol problem.

COUNSELOR: You feel very strongly that drinking isn't an issue for you.

JOSE: Absolutely, and I won't listen to someone telling me that it is an issue when it's not!

COUNSELOR: I hear a lot of irritation in your voice, and I wonder if there have been people in your life who have accused you of having an alcohol problem.

JOSE: Oh, yeah. My mother and my girlfriend. What do they know? They don't drink and they think it's okay to get on my back because I have a few beers on the weekend.

COUNSELOR: We both agree that it's not helpful to make judgments about others and their drinking, and I'm not here to tell you that you have an alcohol problem. We've just met, and I'd like to hear your own perspective and thoughts about alcohol. What are some of the not-so-good things about drinking?

JOSE: Like I said, there's not really anything I don't like. Well, maybe the cost. I only like the good stuff, and after a while it can add up.

COUNSELOR: So, the cost of it is one thing you don't like about drinking. What else?

JOSE: That's it.

COUNSELOR: May I ask you about some things that others have said they don't like about drinking and hear your thoughts on them?

JOSE: Sure. Whatever.

COUNSELOR: Some people don't like how they feel the next day after drinking; they might get very sick, or hung over, or perhaps can't remember everything that happened the night before.

JOSE: Oh, I see what you mean. Of course, I don't enjoy getting hangovers. That doesn't happen too much, so it's not a problem for me.

COUNSELOR: So, let's see if I have it right. There are several things you like about drinking: the taste, having fun with friends, relaxing, celebrating the end of the week, and forgetting about work. On the other hand, however, there are a few things you don't like about drinking, such as the money you spend on alcohol, getting a hangover occasionally, and having to deal with your mother and your girlfriend getting on your case about drinking.

JOSE: You hit the nail on the head. That's about it.

Tran, a 16-year-old Asian male, was admitted to the ER following injuries sustained in a bicycle accident. He perceived the pros of his alcohol use to far outweigh the cons; this was mainly due to the lack of negative consequences from his drinking, as well as the recent onset of his alcohol use (in the past 3 months). The following vignette illustrates how the counselor "tips the balance" to highlight the cons of drinking and thereby increase discrepancy for the teen.

COUNSELOR: So, tell me some of the things you like about your drinking.

TRAN: Oh, you know, like, it's fun. I only drink a few times a week, nothing big.

COUNSELOR: Tell me more about the ways it's fun for you.

TRAN: Uh, well, it's something to do when I'm hanging out with my friends.

COUNSELOR: What else?

TRAN: Uh, I guess I like the taste of it, getting a buzz and all.

COUNSELOR: Okay, what else?

TRAN: Uh . . . I think that's it.

COUNSELOR: What about some of the things you don't like as much about your drinking?

TRAN: There's really nothing I don't like about drinking. It's not like I've been drinking a long time, you know.

COUNSELOR: I see. You're saying that there are a lot of things you like about drinking, like spending time with friends when you're all drinking and getting a buzz from alcohol. On the flip side, there's really nothing at all that you don't like about drinking.

TRAN: Yeah, that's right.

COUNSELOR: You shared with me earlier that you fell off your bike while giving your friend a ride and that you and he had been drinking. How does alcohol fit into what happened to bring you to the emergency room tonight?

TRAN: Oh. I guess that's true, I was drinking a little bit before it happened, but it was only a little bit.

COUNSELOR: So, although you feel you weren't drinking that much tonight, you see that maybe there's a connection between drinking and falling.

TRAN: Yeah, I see what you mean. Not a big connection, though! If my friend knew how to balance on the back, it wouldn't have happened.

COUNSELOR: And what has it been like for you here in the ER?

TRAN: Well, it's sucked. I have a broken arm, it hurts a lot, and the doctors and nurses make you wait forever before one of them even talks to you!

COUNSELOR: So, if I were to sum up the things you like and don't like so much about drinking, the things you like are hanging out with friends when drinking, the taste of alcohol, and the buzz you get from it. On the other hand, you see a link between drinking and having this broken arm and having to spend your evening stuck here in the hospital, which hasn't sounded pleasant for you at all! Do I have that about right?

TRAN: Yeah. This is the only time that I've had something like this happen to me.

COUNSELOR: And it sounds like you want it to be your last bad experience!

TRAN: Totally.

Enhancement of Motivation

The purpose of this section of the MI is to increase teens' understanding of their patterns of alcohol use, to provide information about any indicators of problem drinking, and to promote interest in making positive changes to hazardous drinking patterns. We do this in three ways. We provide personalized feedback from the assessment instruments, including a comparison of the teen's scores to age and gender norms. We also provide information about alcohol and its effects, for example, alcohol's effects on driving skills. Finally, we ask the teens to elaborate on what they imagine the future would be like if they were to change or not change.

Personalized Feedback

Personalized feedback has been identified as a key element of effective brief interventions (Bien, Miller, & Tonigan, 1993) and is a central feature of our intervention. The computer program we have developed generates a printed personalized feedback sheet (see Table 5.2) that summarizes information gathered during the assessment. This feedback provides age- and gender-based normative information (i.e., percentile rank) on drinking frequency and quantity, frequency of drunkenness, and alcohol-related problems with family, friends, and school. Indices of physical and emotional dependence (including signs of tolerance and withdrawal) and risk taking related to alcohol use are also provided. In addition, we provide personalized feedback about the number of strategies the teen used to avoid driving or riding with a drinking driver. A computer program is not necessary in order to provide feedback; information from normative tables and levels of risk can be transcribed or hand calculated.

The assessment feedback can be given to the teen all at once, reserving discussion for the very end, or the separate sections can be discussed as they are presented. Throughout, the counselor determines whether the teen understands the information and elicits reactions and questions. As in other parts of the interview, the counselor must make decisions about what aspects of the feedback to focus on or emphasize. For example, less severe scores on feedback sections might be highlighted as a sign of strength or potential for change or, if the counselor is trying to elicit concern from the teen, might be deemphasized. Once the feedback has been explained, it is useful to ask teens what aspects they were most surprised by and what was most disturbing to them. The counselor should help the teen interpret the meaning of the feedback. For example, teens who are discouraged by the results can be reminded that negative results can improve with behavior change.

In the interest of time, we present an abbreviated version of the feedback to the teen during the MI and give him or her a more detailed version to take home. Language is kept simple and to the point, with risks expressed in a concerned but matter-of-fact way. Including simple graphics to illustrate scores and statistics in the feedback may engage teens and can better facilitate work with those who do not read well. As with text, graphics should be explained.

Corey is a 15-year-old white male brought into the ER after becoming intoxicated at a school dance. He is not only surprised about his personalized assessment feedback but is also challenging the veracity of the information and the counselor's interpretation of the results. Rather than increasing resistance by telling Corey that he's wrong, the counselor instead reflects Corey's disbelief and uses it as a means of developing discrepancy and heightening ambivalence about his alcohol use. The following clinical vignette illustrates the use of reflective listening and rolling with resistance.

COUNSELOR: What I'd like to do now is go over the results of some of the questionnaires you answered with me. How does that sound?

COREY: Okay, I guess.

COUNSELOR: There are a lot of numbers here, but I'll explain each one. Please ask questions or make comments as we go along. On this first section, we compared your drinking with the drinking of other teenage males your age. You drink more than 8 out of 10 of them.

COREY: No way! That can't be right. I have friends who drink way more than I do.

COUNSELOR: So, you don't think these numbers are correct.

COREY: Well, I didn't say that. I just don't drink that much compared to all my friends, that's all.

COUNSELOR: I can see how this might be confusing to you. You don't feel that you drink very much at all, compared to how your friends drink, and yet your drinking rates turn out to be higher than most teenage males your age. It's hard to figure out.

COREY: Definitely! Some of my friends can drink a six-pack no problem, and they're fine. Where did you get these figures?

COUNSELOR: These figures are from a survey of Rhode Island teenagers on drinking levels. I can see why you'd be surprised, because your friends drink more than you do and yet your levels are higher than most teenagers. The reason for this is that the survey reflects a large number of teenagers. Some of them drink more than you do, some drink less, and still others don't drink alcohol at all. This feedback compares you to all of those teenagers.

COREY: But what about my friends? I also know a lot of other guys who drink a lot more than I do. How do you explain that?

COUNSELOR: What happens is that we tend to hang out with people who are similar to ourselves and who like to do the same things. People who drink at higher levels usually have friends who drink at those same levels. So, it can seem like most teenage males your age drink the same as you do, because that's been your experience. In fact, there are more teenage boys your age who drink less than you do.

COREY: Wow, that's really hard to believe. (*Looks surprised, becomes quiet.*)

COUNSELOR: This really doesn't fit with how you see yourself.

COREY: Yeah. I don't know what to think about it. I honestly never thought I drank that much.

Information

When relevant, information about blood alcohol level and metabolization, effects of alcohol on driving, and related topics can be discussed. In our program, teens are tested for their blood alcohol levels at the time they are treated at the hospital, which provides the basis for discussion. Teens are usually receptive to information about the effects of alcohol at different levels, including the fact that even very low levels of alcohol can impair driving. Information about estimating typical and peak blood alcohol content may also be provided (see Dimeff, Baer, Kivlahan, & Marlatt, 1999).

Envisioning the Future

Motivation can be further enhanced by asking teens to imagine the future if their drinking were to remain the same and again if it were to change. This approach is intended to induce teens to consider the further potential negative outcomes of continuing their drinking behavior and also to introduce the idea of making a change that might have a positive outcome. If it is established that there is a discrepancy between a teen's current drinking pattern and his or her goals for the future, such a discrepancy may provide a motivating function and should be highlighted. For example, if a teen has future athletic aspirations, the interventionist could highlight the discrepancy between the aspirations of highly skilled performance and the teen's current pattern of behavior. Some areas to introduce are the possible reactions of family and friends. An example of a prompt might be: "If you decided to make a change, what do you think would become easier in your life?"

Establishing a Plan

Regardless of the setting in which the intervention is conducted or the focus or length of the MI, the counselor and adolescent should leave the session with an understanding of what the teen is willing to do next. For example, if the motivational session is used as a precursor to entering a treatment program, appropriate goals might be to engage in the treatment program by attending a specific number of sessions or contributing at least one comment in each attended group. For other adolescents, one session of MI can be conceptualized as a precursor to self-change. In either case, teens have a greater chance of being successful at changing if they establish a well-considered plan and make a commitment to it.

Prior to discussing a plan, it is a good idea to reassess the teens' interest in changing. Good open-ended questions to use are: "Where does this leave you now?" or "What, if anything, would you like to change?" Clinical tools such as the readiness ruler also can be used. The readiness ruler provides an easily understood basis for talking about the teen's interest in changing. The teen is asked, "On a scale from 1–10, how interested are you in _____?" Follow-up questions such as "what do you think would have to happen to increase that number?" can be used (Rollnick, Mason, & Butler, 1999).

The requirements and/or limitations of any further treatment should be understood and discussed with the teen when creating the behavior change plan. For example, adolescents entering a hospital treatment program likely will be required to abstain from alcohol or drug use, and this may be the expectation as well when they leave the program. In other settings, (e.g., college campuses) abstinence may not be a realistic expectation, and both the counselor and the adolescent may be more comfortable taking a moderation approach in that a reduction in level of drinking and related risk behavior may result in a reduction in harmful consequences. Although having predetermined behavioral expectations such as abstinence may limit the degree to which the MI is experienced as client centered and runs the risk of eliciting counterproductive or resistant responses from the adolescent, it is not an impossible situation. In fact, one of the early promising studies of MI was with adults who were entering a residential treatment program in which abstinence was a primary treatment goal (Brown & Miller, 1993).

The following vignette describes the process by which a counselor helps a 14-year-old ER patient in developing a behavior change plan for refraining from alcohol use. Krystal, an African American female, was found unconscious in a park and was brought to the ER by some concerned neighbors. She reported to the counselor at the ER that she had consumed several shots of tequila with friends in the park, passed out, and woke up to find herself in the ER.

COUNSELOR: So, we've talked about the things you like and don't like so much about drinking, we've covered the results of the assessment. What I'd like to do is talk to you a bit about what you think will happen if you continue to drink the same way.

KRYSTAL: I dunno. . . . I'm not supposed to drink at all, not just because it's against the law, either. I live in a group home, and I could get kicked out for this whole thing. Then I won't have a place to live, and they'll send me back into foster care.

COUNSELOR: So, right now you're worried about what will happen at the group home and whether you'll be allowed to continue to live there.

KRYSTAL: Yeah. (*Looks away, bites nails.*)

COUNSELOR: Clearly, then, if you keep drinking the way you did today, you won't be allowed to live in the group home. There's a good chance that you might have to leave. What else will happen?

KRYSTAL: (*Shrugs shoulders.*) I don't know.

COUNSELOR: May I tell you some of my own concerns as well?

KRYSTAL: If you want, I guess. I don't care.

COUNSELOR: Well, one concern is that your drinking levels are high compared with other females your age. We talked a bit about tolerance, dependence, and withdrawal, and all of those things could worsen if you continue to drink at the same levels. Another concern is what we call "emotional dependence" on alcohol. Your answers indicated that a lot of your drinking has to do with trying to feel better and forget about problems in your life. Generally, if a person keeps drinking for these reasons, it's not uncommon for them to have to drink even more over time to experience the same effects. Drinking at higher and higher levels is also related to experiencing more problems in life, so it can turn out to be a vicious cycle of drinking at higher levels, having more problems, and in turn drinking even more.

KRYSTAL: Hmm. . . .

COUNSELOR: What do you think would be the good things that would happen if you stopped drinking?

KRYSTAL: Um, well, I would be able to keep living in the group home.

COUNSELOR: Yes! That seems important to you. What else?

KRYSTAL: I wouldn't, like, get sick or have any more hangovers.

COUNSELOR: So, physically you'd feel better. What else?

KRYSTAL: My social worker might stop asking me her stupid questions about, like, "substance use."

COUNSELOR: You'd look forward to the end of those questions, because you could tell her that you're no longer drinking. That would be a relief, huh?

KRYSTAL: Big time.

COUNSELOR: What else?

KRYSTAL: That's it.

COUNSELOR: You know, just from our talk, I could imagine one or two more—would you like to hear them?

KRYSTAL: Yeah, sure.

COUNSELOR: One other good thing about stopping drinking is that your emotional dependence on alcohol might also decrease. In other words, by not drinking, you might find other means of feeling emotionally better—healthier ways that wouldn't get you in trouble and wouldn't cause more problems down the road. I can talk to you later about some of those ways to feel better without drinking, if you're interested.

KRYSTAL: Oh, you mean, like, exercising? My social worker wants me to do that.

COUNSELOR: That's definitely one way to feel better, and there are other ways, too. I'd be happy to go over those with you. Now, back to the good things about stopping drinking, from what you've told me it seems that you are not allowed to drink at all, so you feel that you have to stop drinking altogether.

KRYSTAL: I'm not allowed to use anything or drink while I live in the group home. I can't even smoke, it's so bad in there.

COUNSELOR: Let's see . . . what are some ways that you can successfully stop drinking? What would work for you?

KRYSTAL: I have to say that I hate to exercise! I don't want to do that.

COUNSELOR: Okay, so you feel that wouldn't work for you. Like I said, there are lots of strategies that people use. Would you be interested in going over some of the ones that others have tried that work?

KRYSTAL: Um, all right.

COUNSELOR: (*Shows list of strategies to patient, and emphasizes abstinence-based strategies.*) We can use this checklist as a jumping-off point. What do you think about some of these?

KRYSTAL: Uh, well, I think the one about talking to a friend about how I feel might be okay. I like to talk on the phone, so I can try that out.

COUNSELOR: Great! What else?

KRYSTAL: Maybe this one, about reminding myself of all the reasons why I don't want to drink and why I can't drink—like because I'll get kicked out of the group home if I do.

COUNSELOR: Okay, you seem to have a good sense of what you want to try. That sounds like a great plan. Now part of the reason you said you had been drinking today was because you were hanging out with friends who like to drink. What will it be like for you to hang out with these same friends if you're not drinking anymore?

KRYSTAL: It'll be hard, I guess. But I still want to hang out with them.

COUNSELOR: Hmm . . . let's see. What kinds of things can you do to keep yourself from drinking when you're with these friends?

KRYSTAL: I can ask them not to drink around me, but I don't think that they should have to stop what they're doing just because of me.

COUNSELOR: So, you're saying maybe that one might not work. What else could you do?

KRYSTAL: Um . . . I'm not sure.

COUNSELOR: May I suggest a few things?

KRYSTAL: Sure.

COUNSELOR: Sometimes people will ask their friends to do fun things that don't involve alcohol or to go places where alcohol isn't allowed. Other people will spend more time with friends who don't drink and spend less time with friends who do drink, because it's such a tempting situation for them. Which of those ideas might work for you?

KRYSTAL: I could do both of those things. That might work.

COUNSELOR: What might get in the way of you making these changes?

KRYSTAL: Well, if I'm around my friends who drink, and they give me a drink. I can never say no to that!

COUNSELOR: Because you think it might be hard to say "no," what could you do to make it less likely that your friends will offer you a drink?

KRYSTAL: I dunno. . . . Maybe ask them not to give me anything before I even get there, or maybe leave when I know that they're going to start to drink.

COUNSELOR: Those are great strategies!

The counselor should assist the teen in developing short- and long-term goals that are specific, reasonable, and attainable. This should include generating strategies for reducing drinking and risky behavior, determining which methods are acceptable to the teen, and exploring how these can be accomplished. If the adolescent is able to generate appropriate ways to reduce drinking and related behaviors, the counselor's main task is to help the teen specify which strategies to try and when and to imagine how they might work. However, teenagers will often be vague about what they would like to do differently, and counselors must help them develop a list of specific strategies. For example, a teenager might say, "I just won't drink as much." The counselor's task in this case would be to help the adolescent specify a reduction goal that would place the teen at lower risk. Open-ended exploration questions such as, "Tell me how you might do that" can be used. A more direct response would be, "We know that if you were to have no more than one drink an hour, your blood alcohol level would stay at a low level. What do you think about that for a goal?" Depending on the teen, other suggestions about moderate drinking approaches, refusal skills, and alternative coping strategies should be presented. (See Miller et al., Chapter 2, and Waldron, Brody, & Slesnick, Chapter 7, this volume.)

Developing a plan with teens who are clear about not being interested in making any changes to their drinking is more challenging. In most cases there will be some things the teen would like to avoid, like getting hurt after drinking or getting into dangerous circumstances. In these cases focusing on avoiding those harmful consequences rather than alcohol consumption per se can be effective. In other cases teens may be interested in keeping track of their drinking, such as self-monitoring drinks, or calculating how much money they spend on alcohol over a period of time. The purpose of these strategies is to increase the teen's awareness of his or her drinking and possibly raise his or her level of concern. Suggestions for working with adolescents with different degrees of interest and ideas about changing are presented in Table 5.4.

TABLE 5.4. How to Respond to Adolescents at Different Levels of Interest in Changing

Adolescent presentation	Counselor's task
Adolescent is interested in changing and has ideas about things to try	1. Help the adolescent be specific about ways to reduce drinking and risk-related behavior. 2. Identify things that might get in the way of changing: "What might make it hard to cut down your drinking when you are with your friends?" 3. Assess and enhance self-efficacy: "You have a lot of good ideas about what might work for you. What is it about you that makes you feel you will be successful?" 4. Write down the goals and strategies for accomplishing the goals. Include target dates for attempting the goals. Give a copy of the plan to the teenager.
Adolescent is interested in changing but has no ideas or only vague ideas about how to change	1. Ask the teen's permission to give some examples of what other people have tried. If he or she is agreeable, provide a list of goals that vary in intensity. 2. Identify which goals the adolescent would like to try, and discuss how he or she imagines they would turn out. Identify what might get in the way of success. 3. Assess and enhance self-efficacy. 4. Write down the goals and give a copy to the adolescent.
Adolescent is not interested in changing	1. Establish whether the teen is willing to see a list of things that other people who were not interested in changing have tried: "I get it that you don't want to change anything right now. I wonder if you would be interested in seeing some ways to learn more about alcohol in general and your drinking in particular?" 2. Identify goals, such as observing other people's behavior when they are drinking, counting their drinks, reading informational materials. 3. Write down the goals and give a copy to the adolescent.

Brian, an 18-year-old white college student, admitted himself to the ER after sustaining injuries from falling off a porch at a party. His blood alcohol level registered at 0.20, indicating heavy and recent alcohol consumption. During the assessment, Brian reported engaging in several high-risk behaviors while drinking, particularly unprotected sexual activity. (See Brown & Lourie, Chapter 8, this volume, for more detail on an MI approach with this high-risk behavior.) Although Brian was receptive to the intervention, he was reluctant to change his alcohol use altogether. Below is a description of the counselor guiding Brian in developing a harm reduction plan for behavior change.

COUNSELOR: So, we've covered a lot of material together. I'm wondering, where does this leave you?

BRIAN: I have no idea. Like I said, I'm not trying to be difficult, but I don't have an "alcohol problem." I drink just like everyone else at college does. I just had some bad luck tonight, that's all. In the wrong place at the wrong time, you know?

COUNSELOR: Okay, so it's clear that you feel that your drinking isn't the issue here but that being stuck in this situation and having to come to the ER was a stroke of bad luck. Nevertheless, I wonder if there are some things that you could do to prevent something similar from happening again to you, so that you can avoid this unpleasant experience altogether.

BRIAN: You know, the funny thing is that I really didn't have fun at the party. I don't know why I went, really. One of the guys we were with wanted to go there, the idiot. There was a ton of people there and it was way too crowded. That's how I fell off the porch and hurt my leg—someone knocked into me. Now I'll have a nice scar to remind me forever of this miserable night.

COUNSELOR: It sounds like you're saying that going to parties that are very crowded is not fun for you, and it seems like you're leaning toward avoiding those kinds of situations from now on.

BRIAN: Yeah, I think so.

COUNSELOR: You also mentioned that you were concerned about sleeping with people when you had been drinking and without using protection. From what you said, it sounded to me like you tend to do this when you've been drinking more than your usual amount, and typically this happens at parties like the one tonight. Is that right?

BRIAN: Yup.

COUNSELOR: In addition to avoiding crowded parties, what are some other ways to avoid these kinds of situations?

BRIAN: I only do this when I'm really bombed out of my mind. I probably should pay more attention to how much I'm drinking so that I don't go over the edge.

COUNSELOR: How would you be able to tell when you're starting to "reach the edge"?

BRIAN: Well, like, after about three or four beers I'll get a good buzz going, but then I keep drinking anyway, and after about seven beers I'm hammered.

COUNSELOR: So, it sounds like when you limit yourself to three beers, you have a good buzz and you're feeling more in control.

BRIAN: Yeah, pretty much.

COUNSELOR: I think paying closer attention to the amount that you drink sounds good. That will also help in terms of your judgment and remembering to use protection when you have sex with someone.

BRIAN: Oh, yeah, like I told you earlier, if I've been drinking, I don't think at all about condoms. So, I see what you're saying—I should drink less because it'll help me make better decisions about stuff like that.

COUNSELOR: That's one benefit. Also, sometimes when people drink, they do things that they normally wouldn't if they were sober, like sleep with people that they don't know well.

BRIAN: I see. Yeah, I admit, I do sleep with girls that normally I would never give the time of day to when I've been drinking. I'd like to stop that. In fact, one of my friends was telling me that some girl told him that she's pregnant and he's the father, and he, like, has no idea which party he met this girl at. Pretty scary. I'm in college, just trying to have a good time. I'm not into getting strange girls pregnant. That's not what I'm about.

COUNSELOR: Yes, that would be a big deal. So, you think that you probably need to make some changes, given your own experience and that of your friend. You're really thinking about this.

BRIAN: Yeah. I like drinking, but it's not worth getting hammered and having to deal with all this crap. I'm young, and I don't want to have to worry about getting someone pregnant, or getting a disease, or worse.

COUNSELOR: So, you're ready to take the steps necessary to change these things about your drinking and the things that have gone along with it, like having sex without condoms, so that you don't have to worry and can still have a good time with your friends.

One aid that can be used with teens at this point is a list of behavioral change strategies. Specific and clear strategies should be provided, such as,

"After having an alcoholic drink I will have a nonalcoholic drink," or "I won't 'chug' or 'shotgun' drinks." Such a list can be introduced as things that other people have successfully done and should include a variety of change strategies so that adolescents at any level of readiness could find something that they would be interested in trying. We believe that tailoring this kind of intervention (i.e., presenting goals and strategies that seem appropriate to the teen's level of drinking and readiness to change) is promising, but it may also be worthwhile to expose teens to strategies that could be considered more appropriate for more advanced stages. In this way, the teen is not exposed to a limited number of possibilities and may actually select some things to do that may not seem "stage matched" from the counselor's perspective. For example, a teen who had been showing no interest in changing (i.e., who was precontemplative) might select a more action-oriented strategy than might have been anticipated. Those who decide not to attempt behavior change are at least exposed to these ideas and may use them if they become more interested in changing once the session is over. Regardless of their level of interest in changing, teens should not have goals selected for them and should have a variety of options.

Goal setting is most successful when goals are personalized, concrete, behavioral, and simple but well elaborated and include a time line. In order to capitalize on any enhanced motivation as a result of the session, teens should be encouraged to specify a time within the next few days that they will attempt a goal. As with the feedback sheet, one copy of the list of goals and their target dates should be given to the teen, and one copy should be retained by the counselor as a reference for future sessions.

Anticipating Barriers

During the development of the behavior-change plan, the counselor should help the teen imagine how their strategies will work and what barriers might get in the way of being successful at the plan. For example, the counselor could ask how the teen imagines his or her friends would react to his or her deciding not to drive after drinking. Asking the teen to anticipate what might be difficult about implementing the plan will serve to help the teen and the counselor to identify ways to handle challenging situations, to develop further needed details of the plan, and to evaluate and enhance the teen's self-efficacy.

Providing Advice

Giving advice about limiting drinking (vs. recommending abstinence) may be controversial when working with minors. However, providing advice is warranted in some cases, including those in which adolescents are not able to generate ideas, in which they ask for advice, or in which they are not developing appropriate goals.

Abby, a 16-year-old white female, arrived by ambulance at the ER after sustaining a broken arm in a car accident in which she was a passenger. As it turned out, the driver of the car had a positive blood alcohol content, as did Abby. Here, the counselor reframes some misconceptions and misinformation that Abby has about the effects of alcohol and provides her with advice as to how to avoid similar situations in the future.

COUNSELOR: You seem really shaken and upset by this whole experience. How are you feeling about it?

ABBY: Oh, my God, I never want to go through this again. This was a terrible night. I'm just glad my friends are all okay.

COUNSELOR: What a relief that is.

ABBY: Yeah, thank God. Justin seemed okay at the time, you know, we had no idea that he was that drunk when we got in the car.

COUNSELOR: It's really not obvious, is it?

ABBY: No, it's not. At least, not with some guys. With girls, you can always tell if they've been drinking.

COUNSELOR: So, by looking at the way someone's acting, you can tell how much they've had to drink.

ABBY: Yeah, usually.

COUNSELOR: That's one way to judge, but sometimes it can be misleading. Some people get very affected right away, and others don't, or take longer to show effects, depending on how much alcohol they've had and how quickly they've consumed it. It can be tough to tell just how much a person's had to drink, even for a professional. That's why a blood alcohol test is used here in the hospital—it gives the fastest and most reliable information about how much alcohol a person has had.

ABBY: Oh. What was my blood alcohol test?

COUNSELOR: Your reading was .034 when you arrived at the ER. Are you familiar with what that means?

ABBY: Um, well, I think that if it's .10, that means you're drunk, right? I know that you can get a DWI [driving while intoxicated] if your test is higher than that.

COUNSELOR: Actually, you're referring to the legal limit, which for adults in this state is .10 and for anyone under age 21 is .02. So, if you were driving and you got pulled over and your test was .02 or higher, you could be charged with DWI.

ABBY: Oh, wow, I didn't know that. Why is it lower for kids?

COUNSELOR: Because this state has what's called a "zero tolerance law" for underage drinking. For most people, having one standard drink of alcohol raises their blood alcohol level to .02. So, basically, the message is that the police will arrest you if you're driving and if you've had anything at all to drink, even if it's one beer.

ABBY: But that seems ridiculous. One or two beers doesn't do anything to you. I mean, like, I know lots of people who drive after drinking that amount.

COUNSELOR: I can see why this seems confusing, especially if you don't feel the effects of alcohol after one or two beers—why should such a small amount of alcohol be grounds for getting a DWI?

ABBY: Uh huh.

COUNSELOR: Would you be interested in hearing more information about this?

ABBY: Um, okay.

COUNSELOR: Well, alcohol affects motor coordination, such as reaction time, hand–eye coordination, and the ability to pay attention to two or more things at once. This effect can happen at blood alcohol levels starting as low as .02, which is about equivalent to one drink. These effects tend to be more pronounced for younger, less experienced drivers.

ABBY: Oh.

COUNSELOR: Plus, it can be tough for someone to judge not only how much someone else has had to drink but also how intoxicated they themselves are. That's because of three factors. The first is that our judgment is impaired by alcohol. Second, our ability to estimate how intoxicated we are is less accurate when our blood alcohol levels are going down than when they are rising. For example, after you have a drink, your blood alcohol continues to rise for 20 to 30 minutes to its highest point and then begins to fall more gradually. When it begins to fall, people tend to think that they're less intoxicated than they actually are.

ABBY: So, like, you can judge better right away how buzzed you are, but it's harder after you've been drinking for a while.

COUNSELOR: Exactly! Finally, becoming tolerant to alcohol's effects makes us less able to judge how intoxicated we are. If you have a few drinks at a time on a regular basis, your body gets used to it in that you lose some of the ability to feel alcohol's effects. However, your ability to drive is still affected at the same number of drinks as before—you just can't feel it. You temporarily lose some of the "warning system" your body had before.

ABBY: I see. I didn't know that. So that's why my guy friends who drink a lot seem like they're not drunk, but maybe they are?

COUNSELOR: Yes. Would you be interested in hearing about some ways to avoid a situation like getting into a car with a driver who's been drinking or driving after drinking?

ABBY: Yeah, I guess.

COUNSELOR: Here's a list that we can go over together. Let's read off each of these and see which ones might work for you: sleep over, find someone who has not been drinking at all to drive you home, designate a driver beforehand who won't drink at all, call a taxi, take a bus, call a parent for a ride, call another adult for a ride, walk home, only go places where no alcohol is available, don't drink, and don't go out with people who drink.

ABBY: Uh, let me think. . . . I could sleep over, call a taxi, call my cousin for a ride, um, I don't think I want to call my parents, though, because they'll just, like, freak about it if they know I'm at a party where there's alcohol, and, um, maybe designate a driver beforehand.

COUNSELOR: Terrific! How do you think those strategies will work?

ABBY: Okay, I guess. I'd either just sleep over or call my cousin, probably. I don't like buses or taxis, and no way am I walking home late at night.

COUNSELOR: So, the strategies you've picked out should work well in helping you avoid a situation like this in the future.

ABBY: (Nods head.)

Enhancing Self-Efficacy

If the adolescent makes a plan to change, it is critical that he or she feels hopeful about and capable of implementing this plan. So, in addition to being willing to change, we also want the teen to feel confident that he or she can be successful. Therefore, one of the counselor's primary responsibilities is to enhance the teen's sense that he or she can effectively make changes. The counselor can do this by reinforcing promising but realistic ideas, by making supportive statements about the adolescent's strengths, and by being optimistic about his or her future once change is implemented. One of the more important things a counselor can do is to make statements about his or her own belief that the teen has the resources to be successful in carrying out the plan.

Planning Further Contact

Even minimal counselor contact outside of the treatment session has been shown to increase engagement in treatment and participation in ongoing treatment. Therefore, counselors should consider whether further contact is feasible. The purpose of such further sessions would be to reinforce the process of motivation toward behavior change begun in the initial session. The counselor draws upon information from the initial session, including the teen's interest in changing, the pros and cons of drinking, the assessment feedback, and concerns about changing. Progress toward goals should be discussed, problems and barriers identified, and strategies reviewed. Suggestions for responding to different teen presentations are presented in Table 5.5.

TABLE 5.5. Follow-Up Sessions: Three Possible Presentations
and Suggested Responses

1. *Adolescent didn't try anything.* If the adolescent had at the initial meeting set some concrete goals but reports that none were attempted, open-ended questions and reflective listening should be used extensively to understand the teen's situation before continuing. Explore what the interim time period has been like for the teen. Some possibilities are that the goals were not appropriate, that the teen's interest in changing has declined, or that some unanticipated events occurred that made it difficult for the teen to attempt change. As rapport is built in the second session, further information about the teen's pattern of drinking, other behavior, or life circumstances may be revealed. The aim of the session should be maintaining the relationship with the teen, minimizing resistance, and establishing an appropriate course from this point. When appropriate, motivational enhancement strategies (i.e., the discussion of pros and cons of changing and not changing) should be used to attempt to renew the adolescent's commitment to making a change.

2. *Adolescent attempted goals but was not successful.* If the adolescent reports having attempted some goals but had limited success, the strategies should be reviewed, as well as what difficulties the teen had in implementing them. It may be that he or she did not anticipate certain barriers and that the goals and strategies for addressing barriers to change should be discussed at length.

3. *Adolescent attempted change and experienced some success.* For teens who report having met some or all of the goals set at baseline, the counselor would first review this success, asking such questions as "What did you do?" "How did that work?" "How do you feel about making this change?" This is a critical time for the counselor to reinforce self-efficacy by making statements such as, "I'm impressed with how you were able to make this change." After getting a good sense of the teen's experience, the counselor can help him or her determine whether further goals should be set ("What do you think needs to happen next?"). It is also important to pursue discussion of how to prevent a return to the previous behavior pattern ("What would you do if you started drinking?").

OTHER CONSIDERATIONS

The preceding sections describe in some detail the basic elements of our brief MI approach with adolescents. To illustrate our approach, we have provided many examples from among the hundreds of adolescents with whom we have worked. In this section we discuss several additional considerations that have emerged that perhaps can be best described as process/procedural issues.

Counselor Training Recommendations

As is true for all types of therapy, there is no substitute for a well-trained treatment counselor. Because behavioral treatment approaches are sometimes misunderstood as being applied in a "cookbook fashion"—that is, in the absence of careful consideration of the training of the counselor and the unique needs of adolescents—it is of paramount importance that counselors are experienced in therapy skills, as well as in behavioral principles (Monti et al., 1989). Of equal importance, they must have good interpersonal skills that enable them to "connect" with adolescents. In short, they must be credible role models for teens.

A master's degree in a mental health discipline (e.g., child psychology, child development, clinical or counseling psychology) is considered "entry level" for our counselors. We occasionally employ individuals with bachelor's degrees, particularly if they have adolescent-related clinical experiences. One year of clinical experience is the usual minimum required for our counselor training program. Training itself consists of several elements, including: 2–4 months (approximately 75 hours) of one-on-one training, viewing videotaped clinical demonstrations such as those produced by Miller, Rollnick, and Moyers (1998), reading Miller and Rollnick (1991), listening to several hours of audiotaped MIs, in vivo sessions with actors as mock clients, and ongoing weekly supervision. In addition, we recommend that counselors-in-training read Barnett, Monti, and Wood (in press) and Dimeff and colleagues (1999).

Our counselor-training program seems to prepare our counselors adequately in that extensive assessment of our intervention's fidelity has proven its conceptual match to the tenets of MI. Ratings from our adolescents, counselors, and trained observers have provided us with converging evidence that our training has been successful in teaching counselors to consistently adhere to the stylistic and protocol-driven elements of the MI in the context of an empathic interaction with our teens. Interested readers are referred to Barnett, Monti, and Wood (in press) for an elaboration of our intervention fidelity evaluation procedures.

As is the case in other clinical work, use of appropriate self-disclosure and humor can be helpful clinical tools (Monti et al., 1989), especially in dealing effectively with adolescents. One self-disclosure issue that occasionally comes up is the question regarding the drinking and perhaps even the drinking and driving practices of the counselor. As a general guideline to our counselors, we emphasize that it is not so important whether the question gets answered as that the teen feels that he or she is being understood.

The issue of handling personal questions directed at the counselor during the MI can be a thorny one, particularly with questions having to do with the counselor's own experiences with alcohol use and other substances. Below is a vignette illustrating how a counselor fielded such inquiries from Mikal, an 18-year-old African American college male who was found intoxicated in his dormitory room and was brought to the ER by university emergency medical technicians.

MIKAL: So, you keep asking me all these questions about drinking. You must have gone to college to have your job—didn't you drink when you were in school?

COUNSELOR: It seems strange to you that I'd be asking you these questions about drinking, as if I didn't know firsthand what the experience of drinking was like.

MIKAL: Yeah.

COUNSELOR: I can see why you'd wonder that. The reason I ask those questions is because people can have different reactions to drinking and different reasons for liking it. I'm interested to hear about your perceptions and feelings and what you've personally experienced. Plus, I don't want to assume anything about your drinking—I'd rather hear what you think and how you feel about it. You're the expert on you. Sometimes, people ask that question because they're concerned that if the other person has never been drunk or hasn't ever had alcohol, they might not be able to understand or help.

MIKAL: Uh, well . . . yeah, I don't know how someone could be helpful if they've never had a hangover or whatever. I'm not trying to say that you're not good at what you do or anything.

COUNSELOR: But, maybe if I don't drink I won't be able to relate to what it's like being in college and having a few beers with buddies.

MIKAL: Where I go to school, being hungover is pretty normal. Everyone has a wicked hangover on Sunday, that's just a fact.

COUNSELOR: I can see your point. What I'm here to do is to help people to avoid situations where they drink too much, like what happened to you this evening, or drink in situations that are risky or dangerous that increase their chances of getting hurt. So, I help people to take a look at their drinking and make changes in their drinking that are effective, if they're interested. I'm not here to pass judgment on what's normal or not normal, but rather, what it is that you'd like to do about drinking. Again, that's your choice; it's completely up to you.

MIKAL: All right. Fair enough.

Population and Modality

As was mentioned earlier in this chapter, adolescents with whom we have worked range from 13 through 19 years of age and have been enrolled because they are in our ER after having been involved in an alcohol-related incident. Thus the population of teens with whom we have the most experience is fairly restricted and deserves comment. Perhaps the least restricted aspect of this population is the age range that it spans. Initially, we may have been somewhat naive in thinking that our approach would work "across the board" with teens of all ages. However, our clinical experience suggests that development matters and must be seriously considered in designing interventions (see Schulenberg, Maggs, Steinman, and Zucker, Chapter 1, this volume). Some issues that we have come to deal with on a routine basis include the different patterns of drinking and problems seen in younger adolescents versus young adults (i.e., younger adolescents may not have established a pattern of regular drinking), the necessity for parental involvement and perhaps even parental intervention with younger teens, issues of consent and confidentiality that emerge in dealing with parent–child dyads, and the fact that younger teens may require a more structured approach than older teens. Each of these issues requires careful and considerable clinical judgment.

Although it would be valuable to have empirical data on what works best across the teenage years, to date we must rely on a combination of what little there is in the research literature, clinical judgment, and a sensitivity to developmental psychology. However, as is discussed in the final section of this chapter, one of our studies can provide some guidance on this matter. One rather obvious issue is that feedback material must be presented in a format and modality that is sensitive to age and intellect. Our counselors do not assume reading competence. Rather, the entire protocol is implemented in the context of a discussion between the counselor and the teen. Although multimodal presentation is generally preferable, it is especially appropriate when dealing with youngsters. Computerized interventions are appealing to youth and becoming more popular. The chapter by Skinner, Maley, Smith, Chirrey, and Morrison (Chapter 10, this volume) outlines a particularly vivid presentation format in the context of using the

Internet for engaging teens in substance abuse prevention. Although we have not used this modality in our own work, its potential for a variety of settings is intriguing and worthy of further exploration.

Dealing with Other Drugs of Abuse

Although we do not directly address other drugs of abuse in our brief intervention, many of the teens involved in our alcohol projects also report smoking cigarettes and marijuana. We see no clinical reason why an approach similar to that outlined herein, with marijuana as its focus, would not work. Indeed, we have recently pointed out (Monti, 1999) that the effects of our brief alcohol intervention with older adolescents seem to generalize to marijuana use at a 12-month follow-up. Although this effect bears replication, it does suggest that a treatment focused on marijuana use would seem to be warranted. Additional indirect support for the notion of addressing other substances of abuse comes from a study recently conducted by our group in the use of a brief MI with adolescent smokers who were not selected on the basis of their motivation to quit (Colby et al., 1998). Results of this 30-minute intervention (which was similar in form and process to the one described in this chapter) showed encouraging results on quit attempts at a 3-month follow-up. Thus at least one other drug of abuse seems sensitive to a brief MI approach with teens.

EMPIRICAL SUPPORT, CONCLUSIONS, AND FUTURE DIRECTIONS

For several reasons, we have chosen to conceptualize our population of teens as comprising two distinct samples. Developmental differences within the 13- to 19-year-age range, differences in parental involvement necessitated by the "minor status" of those under 18 years of age, and differences in the ERs (adult hospital ER vs. pediatric hospital ER) in which each group was treated all contributed to this decision. When analyzing the effectiveness of our intervention, therefore, we evaluate effects on younger (13- to 17-year-old) teens and older (18- to 19-year-old) teens separately.

The results of the first outcome study produced from our ER intervention program have recently been presented in detail elsewhere (Monti, Colby, Barnett, Spirito, et al., 1999). This study, conducted on the older age group, showed promising effects of our MI on 94 teens who were randomly assigned to receive either MI or standard care, which consisted of assessment and informational handouts. Teens were interviewed 3 and 6 months following their ER visit. Follow-up rates averaged 91% across the two interviews with no differential follow-up rates between groups or by gender. Compared with those who completed follow-up, teens who did not were more likely to have been school dropouts and to have reported less severe drinking at baseline. Interestingly, regardless of group assignment, teens showed a reduction in overall drinking, with the greatest reduction occurring from baseline to the 3-month follow-up interview. It is plausible that the experience of having an alcohol-related ER visit can account for this reduction. However, it should also be noted that our control condition provided somewhat more than typical hospital care in that teens received assessments, handouts, and follow-up. Reactivity to assessment may account for the lack of group differences in alcohol use.

To test whether our MI resulted in reduction in harm associated with alcohol use, its effects on alcohol-related injuries, social problems, and drinking and driving were examined at 6-month follow-up. Results of our interviews showed that teens who received MI had a significantly lower incidence of each of these categories of behaviors. Furthermore, according to Department of Motor Vehicle records, teens who received MI were less likely to have a moving violation in the 6 months postintervention compared with those who received standard care.

The clinical significance of these effects is of particular interest. Indeed, 6 months after their ER visit, the MI group showed a 32% reduction in drinking and driving and had only half the occurrence of alcohol-related injuries of the standard-care group. Thus our brief MI had a meaningful effect on clinically significant sequelae of drinking behavior. Furthermore, harm reduction effects were maintained at 12 months following the alcohol-related event.

The utility of our MI for older teens appears to be its efficacy in producing harm-reduction effects rather than reduced alcohol use. These results are consistent both with those of Marlatt and colleagues (1998), who found smaller effects for use than for problems, and with those of Chick, Lloyd, and Crombie (1985), who found reduction in consumption across the board in primary care settings but harm-reduction effects only with a brief intervention. As we have noted elsewhere (Monti, Colby, Barnett, Rohsenow, et al., 1999), it may be that a more intense intervention—perhaps one that includes booster sessions at certain target points after the intervention—would result in differential reductions in alcohol use. Because the older teens showed the greatest reduction in use during the first 3 months following the ER visit, with little reduction thereafter, perhaps boosters toward the end of this period might prove useful. Such boosters could include discussion of the original event and relevant things that have happened in the teen's life since the event. These sessions might serve to prolong any changes that the adolescent might have implemented (Barnett, Monti, & Wood, in press) and would be consistent with clinical guidelines (U.S. Department of Health and Human Services [USDHHS], 1993) that recommend this type of contact. Enhancing our MI with booster sessions is an idea that we are pursuing in our ongoing work with older adolescents.

As in our trial with older adolescents, we found that among younger alcohol-positive patients, drinking decreased significantly in the 3 months following the alcohol-related incident that required treatment (Colby et al., 1999). Drinking reductions were again the same regardless of whether participants had received standard care or MI. However, there was an effect of MI on drinking and driving behavior. Teens who had received standard care in the ER were three times more likely to be drinking and driving at 3-month follow-up than teens who received MI.

It appears that younger adolescents who are resistant to changing their behavior may differentially benefit from MI. Among a subgroup of teens in the precontemplation stage, those who received MI reported significantly more cognitive and behavioral benefits at 3-month follow-up than teens who received standard care. Specifically, they expressed more motivation to moderate their drinking and reported less drunkenness and fewer instances of driving after drinking. Conversely, teens who were already motivated to decrease their drinking at baseline received no additive benefit from MI. Preliminary long-term follow-up results indicate that the reductions in drinking persist for 1 year after the initial incident. Also, the effect of MI on drinking and driving is still detected 1 year postintervention.

These results confirm that alcohol-related incidents that require medical treatment appear to enhance motivation for change among younger adolescent drinkers, as both groups substantially reduced their drinking after the incident regardless of which intervention they received. Importantly, MI seems to turn the event into a teachable moment for those adolescents who initially appear unmoved by the experience as well.

We have been encouraged by the results of our clinical trials to date. Motivational interviewing seems to have shown harm-reduction benefits for both older and younger adolescents, particularly those who are more resistant to changing their behavior. Treatment effects seem to be holding up to 1 year postintervention for both groups. Indeed, among the older adolescents, treatment effects seem to have generalized to their marijuana use as well.

Such generalization begs the question as to whether a treatment focused on marijuana use, on some other drug of abuse, on some other abusive behavior, or on some combination of these could benefit from an MI approach similar to that outlined herein. The results of our smoking study (Colby et al., 1998), reviewed previously, is suggestive in this regard. Although there is a dearth of data on other behaviors, other possible foci of interest are sexual risk behavior (see Brown & Lourie, Chapter 8, this volume) and other drugs of abuse. However, a cautionary note is in order here in that, although our MI is a promising approach for ER settings and perhaps other settings in which there is the potential for a teachable moment, older adolescents and young adults who are severe problem drinkers and/or drug abusers may not respond with so little intervention. Our series of studies does not directly address the issues of whether an MI would be effective or of how long treatment should be for a more seriously impaired adolescent population under other circumstances (see Myers et al., Chapter 9, and Waldron et al., Chapter 7, this volume, for information on treating more severely impaired adolescents).

One interesting possibility might be to use MI as a preparation for standard adolescent treatment programs, as this has been found with adults to facilitate compliance and treatment outcomes for alcohol and cocaine problems (Brown & Miller, 1993; Monti, Rohsenow, & O'Leary, 1997). Possible differences in readiness to change should be considered in any such front-end design, as teens in both our older and younger age groups changed in response to MI, even when they said they were not interested in changing. In contrast, teens in our younger standard-care group changed only if they had already planned to. Matching MI to teens who show no interest in change in a combined MI and additional-treatment design is certainly worth researching with more severely impaired adolescent populations.

In sum, our work to date suggests that the brief MI outlined in this chapter, when introduced at what is perhaps best described as a "teachable moment," is particularly effective in reducing harmful behaviors such as drinking and driving, alcohol-related injuries, alcohol-related problems, and traffic violations among older adolescents and drunkenness and driving after drinking among younger adolescents. Developmental differences and the broad range of adolescents we have treated are likely to account for the different patterns of results. Although we have found less impressive effects on actual drinking per se, we feel that timely booster sessions and increased focus on reducing alcohol consumption could potentially remedy this situation. The addition of booster sessions; more systematic study of developmental considerations and their interaction with MI treatment; possible matching, particularly with more severely impaired adolescents; and combining MI with other forms of compatible adolescent treatment are all possibilities for extending motivational enhancement effects with alcohol-involved adolescents.

REFERENCES

Babor, C. F., & Grant, M. (1992). *Project on identification and management of alcohol-related problems. Report on Phase II: A randomized clinical trial of brief interventions in primary health care.* Geneva, Switzerland: World Health Organization.

Babor, T. F., Longabaugh, R., Zweben, A., Fuller, R. K., Stout, R. L., Anton, R. F., & Randall, C. L. (1994). Issues in the definition and measurement of drinking outcomes in alcoholism treatment research. *Journal of Studies on Alcohol, 55*(Suppl. 12), 101–111.

Barnett, N. P., Monti, P. M., & Wood, M. D. (in press). Motivational interviewing for alcohol-involved adolescents in the emergency room. In E.F. Wagner & H. B. Waldron (Eds.), *Innovations in adolescent substance abuse intervention*. New York: Elsevier.

Barnett, N. P., Spirito, A., Colby, S. M., Vallee, J. A., Woolard, R., Lewander, W., & Monti, P. M (1998). Detection of alcohol use in adolescent patients in the Emergency Department. *Academic Emergency Medicine 5*(6), 607–612.

Bien, T. H., Miller, W. R., & Tonigan, J. S. (1993). Brief interventions for alcohol problems: A review. *Addiction, 88*, 315–336.

Botvin, G. J., Schinke, S. P., Epstein, J. A., Diaz, T., & Botvin, E. M. (1995). Effectiveness of culturally focused and generic skills training approaches to alcohol and drug abuse prevention among minority adolescents: Two-year follow-up results. *Psychology of Addictive Behaviors, 9*(3), 183–194.

Brown, J. M., & Miller, W. R. (1993). Impact of motivational interviewing on participation and outcome in residential alcoholism treatment. *Psychology of Addictive Behaviors, 7*(4), 211–218.

Chick, J., Lloyd, G., & Crombie, E. (1985). Counseling problem drinkers in medical wards: A controlled study. *British Medical Journal, 290*, 965–967.

Chung, T., Colby, S. M., Barnett, N. P., Rohsenow, D. J., Monti, P. M., & Spirito, A. (2000). Screening adolescents for problem drinking: Performance of brief screens against DSM-IV alcohol diagnoses. *Journal of Studies on Alcohol, 61*, 579–587.

Cohen, T. P., Cohen, J., Kasen, S., Velez, C. N., Hartmark, C., Johnson, J., Rojas, M., Brook, J., & Streuning, E. L. (1993). An epidemiological study of disorders in late childhood and adolescence: 1. Age- and gender-specific prevalence. *Journal of Child Psychology and Psychiatry, 34*, 851–867.

Colby, S. M., Monti, P. M., Barnett, N. P., Spirito, A., Myers, M., Rohsenow, D. J., Woolard, R. H., & Lewander, W. J. (1999, June). Effects of a brief motivational interview on alcohol use and consequences: Predictors of response to intervention among 13- to 17-year-olds. In R. Longabaugh & P. Monti (Chairs), *Brief motivational interventions in the emergency department for adolescents and adults*. Symposium conducted at the annual meeting of the Research Society on Alcoholism, Santa Barbara, CA.

Colby, S. M., Monti, P. M., Barnett, N. P., Rohsenow, D. J., Weissman, K., Spirito, A., Woolard, R. H., & Lewander, W. J. (1998). Brief motivational interviewing in a hospital setting for adolescent smoking: A preliminary study. *Journal of Consulting and Clinical Psychology, 66*, 574–578.

Cook, T. J., & Moore, M. J. (1993). Drinking and schooling. *Journal of Health Economics, 12*, 411–429.

Dimeff, L. A., Baer, J. S., Kivlahan, D. R., & Marlatt, G. A. (1999). *Brief Alcohol Screening and Intervention for College Students (BASICS): A harm reduction approach*. New York: Guilford Press.

Farrow, J. (1989). *Reducing adolescent drinking and driving*. Seattle: University of Washington.

Fleming, M. F., Barry, K. L., Manwell, L. B., Johnson, K., & London, R. (1997). Brief physician advice for problem alcohol drinkers: A randomized controlled trial in community-based primary care practices. *Journal of the American Medical Association, 277,* 1039–1045.

Glynn, C. J., Anderson, M., & Schwartz, L. (1991). Tobacco-use reduction among high-risk youth: Recommendations of a National Cancer Institute expert advisory panel. *Preventive Medicine, 20,* 279–291.

Gould, M. S., King, R., Greenwald, S., Fisher, T., Schwab-Stone, M., Kramer, R., Flisher, A. J., Goodman, S., Canino, G., & Shaffer, D. (1998). Psychopathology associated with suicidal ideation and attempts among children and adolescents. *Journal of the American Academy of Child and Adolescent Psychiatry, 37,* 915–923.

Harrell, A. V., & Wirtz, P. W. (1985). *The Adolescent Drinking Index Professional Manual.* Odessa, FL: Psychological Assessment Resources.

Hester, R. K., & Miller, W. R. (Eds.). (1995). *Handbook of alcoholism treatment approaches* (2nd ed.). Boston: Allyn & Bacon.

Hicks, B., Morris, J., Bass, S., Holcomb, G., & Neblett, W. (1990). Alcohol and the adolescent trauma population. *Journal of Pediatric Surgery, 25,* 944–949.

Institute of Medicine. (1990). *Broadening the base of treatment for alcohol problems.* Washington, DC: National Academy Press.

Jelalian, E., Spirito, A., Rasile, D., Vinnick, L., Rohrbeck, C., & Arrigan, M. (1997). Risk taking, reported injury, and perception of future injury among adolescents. *Journal of Pediatric Psychology, 22*(4), 513–531.

Johnston, L. D., O'Malley, P. M., & Bachman, J. G. (1999). *National survey results on drug use from the Monitoring the Future Study, 1975–1998.* Rockville, MD: National Institute on Drug Abuse.

Leccese, M., & Waldron, H. B. (1994). Assessing adolescent substance use: A critique of current measurement instruments. *Journal of Substance Abuse Treatment, 11,* 553–563.

Maio, R. F., Portnoy, J., Blow, F. C., & Hill, E. M. (1994). Injury type, injury severity, and repeat occurrence of alcohol-related trauma in adolescents. *Alcoholism: Clinical and Experimental Research, 18,* 261–264.

Marlatt, G. A., Baer, J. S., Kivlahan, D. R., Dimeff, L. A., Larimer, M. E., Quigley, L. A., Somers, J. M., & Williams, E. (1998). Screening and brief intervention for high-risk college student drinkers: Results from a two-year follow-up assessment. *Journal of Consulting and Clinical Psychology, 66*(4), 604–615.

Miller, W. R. (1995). Increasing motivation for change. In R. K. Hester & W. R. Miller (Eds.), *Handbook of alcoholism treatment approaches* (2nd ed., pp. 89–104). Boston: Allyn & Bacon.

Miller, W. R., & Rollnick, S. (1991). *Motivational interviewing: Preparing people to change addictive behavior.* New York: Guilford Press.

Miller, W. R., Rollnick, S. (Producers), & Moyers, T. B. (Director). (1998). *Motivational interviewing* [Videotape series]. (Available from Delilah Yao, Department of Psychology, University of New Mexico, Albuquerque, NM 87131)

Monti, P. M. (1997, July). Motivational interviewing with alcohol-positive teens in an emergency department. In E. Wagner (Chair), *Innovations in adolescent substance abuse intervention.* Symposium conducted at the annual meeting of the Research Society on Alcoholism, San Francisco.

Monti, P. M. (1999, June). Brief intervention for harm reduction with alcohol-positive older adolescents in a hospital emergency department. In R. Longabaugh & P. Monti (Chairs), *Brief motivational interventions in the emergency department for adolescents and adults.* Symposium conducted at the annual meeting of the Research Society on Alcoholism, Santa Barbara, CA.

Monti, P. M., Abrams, D. B., Kadden, R. M., & Cooney, N. L. (1989). *Treating alcohol dependence: A coping skills training guide.* New York: Guilford Press.

Monti, P. M., Colby, S. M., Barnett, N. P., Rohsenow, D. J., Spirito, A., Woolard, R., Myers, M., & Lewander, W. (1999, June). Brief intervention for harm reduction with alcohol-positive older adolescents in a hospital emergency room. In R. Longabaugh & P. M. Monti (Chairs), *Brief motivational interventions in the emergency department for adolescents and adults.* Symposium conducted at the annual meeting of the Research Society on Alcoholism, Santa Barbara, CA.

Monti, P. M., Colby, S. M., Barnett, N. P., Spirito, A., Rohsenow, D. J., Myers, M., Woolard, R., & Lewander, W. (1999). Brief intervention for harm reduction with alcohol-positive older adolescents in a hospital emergency department. *Journal of Consulting and Clinical Psychology, 67,* 989–994.

Monti, P. M., Rohsenow, D. J., & O'Leary, T. (1997). *Treating substance abusers with coping skills training and motivational interviewing.* Invited institute presented at the annual meeting of the Association for Advancement of Behavior Therapy, Miami, FL.

National Institute on Alcohol Abuse and Alcoholism. (1995). *Assessing alcohol problems: A guide for clinicians and researchers* (NIH Publication No. 95–3745). Bethesda, MD: U.S. Department of Health and Human Services.

Reinhertz, H. Z., Giaconia, R. M., Lefkowitz, E. S., Pakiz, B., & Frost, A. K. (1993). Prevalence of psychiatric disorders in a community population of older adolescents. *Journal of the American Academy of Child and Adolescent Psychiatry, 32,* 369–377.

Rollnick, S., Mason, P., & Butler, C. (1999). *Health behaviour change: A guide for practitioners.* Edinburgh, Scotland: Churchill Livingstone.

Shaw, D. S., Wagner, E. F., Arnett, J., & Aber, M. S. (1992). The factor structure of the Reckless Behavior Questionnaire. *Journal of Youth and Adolescence, 21,* 305–323.

U.S. Department of Health and Human Services. (1993). *Guidelines for treatment of alcohol and other drug-abusing adolescents* (Treatment Improvement Protocol Series Pub. No. 93–2010). Rockville, MD: Center for Substance Abuse Treatment.

Wilk, A. I., Jensen, N. M., & Havighurst, C. C. (1997). Meta-analysis of randomized control trials addressing brief interventions in heavy alcohol drinkers. *Journal of General Internal Medicine, 12,* 274–283.

World Health Organization. (1996). A cross-national trial of brief interventions with heavy drinkers. *American Journal of Public Health, 86,* 948–955.

6

Alcohol Skills Training for College Students

ELIZABETH T. MILLER, JASON R. KILMER,
ELEANOR L. KIM, KENNETH R. WEINGARDT,
and G. ALAN MARLATT

In a recent survey of more than 17,000 college students across the country, 90% of them reported consuming alcohol and 40% reported consuming five or more drinks in a row during the previous 2 weeks (Weschler, Davenport, Dowdall, Moeykens, & Castillo, 1994). However, although most college students consume alcohol, not all of those who drink experience the alcohol-related problems seen on college campuses (e.g., impaired academic performance, violent behavior, and unplanned or risky sexual behavior). Furthermore, not all college students who abuse alcohol during their college years go on to develop alcohol dependence in adulthood. In fact, research suggests that most go on to become moderate social drinkers (Johnston, O'Malley, & Bachman, 1995). Despite decades of prevention efforts and attempts to prohibit or regulate access to alcohol on campus, these rates have remained remarkably constant since the early 1950s (Strauss & Bacon, 1953). The Alcohol Skills Training Program (ASTP) is unlike most alcohol programs because it acknowledges that college students drink, and, rather than try to impose abstinence on college students, it acknowledges that any steps toward reduced risk are steps in the right direction. As a result, this innovative program engages students who would otherwise "just say no" to alcohol programs that emphasize complete abstinence.

The ASTP acknowledges that episodic heavy drinking in this population is generally normative and transitional and views the college years as a window of risk through which students pass. Most students pass safely through this period of risk without experiencing serious alcohol-related problems. The ASTP was designed to provide drinkers and nondrinkers with information regarding alcohol use and associated negative consequences and with the skills to reduce risky use and/or abstain from use altogether. Students who feel that abstinence is the best route for them are provided with techniques and strategies for achieving this goal. Students who acknowledge that they have experienced some negative consequences but do not want to stop drinking are provided with strategies for drinking to a lower blood alcohol level when they do drink, allowing for a reduction in risk and potential harm.

The ASTP is not intended to be used to treat those who meet criteria for alcohol dependence, nor for those students who are most at risk for continued alcohol problems associated with chronic heavy alcohol use. By including an initial assessment phase in the ASTP program, the clinician can quickly identify those students who are in need of more intensive clinical services and provide them with the appropriate referrals for treatment.

THE MOTIVATIONAL APPROACH: MEETING STUDENTS WHERE THEY ARE IN TERMS OF READINESS TO CHANGE

Information or Motivation?

Traditional alcohol programs offered in the college setting often respond to excessive alcohol use through education. The information-based programs assume that increased knowledge about alcohol and the negative consequences is sufficient to change behavior. However, research has long established that information alone does not necessarily change behavior (Engs, 1977). In fact, students can often speak quite intelligently about how long it takes to oxidize a drink and list the negative consequences of drinking without showing any evidence of the information changing their own behavior.

Unlike more traditional approaches, the ASTP uses information about alcohol as the foundation of a more comprehensive intervention. Problematic college student drinking is conceptualized as both a skills-based and motivational problem. The goal of the ASTP is to educate students about alcohol-related behavior while increasing the students' interest in critically examining their drinking patterns and eventually implementing the skills they learn. In doing so, students can learn to recognize high-risk situations and to minimize the potential negative consequences through preventive action, reduced consumption, or abstinence. This chapter provides the empirically validated techniques and some of the theory used by facilitators to move students in this direction. First, we introduce a conceptual framework for understanding and recognizing how college students differ in their readiness to change their behavior. We also provide the key elements of a practical stylistic tool called motivational interviewing, which was developed to assist professionals in moving individuals in a direction of increased motivation to change their problematic behaviors. This stylistic tool has been extended to our work with college students in a group format.

Sensitivity to Stages of Change

Applying the conceptual framework of the stages of change model (see Prochaska & DiClemente, 1986, for a review) has been a helpful tool in facilitating behavioral change among college students. According to this theory, an individual's behavioral change process involves progression through six stages. These six stages of change are as follows: precontemplation, contemplation, preparation, action, maintenance, and relapse (see Chapter 2). An important point to keep in mind is that students commonly cycle in and out of these stages, not necessarily going through them in a strict step-by-step manner. By asking a few key questions, the clinician can assess at what point each of the students is in the stages of change model. We suggest incorporating a brief version of the University of Rhode Island Change Assessment (URICA; DiClemente & Hughes, 1990) or the Stages of Change Readiness and Treatment Eagerness Survey (SOCRATES; Miller & Tonigan, 1994; Miller et al., 1990). With this information, you can begin to meet them where they are in the process of looking at the way drinking and drinking-related problems fit into their lives.

Facilitating Change with Motivational Interviewing Techniques

Motivational interviewing (Miller, 1983) is a nonjudgmental and non-confrontational style of interacting that allows for flexibility and acceptance of an individual's ambivalence about change. It is assumed that college students are in a natural state of ambivalence regarding their own alcohol use and must arrive at their own decisions regarding whether to change their drinking habits (see Marlatt et al., 1999, for a review). The primary strategy utilized in the ASTP involves developing discrepancies between how students perceive themselves and/or their alcohol use and more objective measures of use and consequences. One technique for successfully implementing this strategy is getting students to articulate the types of negative consequences they or their peers have experienced.

The five core principles of a motivational interviewing approach are summarized as follows:

1. *Express empathy.* Through the expression of empathy, you let the student know that you understand him or her or that you are working toward an understanding of his or her situation. Empathy can be expressed through acceptance, reflective listening, and understanding the student's potential ambivalence toward wanting to make changes. For example, understanding how alcohol fits into a student's life and being able to acknowledge this communicates that you can understand and acknowledge the ambivalence and difficulty a student may have in considering a change in behavior.

2. *Develop discrepancy.* Miller and Rollnick (1991) suggest that motivation for change occurs when people perceive a discrepancy between where they are and where they want to be. By raising students' awareness of the consequences of their alcohol consumption, as well as by highlighting the negative consequences that can be reduced by drinking in a more moderate way, a counselor can develop discrepancies between how students see themselves and what they may actually be experiencing. For example, when presenting information on the way alcohol can influence the sleep cycle, the program presenter can discuss consequences of this sleep cycle disruption. If an individual is given the opportunity to articulate the discrepancy him- or herself, the information will be integrated more readily.

3. *Avoid argumentation.* By engaging in an interactive, nonjudgmental exploration of drinking and its related consequences, the facilitator can meet students where they are in terms of readiness to change and provide a place where students can bring the concerns they may have about their drinking. For example, a counselor may brainstorm and subsequently explore the things that the group likes about drinking (e.g., taste, way of celebrating, etc.) and the things that they don't like (e.g., hangovers, dizziness, etc.). Acknowledging both sides of the coin provides an opening to discuss how students can move toward maximizing what they like and minimizing what they don't like about drinking.

4. *Roll with the resistance.* Acknowledging the students' reluctance and ambivalence as typical aspects of the process of change rather than responses that need to be broken down is important in promoting change. Although the responsibility for change is the students', the facilitator can take an active role in generating a menu of possible options (e.g., asking the group to brainstorm ideas) for why and how this change might and can happen. For example, you might ask a group to generate ways to refuse alcohol at an event where alcohol is being served.

5. *Support self-efficacy.* Providing skills-training information about ways to drink in a less dangerous or risky manner is the foundation for achieving change. A presenter can help students to see how they can be suc-

cessful in coping with a particular situation and to stick to their goals. This might involve examining the skills that the student already has, generating a toolbox of skills to use in certain situations, and practicing the skills in the program. Supporting self-efficacy also involves recognizing and commending changes that have already occurred. Finally, the presenter may choose to normalize some frustrations students may experience in order to minimize the likelihood that they will interpret a situation as reflecting their inability to change.

Motivational techniques are continuously woven into the framework of our program. After an initial assessment, the facilitator will have an idea of the individual drinking levels, as well as where the students are along the continuum of "readiness to change." The diversity of the group requires that the facilitator act as a guide who interacts with the group as a whole (while at the same time being mindful of each individual and where he or she is on the continuum). It requires the facilitator to use his or her own influence, as well as the influence of the group members, skillfully. In doing so, he or she creates a dynamic setting in which peers are answering and challenging the thoughts and behaviors of others. It is extremely important that the facilitator model a supportive, nonjudgmental, and nonconfrontational manner for students in the group.

Program Overview

The ASTP consists of 10 conceptually distinct, stand-alone components, which we have divided into two sessions. Although progression through the 10 components in a sequential fashion is recommended, the components are designed to allow for customization (e.g., unusual scheduling demands). In addition, there may be specific aspects, resources, and/or ideas relevant to each college's culture, organization, or environment that should be incorporated into the presentation.

COMPONENTS OF THE ASTP

Component 1: Orientation and Building Rapport

Goals

- Establish rapport.
- Assess drinking behavior of group members.
- Describe the ASTP philosophy.
- Offer abstinence as an option.
- Describe program structure.

- Discuss confidentiality.
- Engage students and build motivation to engage in the program.

Step by Step

BUILDING RAPPORT

Motivational interviewing is a tool that is important in setting the stage for establishing and maintaining rapport with the group throughout the program. However, the other basic building blocks are as follows:

1. *Conveying a message.* Clothing, setting, presentation style, and language convey a message to an audience. Students tend to dress very casually; therefore, a suit and tie may create increased distance between you and the students. Be creative in organizing a room to be more conducive to open discussion. Be natural and present; discuss material casually, yet professionally; use your own language; and, most important, be clear and concise when describing information or responding to a student's question.

2. *Approachability.* Acknowledging students as more than just warm bodies is important in establishing rapport from the beginning. Given the nature of the topic, you may be viewed as "just another alcohol/drug abuse prevention counselor." Thus it is critical to convey approachability from the beginning, through the utilization of motivational interviewing techniques.

3. *Discussion versus lecture.* A discussion rather than a lecture format is critical to successful engagement. As mentioned previously, it is most useful when the majority of the information and skills are delivered in response to the students' own experiences.

4. *The student social scene.* Being in tune with the student social scene is a good way to demonstrate genuine interest. What types of alcohol are students drinking, where does that drinking occur, what events are popular drinking occasions, and what are the popular drinking games? Being in the know can boost your credibility, as well as improve your ability to tailor the skills-training components of the program.

5. *Authenticity and boundaries.* College students can see through a facilitator's attempt to be something he or she is not in an effort to "get in" with them. Being approachable while maintaining boundaries communicates the importance and seriousness of the problems associated with hazardous alcohol use among students. Facilitation is a job, albeit a fun one.

6. *Creativity.* The ASTP has the flexibility to allow facilitators to be creative, energized, and dynamic about the presentation. For example, incorporating role playing into some of the skills-training components is an effective way for students to rehearse refusing drinks. Using different types

of visuals is also a good way to increase understanding of information. Bringing snacks may increase follow-up attendance.

GROUP ASSESSMENT

Significant differences in drinking levels (e.g., from abstainer to problem user) among group members are important to know at the outset. The abstainer may experience participation in a group of drinkers as uncomfortable because he or she is the only representative from a particular category of drinking. Asking students to imagine what other types of drinkers would say or think, rather than singling out the only representative of a particular group, may minimize the discomfort.

DESCRIPTION OF THE ASTP PHILOSOPHY—NOT A "JUST SAY NO," BUT NOT A "JUST SAY YES" APPROACH

The goal is to help students, particularly underage students, appreciate that this program will treat them as responsible adults with regard to their alcohol consumption. Although it is important to remind underage group members that it is against the law for them to drink, it is even more important for students to understand that you are not there to enforce the law and that you support each individual student's decision about his or her drinking. This is not, however, a "Just say yes" program. The purpose of this program is to help those students who do choose to drink make informed decisions about their drinking that may allow them to do so in a less dangerous or less risky way while being careful not to communicate that any drinking is safe.

One way to include nondrinkers in the group is by stating that the information and skills may be helpful for a friend or for future reference if they or anyone they know chooses to drink.

A NOTE ON ABSTINENCE

The ASTP philosophy essentially empowers students to make informed decisions about their own drinking. When introducing the program, it is important to emphasize that students who choose to abstain from alcohol are highly respected and supported in that decision. The ASTP philosophy is based on acceptance, both of those who choose to drink and those who choose not to.

DESCRIPTION OF THE STRUCTURE OF THE ASTP

Discuss times and places for the groups to meet (e.g., current location for 90 minutes today and 90 minutes next week). Outline program content:

Week 1
What your drinking looks like in comparison with college student norms.
The physiological and psychological effects of alcohol.
How to monitor your drinking.

Week 2
How to get more of what you want from drinking (and less of what you don't).

DISCUSSION OF CONFIDENTIALITY

"Everything said here stays within these four walls." Because this program is peer-based and because students are encouraged to discuss sensitive issues such as underage drinking, it is of utmost importance for students to understand that specific discussions will not be shared with anyone outside of the group. Explain that these rules are intended to help everyone feel that the group is a safe place to talk about their experiences without having to worry about who might find out about it. Offering this kind of environment is intended to promote a safer atmosphere so the students feel free to discuss things they might not otherwise discuss.

Key Points

- Philosophy and structure of the ASTP
- Everything is confidential

Component 2: Assessment of Use

Goals

- Identify discrepancies between students' present drinking behavior and their important personal goals.
- Discuss how students' reported levels of alcohol use compare to those of most college students.
- Identify drinkers who are dependent on alcohol so that you can offer additional referrals at end of session.

Step by Step

EXPLANATION OF A "STANDARD" DRINK

It may surprise you to hear from a student that he or she gets drunk on one beer—until you find that out the student is talking about a 40-ounce bottle rather than a 12-ounce glass. Conversely, it may shock you to learn that a student reports drinking six glasses of wine with dinner—until you discover that those "glasses" are champagne flutes that hold 2 ounces at a time.

In order to help students critically examine their drinking patterns, you first need to make sure that there is a common metric from which to measure. The "standard drink" is any beverage that contains ½ oz of ethyl alcohol. Although the alcohol content of beer can vary depending on the brand, the following beverages all contain roughly the same amount of alcohol:

- 12 oz beer
- 10 oz microbrew
- 8 oz ice beer or malt liquor
- 4 oz wine
- 2½ oz fortified wine
- 1¼ oz 80-proof alcohol
- 1 oz 100-proof alcohol

Drinking out of a container (a can or bottle) makes it easier to know how much alcohol is consumed. Often, however, students have to do a bit of estimation to convert the amount that they remember consuming into standard drinks. For example, a student who reports drinking three 16-ounce pints of beer at a party would actually have consumed four "standard" 12-ounce beers. It may be useful to ask students what types of drinks they usually have and to work together as a group to convert the amounts into standard drinks.

DISCUSSION OF COLLEGE STUDENT DRINKING NORMS

Ask all students to think of the occasion on which they each drank the most during the past month. If some did not drink during the month, they can think of in the past year. If they abstained for the past year, they can think of the amount they observed someone else drink. Give them some time to recall and record the information. Ask them to share the amounts if they feel comfortable. Then ask them to guess how the typical college student would have responded to that question. You can share with them that, according to a study conducted at the University of Washington, on average 90% of college students drink and that of those who drink, the average number of drinks per week is 10. Ask them what they think about those statistics.

Often students who guess toward the lower end of the spectrum will discuss their responses with students who guess in the upper range. If they do not, ask some questions to spark the conversation. Discuss how people's perceptions of what is "average" or "typical" drinking can be distorted:

1. Some students are surrounded by a group of friends who drink heavily, and thus heavy drinking may seem more "normal" to them than it really is.
2. Everyone has heard the tales of heavy partying, but rarely do people brag about the times that they only drank one or two drinks.

Key Points

- Not all students drink
- Definition and calculation of the "standard drink"
- College student drinking norms (if the statistics are available for your school, include them)

Component 3: Alcohol 101—Alcohol and the Body

Goals

- Describe basic information about the way alcohol is absorbed, processed, and eliminated.
- Define tolerance.
- Define potentiation.
- Define cross-tolerance.

Due to the amount of information that has to be presented in a short time, this component is designed to be mainly didactic (i.e., delivered in lecture format). Although many students have probably been exposed to this basic information during other prevention programs, it is important to go through it again. Asking questions of those students who demonstrate knowledge can keep them involved and keep other group members listening (e.g., "Does anyone know some of the factors that influence how fast the alcohol that you drink enters your bloodstream?"). Outlining the main points on a blackboard or easel as you go through them is recommended.

Step by Step

WHAT IS ALCOHOL?

Alcohol is a central nervous system depressant. The term "depressant" often gets misused. In short, alcohol depresses, or slows down, the central nervous system. As one's blood alcohol level goes up, the depressant effects get more pronounced. Because the brain is a part of the central nervous system, we see the deficits in cognitive processing and motor coordination increase as an individual gets more intoxicated.

Recall that a standard drink is any beverage that contains ½ oz of ethyl alcohol. Most often the amount of ethyl alcohol in a beverage is expressed by the "proof," which is two times the absolute percentage of ethyl alcohol. So 80-proof hard alcohol contains 40% ethyl alcohol. To get ½ oz of ethyl alcohol, one would need 1¼ oz of 80-proof liquor and 1 oz of 100-proof alcohol—the standard drink for 80-proof alcohol described previously.

HOW DOES ALCOHOL GET INTO YOUR SYSTEM?

When you swallow a drink, the alcohol first travels to the stomach. There, some of the alcohol (approximately 20%) begins going through the stomach wall and into your bloodstream through a process called *absorption*. The rest of the alcohol then travels to the small intestine, where it enters the bloodstream rapidly and completely, regardless of the food content in it. Therefore, once the alcohol reaches the intestine, the rate of absorption is fairly standard.

WHAT INFLUENCES THE RATE OF ABSORPTION?

How fast alcohol is absorbed from your stomach and intestine into your bloodstream will determine how quickly you will feel intoxicated. This rate of absorption is determined by a number of things that you may already know about:

1. *The higher the concentration of alcohol* in your beverage, *the faster it is absorbed* into your bloodstream. For example, shots of liquor are absorbed faster than a bottle of beer. Also, beverages with effervescence trigger the muscle between the stomach and the small intestine, called the pylorus sphincter, to open and thus will reach the small intestine quickly, resulting in faster intoxication.
2. *When you have eaten recently* and there is still food in your stomach, the movement of alcohol from the stomach to the small intestine will be delayed, and thus *absorption of alcohol will be slower* than if you are drinking on an empty stomach.
3. And of course, *the faster you drink, the faster the alcohol will get into your bloodstream*.

HOW DOES ALCOHOL LEAVE THE SYSTEM?

Approximately 90% of alcohol is broken down, or *metabolized*, in the body primarily by the liver and to a lesser extent in the stomach lining. When alcohol is metabolized, it is first changed into a toxic chemical called acetaldehyde but is quickly changed into a less toxic chemical called acetate. Eventually acetate is changed to carbon dioxide and water, which are returned to the bloodstream to be filtered out by the kidneys and eventually excreted as urine. The 10% of alcohol that is not oxidized in the liver gets out of the body through sweat, breath, or directly through urine.

THE RATE OF METABOLISM

TIP: Ask the group what people do to "sober up."

Compared with how quickly your body can absorb alcohol, the rate of metabolism is very slow; the liver can metabolize alcohol only at a rate of 0.016% of blood alcohol level per hour. The rate of metabolism can be thought of as the speed of "sobering up." When students view their personalized blood alcohol level charts, this number will make more sense. It is extremely important to emphasize 0.016 per hour as the take-home message! There are no significant differences in the rate of alcohol metabolism among individuals. Even more important, *this process cannot be speeded up.* Contrary to popular beliefs, neither several cups of strong coffee nor a cold shower nor exercise will sober up an intoxicated person. For example, if someone reaches a blood alcohol level of 0.080, it will take this person 5 hours to return to a blood alcohol level of 0.000. Because alcohol is primarily metabolized by the liver, excessive drinking damages the liver.

On a related note, some people think that making themselves vomit will get the alcohol out of their systems quickly. This is also a myth. Absorption happens so quickly (usually within 10 minutes) that by the time a person is vomiting, most of the alcohol consumed is already in the bloodstream. Vomiting, in fact, can be dangerous, particularly if enough alcohol has been ingested to disrupt motor behavior (e.g., choking on vomit can occur).

Key Points

- Once the alcohol is in the system it has to work its way through the system to get out—there are no shortcuts
- The myths about "sobering up"
- 0.016 per hour

Component 4: Blood Alcohol Level

Goals

- Define Blood Alcohol Level (BAL).
- Identify factors that influence BAL.
- Explain alcohol effects at various BALs.

- Highlight gender differences in BAL.
- Communicate how to maximize the positive effects of alcohol while minimizing the negative effects.
- Emphasize that reaction time is impaired from the moment alcohol gets into the bloodstream, regardless of tolerance and perceived effects.

Step by Step

DEFINITION OF BLOOD ALCOHOL LEVEL

TIP: Ask the group what BAL and BAC stand for.

- BAL = BAC (Blood Alcohol Content).
- BAL is defined as the ratio of alcohol to blood in the bloodstream and is determined by calculating the milligrams of alcohol in a person's body per 1000 milliliters of blood.
- BAL is usually calculated as a percentage. Thus an individual who achieves the legal limit of .008% BAL has a concentration of alcohol in the bloodstream equal to 0.8 parts alcohol for every 1,000 parts of blood.
- Identify the well-known legal limit for driving while intoxicated as 0.08% (0.10% in some states, 0.02% for minors).
- What it definitely is not: *the number of drinks a person consumes.*

IDENTIFICATION OF FACTORS THAT INFLUENCE BAL

TIP: Ask the group what affects BAL?

1. *Quantity.* The more alcohol you drink, the higher your blood alcohol level will be.

2. *Rate.* The faster you consume alcohol, the higher your blood alcohol level will be. Your liver is the principal means by which alcohol is removed from the bloodstream. It can break down no more than 0.016% BAC per hour; many people have heard this described as one drink per hour, which is not completely accurate but is a rough estimate for an average-sized man. If you drink more than this amount, you put alcohol into your body faster than it can be removed. Thus drinking four beers in 1 hour will result in a higher blood alcohol level than drinking one beer every hour for 4 hours. You cannot maintain a set rate without seeing an eventual rise in BAL.

3. *Weight.* The less you weigh, the higher your blood alcohol level will be. Your weight reflects the volume of fluid in your body. Because BAL represents the ratio of alcohol to overall fluid volume, a person who weighs 200 pounds and drinks one beer will have a lower concentration of alcohol in the bloodstream than a person who weighs 100 pounds and also drinks one beer.

4. *Time.* Over the course of a drinking occasion, the amount of alcohol you can consume per hour to maintain a constant BAL will decrease. Your BAL drops at a steady rate of 0.016% per hour, but your BAL may rise at a rate faster than your liver can metabolize. Thus some of the effects of each drink accumulate.

5. *Gender.* A woman will get more intoxicated than a man of the same weight who is drinking at the same rate. Why is this the case? Details are provided in an upcoming section.

Drinking coffee and engaging in physical activity do not affect BAL.

EXPLANATION OF ALCOHOL EFFECTS AT VARIOUS LEVELS OF BAL

- Remember that BAL is the percentage of alcohol in the blood. For example, someone with a BAL of 0.10% would have 1 part alcohol for every 1,000 parts of blood.
- These numbers won't really mean anything to students unless they know what effects they can expect to feel at each BAL.
- Present Figure 6.1 and discuss the effects at each level, being sure to point out the BAL limit for legal intoxication in your state or locality. Discuss the differences between MIP (minor in possession), Minor DUI (driving under the influence), and DUI (driving under the influence).
- Let students know if you will provide personalized BAL charts, generated specifically for each of them, in the next session (see Component 6).

0.02	A person will begin to feel relaxed. Even though the impairment is minimal, reaction time declines as BAL goes up.
0.04	Feeling of relaxation grows, buzz starts to develop.
0.06	Decrease in cognitive judgment, alcohol is affecting the brain's ability to process information.
0.08	Decrease in motor coordination. Nausea is possible at this level.
0.10	Clear deterioration of cognitive judgment and motor coordination.
0.15–0.25	Person is at risk for blacking out.
0.25–0.35	A person may lose consciousness. Death becomes possible.
0.40–0.45	Generally considered the lethal dose.
	REACTION TIME IS ALWAYS IMPAIRED

FIGURE 6.1. Effects chart.

GENDER DIFFERENCES IN BAL

TIP: Ask students to estimate the BALs attained by the "average" 160-pound male and "average" 120-pound female who have both consumed five drinks over 3 hours. This is a dramatic example, because the woman in this scenario attains a BAL twice that of the man.

The same quantity and frequency of alcohol use will result in different BALs for men and women of the same weight. There are a number of reasons for this.

- *Different fluid volume.* It is estimated that, whereas an average male body is composed of approximately 60% water, an average female body is only 50% water. Lower fluid volumes in women result in higher concentration levels of alcohol in the bloodstream.
- *Different enzyme levels.* Levels of gastric alcohol dehydrogenase, an enzyme that aids in the decomposition of alcohol, are significantly lower in women than in men.
- *Different hormone levels.* The hormone levels change during the luteal phase of a woman's menstrual cycle such that she will get more intoxicated and will stay intoxicated longer. This is true for woman taking oral contraceptives, as well.

Key Points

- Clarification of BAL
- Factors that influence BAL
- Reaction time is always impaired

Component 5: Biphasic Effects of Alcohol and Tolerance

Goals

- Debunk the cultural myth that "more alcohol is better."
- Describe the biphasic response to alcohol.
- Identify the point of diminishing returns as an optimal moderation goal.
- Discuss tolerance, how it can be problematic, and how it can be reduced.
- Explore the dangers of drug interaction effects, including potentiation and cross-tolerance.
- Define alcohol myopia.

Step by Step

THE CHANGING EFFECTS OF ALCOHOL OVER TIME

Get people thinking about their drinking practices and experiences. Does the "buzz" change over time? What negatives do they experience and when do they occur? Ask students whether they notice any changes in the effects of drinking over the course of the evening. How do they feel after the first drink? The second drink? The fifth drink?

THE BIPHASIC CURVE

As mentioned previously, alcohol is a depressant to the central nervous system. Although it is a depressant, its initial effects may be energizing—a "buzz" develops, and people start "feeling good." The body's experience of alcohol, even with these energizing effects, also includes a depressant component with every sip. This reflects alcohol's biphasic (two-phase) effect—the body experiences an energizing, perhaps "positive," component followed by the introduction of the depressant, "negative," effects of alcohol. Each time alcohol is introduced into the system, this biphasic effect, or "biphasic curve," occurs. Early into a drinking occasion, the positive experiences and sensations are maximized, and the negative sensations and consequences are minimized. A person may feel energized, relaxed, and pleasantly high. Yet the depressant and negative components are also occurring. The relaxation comes from the depression of the central nervous system. As alcohol goes through the bloodstream and into the brain, the brain's ability to process information decreases, so reaction time, for example, will diminish. Alcohol is a toxic substance to cells in the body, and the "blow" to the cells of the body from the presence of alcohol, albeit minimal at lower doses, is still occurring. At low BALs, the balance between positive and negative remains on the positive side. However, each successive drink adds less to the positive experiences and more to the negative experiences. Therefore, above a certain blood alcohol level, the body's experience of alcohol will begin to change. The positive sensations and feelings one gets will be less positive, and the negative sensations, consequences, and reactions will get more negative. At this point, any additional drinks will result in a continued shift in the body's experience of alcohol. The negative effects get more and more pronounced in the face of minimal positive sensations as one's BAL continues to go up. Get people thinking about this and their experiences. When they lose their "high" and try to get it back by drinking more, do they ever really recapture those initial feelings? Do they notice a point at which their bodies seem to be having a different experience? What if people want to make the choice to drink but want to minimize the negative feelings and consequences associated with their alcohol use? All are

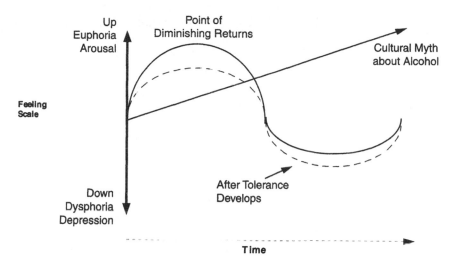

FIGURE 6.2. The biphasic response to alcohol.

good questions, and the answers lie in examining the point at which the effects of alcohol change.

The cultural myth about alcohol is that the more we drink, the better we'll feel. However, the biphasic effect demonstrates that this is not the case. Feeling good involves not feeling bad. Some people who report that they had a great time drinking may acknowledge that this drinking was accompanied by blacking out, vomiting, getting in a fight, or other problems. None of this information is designed to suggest that any drinking is safe or can be problem-free. Rather, there is a point at which one can minimize the negative consequences associated with drinking.

THE POINT OF DIMINISHING RETURNS

This is the point at which the positives have been maximized and the negatives have been minimized—one more drink will not do a person any more good (i.e., there will be diminishing returns from that point on). This change in the body's experience of alcohol occurs at or below a blood alcohol level of between 0.05% and 0.06%. What does this mean for college students and their drinking? Students who currently drink at or below this point of diminishing returns should stay at this point if they haven't had problems associated with drinking. They are clearly less impaired at 0.02, for example, than at 0.05 or 0.06. Most important, everyone has to find his or her own limit based on what he or she wants to get out of drinking. This information is provided for the many students whose drinking results in a

BAL in excess of this limit and who experience negative consequences. The only way not to experience any negative consequences is not to drink. For those aiming to reduce their negative consequences, this information can be helpful.

TOLERANCE

Many students view tolerance as a sort of status indicator, and many may see it as a positive thing. In fact, however, tolerance results in increased negative health risks. When someone develops tolerance, it means that over time he or she has to drink more alcohol to get the effects one would normally expect at a lower BAL. Or, consequently, the same amount of alcohol does not produce the effects it did in the past. Even the environment can affect this process. If a person's drinking occurs over and over in the same environment, stimuli in the environment become cues associated with drinking. In the presence of these cues, the body may experience an anticipatory compensatory response to the drug effects before the drug is actually present (Diaz, 1997), resulting in a need for greater consumption to get the same effects.

Tolerance is not the same as BAL. Two people of the same weight and gender who have been drinking at the same rate will reach the same blood alcohol levels, even if one has developed tolerance and the other hasn't. Despite the status that "holding one's liquor" may bring, tolerance is not an advantage. In fact, there are a number of disadvantages to having developed tolerance:

• When people with a low to average level of tolerance have too much alcohol, their bodies let them know (by getting dizzy or nauseous). In essence, they have a built-in warning system that prevents them from doing serious damage to their bodies. Because people who have developed tolerance don't experience these negative reactions, they drink without the cues that would alert many to stop.

• Tolerance can give people a false sense of security. People with tolerance may be unaware of how impaired they really are and may drink to a near-lethal or lethal limit without getting the cues that would normally prompt a person to stop. Additionally, even though tolerance may result in a person seeming less physically impaired, he or she will still experience the reaction time deficits any nontolerant person would experience. Thus the person with tolerance may feel "OK" to drive, but he or she is just as impaired as someone at the same BAL without tolerance.

• It's more expensive to drink five drinks to feel a buzz than it is to get a buzz from two drinks.

• Tolerance results in an increase in negative health risks, as the toxic effects of alcohol on the cellular level are as pronounced in tolerant as in nontolerant individuals.

TOLERANCE AND THE BIPHASIC EFFECT

Negative health risks increase as tolerance develops. A person with tolerance drinks to a higher blood alcohol level in search of the effects he or she previously experienced and, consequently, has alcohol in his or her system for a longer amount of time. The biphasic effect described previously is also influenced. As tolerance develops, the initial positive phase is less positive than it was prior to the development of tolerance, and the subsequent negative phase is more negative. With a more pronounced depressant or negative phase comes more negative health risks. Regardless of what the person feels, the body's experience of alcohol is a more negative one.

Tolerance and all the health risks that are associated with it can be gradually reduced either through moderating the quantity and frequency of drinking or taking a break from alcohol for a few weeks.

DRUG INTERACTION EFFECTS

There are two serious concerns related to mixing alcohol with other drugs:

• *Potentiation.* Potentiation refers to the interaction that results from the combination of two drugs that act in the same direction and is most easily summarized through the mathematical expression: $1 + 1 > 2$. For example, alcohol potentiates, or multiplies, the effects of central nervous system depressants (e.g., barbiturates) and can lead to an overdose when combined with them, even if the dose is typical of previous doses consumed.

• *Cross-tolerance.* This is the interaction that occurs when two drugs affect the central nervous system in opposite ways (e.g., a depressant and a stimulant). Consuming drugs in this way puts the central nervous system in a physiological "tug of war." This in and of itself can result in lethal consequences. A cross-tolerance interaction results because the alcohol works against the effects of the other drugs and increases tolerance for each of the drugs. For example, someone who drinks alcohol while using cocaine can ingest large amounts of each without feeling the full negative effects of either. Cross-tolerance can lead to a potentially lethal situation due to the lack of an operative warning system (e.g., alcohol, a depressant, and cocaine, a stimulant, when combined equalize the effects of each other). Further, even if a person controls the intake of each substance, the person cannot control the way in which each drug leaves the body. If one drug leaves the system more quickly than the other, a person may be left with a lethal dose of one of the drugs.

Myopia means nearsightedness. Alcohol myopia refers to the phenomenon that affects cognitive processing and that occurs as a person's BAL increases, resulting in a narrow focus on just the "here and now." The usual concerns, values, thoughts, or rules may be out of "focus" at high blood alcohol levels. For example, the person who knows not to drink and drive and espouses the virtues of calling a cab may only focus on the fact that he or she is cold, tired, and wants to go home when very impaired. The result is that people may make choices that, when sober, they would not normally make.

Key Points

- Biphasic response to every sip of alcohol
- Effects of tolerance in relation to BAL and alcohol use in general
- Interaction effects of alcohol and other drugs
- Definition of alcohol myopia

Component 6: Monitoring Drinking Behavior

Goals

- Provide a rationale for monitoring drinking behavior.
- Review the advantages and disadvantages of self-monitoring drinking.
- Explain how to monitor drinking behavior.
- Clarify that this exercise is not a mandate for students to drink.

Step by Step

RATIONALE FOR MONITORING DRINKING BEHAVIOR

After people engage in a particular behavior for weeks, months, or years, they may become less and less aware that they are doing it. For example, driving the same route on a regular basis becomes so familiar that making the left turn, stopping at the stop sign, keeping an eye out for pedestrians, and so forth occur without much thought. Similarly, the same thing can happen with drinking. Drinking under the same circumstances, with the same friends, in the same bars, and so forth may decrease awareness of how much or how quickly alcohol is being consumed. One way of becoming more aware of how much and how often drinking occurs is to monitor drinking behavior. Self-monitoring means paying close attention to your drinking as it happens and keeping track of it as you go.

For this exercise to be meaningful, it will be important for students to record their drinking behaviors on monitoring cards. This exercise will ensure that reading and understanding the personalized BAL charts in the next session will be personally relevant. *The key is that this is not an assignment to drink.* Rather, if students do make the choice to drink in between sessions, the monitoring of their drinking data will make the interpretation of the BAL chart more meaningful.

ADVANTAGES OF MONITORING DRINKING BEHAVIOR

TIP: Suggest that students get their friends to do it with them. Those who choose not to drink can monitor friends who do or can monitor another behavior (sugar intake, exercise, smoking, etc.).

The important considerations of this exercise:

- *Increased awareness.* Some potential advantages include becoming aware of how often drinking occurs, how much alcohol is consumed, which people are associated with drinking, which places are associated with drinking, which moods are associated with drinking
- *Possible behavior change.* Sometimes when people self-monitor their drinking behaviors, they become aware of patterns that they want to change.

DISADVANTAGES OF MONITORING DRINKING BEHAVIOR

- *Time consuming.* Recording behaviors takes time. One way of making the process more streamlined is to use prepared self-monitoring cards.
- *Awkward exercise.* Students sometimes say that they don't want to carry around the monitoring cards while they are drinking. Two suggestions include telling friends that it is a school assignment or experiment or mentally keeping track of the information until there is time to write it down in private.
- *Unwelcome information.* Some students find the reality of their alcohol patterns a little disconcerting. It will be reassuring to mention this reaction at the outset and encourage discussion. Reiterate that this is a good opportunity to get a closer look and a better understanding of how alcohol fits into their lives.

HOW TO SELF-MONITOR

Although it is fairly straightforward, it is safe to say that most students have not had experience with this process, so it is important to explain it as clearly as possible, being sure to use concrete, specific examples. Pass out the monitoring cards before describing the exercise. Instruct students that every time they drink or have the urge to drink, they should pick up the card and write the following:

- Date, time, and location
- With whom and what their mood was like
- Type of drink (beer, wine, margarita, rum and coke, etc.)
- How much alcohol was in each drink

CLARIFICATION OF THE GOALS OF THE ASSIGNMENT

Before completing this component, it is a good idea to review the purpose of the self-monitoring exercise with the group. Can they summarize the rationale? Remind students that this is not an assignment to drink. Rather, it is an opportunity to better understand what happens when they do drink or have the urge to drink. For those who abstain from alcohol, it is a chance to focus on other behaviors that they would like to understand better (e.g., eating, studying, watching TV).

Key Points

- Clarification of monitoring exercise
- Identification of potential obstacles and solutions
- Obtain students' weight and gender for the purpose of generating personalized BAL charts

Note. Generate personalized BAL charts for each student, to be handed out the following week. If you do not have access to the algorithm, you can log on to the Addictive Behaviors Research Center Website to create the charts: *http://abrc.psych.washington.edu/~abrc/*

Component 7: Feedback—Drinking

Goals

- Debrief self-monitoring exercise
- Distribute personalized BAL charts
- Relate self-monitoring data to peak BAL and the biphasic response

Overview

This first component of Session 2 is an opportunity to reestablish rapport, to review the concepts covered in the first session, and to relate those concepts to students' own drinking experiences during the previous week.

Step by Step

DISCUSSION OF THE SELF-MONITORING EXERCISE

- If there are any students who did not fill out the self-monitoring cards, give them a few minutes prior to the discussion to try to reconstruct their drinking over the previous week.
- What was filling out the cards like? Was it difficult? How did they explain it to their friends? Did they find out anything about their drinking patterns that they didn't know before?
- Have the list of pros and cons from the previous session (on the board or as a poster), as well as the biphasic curve. Ask students to recall the previous week—do they want to add any other pros or cons? Ask them to identify the episode when they drank the most on one day. For those who did not drink, ask them to recall a similar experience from the previous month. For those who abstain, ask them to consider a friend's recent experience.
- Did their drinking experiences match the description of the biphasic curve? At what point during the drinking episode did they reach the "point of diminishing returns"—how many standard drinks, how much time? Did they drink beyond that point? Why? What was going on for them? What were they thinking or feeling (situational effects)? Did they feel the effects of tolerance? Did they have a hangover the next day?

INTRODUCTION OF BAL CHART

Put the nuts-and-bolts version of the BAL effects chart (see Figure 6.1) on the board. This chart can act as a way to review the effects of alcohol and the relation to BAL.

- *The effects of each drink on BAL are cumulative.* Most people require more than 1 hour to metabolize one drink. The reason for this is that the liver can metabolize only a small amount of alcohol each hour, and it typically falls slowly behind. Likewise, the number of drinks per hour one needs to consume to maintain a constant BAL decreases with each hour.
- *BAL is specific to gender and weight.* Gender and body weight affect BAL. Therefore, it is important to use a chart appropriate for each individual's weight and gender.
- *BAL tables are estimates only.* Calculating BALs from charts result in estimates only. The personalized BAL charts are only an approxima-

tion—the exact level depends on everything in combination—sex, food intake, muscle-to-fat ratio, amount of alcohol, and so forth. Therefore, the charts should not be used to determine whether or not someone should drive, for example.

DISTRIBUTION AND DISCUSSION OF PERSONALIZED BAL CHARTS

- *Compare self-monitoring with assessment data.* Compare the drinking patterns from the assessment results with the self-monitoring cards. Were the previous estimates close to the actual amounts consumed? Was the previous week a "typical" week with regard to alcohol consumption?
- *Calculate peak BAL for previous week.* Students can calculate their peak alcohol consumption for the previous week by looking at their individualized BAL charts and their self-monitoring cards. What is the peak BAL? How were they feeling at the time?
- *Relate self-monitoring data to the biphasic effect.* Did students drink beyond the "point of diminishing returns" (BAL of 0.055)? What were their experiences? What do "buzz" and "drunk" mean to them? How does that point of being "buzzed" or "drunk" relate to the 0.055 recommended maximum limit? Does it seem like a reasonable goal to keep within that limit? If not, why not? Were students able to get what they wanted out of drinking while minimizing the negative effects? What can those who choose to drink do to make drinking a pleasurable, yet safe, experience? What are risky situations for each student? Suggest to students that they think about how to handle these situations before they occur—prior preparation. Ask students to recompute the same number of drinks over a longer period of time, or fewer drinks during the same period of time, to see if "moderate drinking" goals seem attainable for them. Remind students of the impact of tolerance on their experience of pleasurable effects and of the need to reduce tolerance to really maximize pleasurable effects of moderate drinking.

Key Points
- Personalized BAL charts

Component 8: Feedback—Expectancies
Goals

- Discuss beliefs students hold about the effects of alcohol.
- Challenge the perception that alcohol is directly responsible for these effects.

- Introduce the role of psychological expectations (set).
- Explore how the environment plays a role in the expectations of alcohol use (setting).

Step by Step

EXPECTATIONS FROM ALCOHOL

In component 5, students were asked to generate a list of positive and negative effects of drinking. Put this list up once again and ask students if they can think of anything else to add to it. The goal in this component is to rule out alcohol as the cause of positive social effects. If students think alcohol is the cause of these effects, they are less willing to explore reduced consumption; therefore, this is an important message to convey.

- *Enjoyable aspects of drinking.* What kinds of positive things do they associate with drinking? How do their feelings about themselves change when they drink?
- *Negative aspects of drinking.* What are some less desirable things that can happen when they are drinking? Have they said or done things when drinking that they would not have under different circumstances?

DISCUSSION OF THE PERCEPTIONS OF ALCOHOL'S EFFECTS ON MEN VERSUS WOMEN

- Do men and women respond to alcohol differently?
- Stereotypically, what are men like when they drink?
- Stereotypically, what are women like when they drink?
- However, doesn't alcohol affect people the same way?
- What could explain the differences (social expectations, etc.)?

INFLUENCES OF SET AND SETTING

- Can alcohol have different effects depending on the environment?
- Are the effects of alcohol the same in different environments or with different people?
- Do they feel the same after a couple of beers at a party as they might when having a couple of glasses of wine at dinner with a small group of close friends?
- Do they feel any different if they are drinking at a football game, compared with watching it on TV?

TIP: It is really more about what's in your head than what's in your cup.

THE BALANCED PLACEBO DESIGN

- This experiment helps to separate the chemical effects of alcohol from the psychological effects of drinking.
- A *placebo* is a substance having no medication that is administered for its psychological effect (like a sugar pill in a clinical trial).
- The balanced placebo design involves two conditions in which participants (college-age students) received a beverage that was not what it seemed. Some expected to receive alcohol, and others expected nonalcoholic drinks.
- There are four conditions in the balanced placebo design. These four conditions correspond to the numbers in Figure 6.3.
  1. Participants expected to drink alcohol and actually received alcohol.
  2. Participants expected to drink tonic water but actually received alcohol. (Drinks contained enough alcohol to get the participant to a BAL of 0.05–0.07. Lime juice was used to cover the taste of the vodka.)
  3. Participants expected alcohol and received tonic water (with alcohol only on the rim of the glass).
  4. Participants expected tonic water and received tonic water.

- *Predicted responses?* How do the students think participants responded in Conditions 2 and 4 (in which they received something different from what they were expecting)?
- *Actual responses*
  In Condition 1, in which participants expected to receive alcohol and did receive alcohol, they acted pretty much the way we would think they might act. The students became more talkative, louder, and more flirtatious with each other.
  In Condition 4, in which students expected to receive tonic water and did receive tonic water, they also acted much as we would expect them to. This group primarily kept to themselves, were fairly quiet, and did not exhibit much socialization.

| | | Subject Expects | |
		Alcohol	Tonic
Subject Receives	Alcohol	1	2
	Tonic	3	4

FIGURE 6.3. The balanced placebo design.

Condition 3 is our first introduction to the powerful impact of expectancies. Students who thought they were being served alcohol, *even though they weren't,* began showing many of alcohol's social effects—they became louder, more verbal, and more flirtatious.

In Condition 2, students who thought they were drinking only tonic water but received alcohol did not exhibit the social effects one may expect from alcohol. The effects of alcohol were beginning to kick in (i.e., they reported feelings of fatigue, flushing, lack of coordination), but students made attributions about what they were experiencing to things other than alcohol (e.g., being tired, being clumsy, etc.).

THE EXPECTANCY EFFECT IS MORE POWERFUL THAN THE CHEMICAL OR PHYSIOLOGICAL EFFECTS OF ALCOHOL

- The social effects of drinking depend less on the actual alcohol content of the drink than on the prior perceptions and expectations that we bring to a drinking situation and on the situation itself.
- Reaction time, cognitive judgment, and motor control all decrease due to alcohol use because they are actual physiological effects.

Key Points

- Positive and negative expectancies from alcohol
- Set and setting
- What's in your cup versus what's in your head

Component 9: Risk Reduction Tips

Goals

- Outline safe drinking guidelines.
- Provide specific strategies students can use to reduce their risk from drinking.

Step by Step

MODERATE DRINKING GUIDELINES

- Hopefully, by this point in the program, students have become motivated not to drink to excess. They have learned how to estimate their BAL and to monitor their drinking behavior.

- Various health authorities have determined that for those who drink, there is a drinking guideline: 0.05–0.06.
- Those who choose to drink and who exceed a BAL of 0.06 should consider setting a limit of 0.05–0.06 in order to maximize the positive effects of alcohol and minimize the negative effects.

MODERATE DRINKING STRATEGIES

Ask group members to discuss ways in which they can keep the amount that they choose to drink within safe drinking guidelines. This discussion might include ideas about how to limit the number of drinks that they consume during a drinking episode, as well as about nondrinking social activities that they might enjoy during those days of the week when they choose not to drink.

TIPS FOR REDUCING THE RISK OF NEGATIVE CONSEQUENCES ASSOCIATED WITH HEAVY ALCOHOL USE

It is hard to know who will be participating in your group; however, there will undoubtedly be some who are interested in learning how to reduce their risk, and they need specific directions for doing this safely and effectively. Brainstorm ideas for reducing risky drinking practices by asking students what they would suggest to a friend who asked for advice on this topic. The following are some practical and realistic tips to include in your discussion. By experimenting with these, a person can figure out which ones work for him or her and which ones do not.

- *Set your drinking limit before a social drinking occasion.* It is more difficult to set a limit when under the influence of alcohol or social pressures. Also, it is easier to forget why there is a limit when under the influence.
- *Keep track of how much you drink.* Keeping bottle caps in a pocket is a creative way to keep count—and taking count throughout the night is important so as not to go over the limit.
- *Space your drinks.* Spacing drinks over longer periods of time allows for more control over the situation and BAL. A time limit can be set per drink or per drinking episode.
- *Alternate alcoholic drinks with nonalcoholic beverages.* This is a great way to keep a steady and comfortable BAL and to decrease the chances of having a hangover the next day.
- *Drink for quality, not quantity.* Replacing the cheaper and less tasty beers and wines with some that are more appealing to the palate is a good way to decrease the amount of alcohol consumed.
- *Avoid drinking games.* Drinking games are a sure way to lose track of how much alcohol is consumed and to increase the risk of a BAL that

rises too quickly without warning. This can lead to nausea and vomiting, blacking out, and so forth.

- *Learn drink refusal skills*. This can be harder than it sounds. For example, some people don't accept "no thanks" and will continue to pressure you to drink. Also, some people will not feel comfortable just saying "no thanks." So there are some other ways to say no: "I have a commitment early tomorrow morning," "I am on medication that requires I do not drink," "I am coming down with a cold," "I just finished one, maybe in a little while," "I haven't decided yet," and so forth; or accept the drink and just put it down somewhere without actually drinking it.
- *Find other things to do*. There are always lots of activities to get involved with around the community individually or with a group of friends. Examples include a late-night game of baseball, flag football, or kick the can or going out for pizza, a movie, or a play. Engaging in hobbies such as writing, gardening, collecting, exploring, or hiking are additional alternatives.
- If you choose to drink, drink slowly and in a safe environment.

TIPS FOR REDUCING RISKS OF NEGATIVE CONSEQUENCES ASSOCIATED WITH ALCOHOL AND SEX

TIP: Keep this gender nonspecific—don't alienate or insult anyone.

- Unwanted or unprotected sex often occurs under the influence of alcohol. More than 75% of acquaintance rapes involve alcohol.
- On initial dates or in larger parties, being selective about when and how much you drink is important.
- Alcohol doesn't improve sexual performance or enjoyment.
- Watch out for friends—a friend who has been drinking may have impaired judgment and may need help to avoid making poor decisions about sex.

TIPS FOR REDUCING RISKS OF NEGATIVE CONSEQUENCES ASSOCIATED WITH DRINKING AND DRIVING

- Arrange for all transportation needs well in advance of a party or drinking occasion.
- Select a reliable designated driver who agrees to stay sober throughout the party.
- Leave the car keys at home or in the possession of the designated driver.
- Bring enough cash, just in case a cab is needed in order to get home.
- A student under age 21 can be cited for driving under the influence (DUI) or minor in possession (MIP), even if his or her BAL is below the legal limit. In fact, even those over 21 can be cited for DUI with a BAL as low as 0.07 if the officer believes his or her driving appears at all impaired.

Key Points

- Alcohol clearly changes the situation
- Tips for reducing negative consequences associated with alcohol use, alcohol and sex, and alcohol and driving

Component 10: Goals and Wrapping It Up

Goals

- Summarize program goals and answer any remaining questions that students may have.
- Provide students with a forum to ask other questions that they have about alcohol and/or other substance use.
- Ask students to think about the future and how they would know if their drinking was at a point at which they might want to make changes.
- Ensure that students know how and who to contact if they desire more information, evaluation, or assistance.
- Solicit feedback from students about the program.
- Discuss referral options.

Step by Step

SUMMARY

Remind students about the main goals of the ASTP. One of the most important messages is that alcohol consumption is a complicated issue with positive and negative consequences. The choice of whether to drink or not to drink is really up to them and only them. Thus the approach cannot be simplified to a "just say no" method, but each student must evaluate the risks and benefits associated with drinking; that is, a harm reduction approach. On the one hand, alcohol is often viewed as a means of socialization and an integral part of college partying. On the other hand, the students have learned about the biphasic effects of alcohol and subsequent ways to ensure a positive and less risky experience by drinking moderately. The specific tips from Component 9 addressed the issue of impaired judgment and what students can do to avoid drinking and driving, unplanned sex, and alcohol overdose.

QUESTIONS AND ANSWERS

Solicit any questions that group members may have. If there are questions that you are unable to answer, ask group members to write down their names and e-mail or postal addresses so that you can send them a response to their questions later.

DISCUSSION OF THE FUTURE

Few students will identify themselves as having a "problem" with alcohol or needing help to change behavior in the group setting. Further, for many students who may be "contemplative" about alcohol, it can be helpful to engage in a brief discussion about what signs might lead them to feel concern in the future. Typically, students reply that if they were drinking alone or drinking to medicate depression, that would mean it is a problem. This response allows for further questions about the more subtle signs that might be observed. It is important to emphasize that there is no reason for alcohol to interfere with functioning at all. Issues of grades, accidents, and embarrassment can be raised again as signs that risk reduction would be appropriate.

SOLICIT FEEDBACK ABOUT THE PROGRAM

Ask students how they liked the program. What parts about it did they like? What parts didn't they like?

DISCUSS REFERRAL OPTIONS AND HAND OUT REVIEW/REFERRAL SHEET

It is important when concluding the program to provide information so that those who are interested in more support know how and who to contact when and if they want additional information or help. Some students may have identified themselves or friends or family members who might benefit from additional assistance. Provide referral information.

ELICIT QUESTIONS AND ANSWERS

Key Points

- Feedback
- Evaluation of program
- Referral forms, if appropriate

SUMMARY

The ASTP has demonstrated effectiveness in reducing drinking quantity, frequency, and associated consequences when delivered in an eight-session group, a six-session group, and a 1-hour individual-feedback session. In response to the changing climate of increased attention on college student drinking, the current two-session, peer-facilitated, group-delivered ASTP intervention was designed to provide an efficacious, cost-effective, universal prevention alternative.

This condensed version of the ASTP was evaluated within a larger effectiveness study comparing the ASTP to a CD-ROM-based brief intervention and to two assessment-only control groups: a 6-month follow-up single-assessment-only control group and a multiple three-assessment-only control group (Miller, 2000). Upper-class undergraduate peers facilitated the groups of 4 to 14 students (college freshmen). The interventions were conducted early in the first quarter of the freshman year in order to address the increase in drinking rates that occurs upon entrance to the college environment. The content of the two 90-minute sessions was didactic in outline, with intervening discussion to illuminate ideas, information, and the development of new skills. Facilitators were instructed to present information and to challenge students' beliefs regarding the effects of alcohol during group discussions in an open manner, employing nondirective questioning and reflective listening techniques to allow the students to evaluate their own risks and to contemplate change. The peer facilitators were trained to present program content using reflective listening skills in a nonconfrontational, nonjudgmental manner to facilitate group discussion and the development of discrepancies (i.e., motivational interviewing; Miller & Rollnick, 1991). All students completed Web-based assessments.[1]

Preliminary results indicate that both interventions (ASTP and CD-ROM) and the multiple-assessment-only control group were successful at preventing significant increases in alcohol use and associated consequences as compared with the single-assessment-only control group. However, the advantages of the ASTP in comparison with the other conditions include higher satisfaction ratings from students and increased motivation to reduce alcohol use in the future. When universities are faced with the challenge of selecting the most effective prevention approach, we recommend that the audience (e.g., "light" to "moderate" drinking freshmen vs. "heavy" problem drinking males) and the ultimate goals (e.g., reduction of use and associated consequences vs. abstinence) be clearly identified prior to program implementation. These results suggest that utilization of brief peer-led interventions may be one possible means of allowing universities to balance the need to implement an effective intervention with the need for a cost-effective framework. Additional research regarding the effectiveness of the ASTP intervention among more diverse drinking and age-related populations and of form of delivery (e.g., peer facilitation, number of sessions, incorporation of technology) is recommended.

---

[1]DatStat.com provides research consulting and Web-based data collection, management, and analysis services; *http://www. datstat.com.*

ACKNOWLEDGMENTS

Special thanks to Mary Larimer, John Baer, Leah Era, Jane Metrik, Jill Carlsen, and Rebekka Palmer, and Britt Anderson for editorial contributions. Preparation of this chapter was supported by a grant from the National Institute on Alcohol Abuse and Alcoholism (No. 5R3A AA05591) awarded to G. Alan Marlatt.

REFERENCES

Diaz, J. (1997). *How drugs influence behavior: A neurobehavioral approach.* Upper Saddle River, NJ: Prentice-Hall.

DiClemente, C. C., & Hughes, S. O. (1990). Stages of change profiles in outpatient alcoholism treatment. *Journal of Substance Abuse, 2,* 217–235.

Engs, R. C. (1977). Drinking patterns and drinking problems of college students. *Journal of Studies on Alcohol, 38*(11), 2144–2156.

Johnston, L. D., O'Malley, P. M., & Bachman, J. G. (1995). *National Survey Results on Drug Use from the Monitoring the Future Study, 1975–1994.* Rockville, MD: National Institute on Drug Abuse.

Marlatt, G. A., Baer, J. S., Kivlahan, D. R., Dimeff, L. A., Larimer, M. E., Quigley, L. A., Somers, J. M., & Williams, E. (1999). Screening and brief intervention for high-risk college student drinkers: Results from a two-year follow-up assessment. *Journal of Consulting and Clinical Psychology, 66*(4), 604–615.

Miller, E. T. (2000). Preventing alcohol abuse and alcohol-related negative consequences among college students: Using emerging computer technology to deliver and evaluate the effectiveness of brief intervention efforts. *Dissertation Abstracts International, 61*(8).

Miller, W. R. (1983, April). Motivational interviewing with problem drinkers. *Behavioural Psychotherapy, 11*(2), 147–172.

Miller, W. R., & Rollnick, S. (1991). *Motivational interviewing: Preparing people to change addictive behavior.* New York: Guilford Press.

Miller, W. R., & Tonigan, J. S. (1994). *Assessing drinkers' motivation for change: The Stages of Change Readiness and Treatment Eagerness Scales (SOCRATES).* Unpublished manuscript, Center on Alcoholism, Substance Abuse, and Addictions, University of New Mexico, Albuquerque.

Miller, W. R., Tonigan, J. S., Montgomery, H. A., Abbott, P. J., Myers, R. J., Hester, R. K., & Delaney, H. D. (1990, November). *Assessment of client motivation for change: Preliminary validation of the SOCRATES instrument.* Paper presented at the annual meeting of the Association for the Advancement of Behavior Therapy, San Francisco.

Prochaska, J. O., & DiClemente, C. C. (1986). Toward a comprehensive model of change. In W. R. Miller & N. Heather (Eds.), *Treating addictive behaviors: Processes of change* (pp. 3–27). New York: Plenum Press.

Strauss, R., & Bacon, S. D. (1953). *Drinking in college.* New Haven, CT: Yale University Press.

Wechsler, H., Davenport, A., Dowdall, G., Moeykens, B., & Castillo, S. (1994). Health and behavioral consequences of binge drinking in college. *Journal of American Medical Association, 272*(21), 1672–1677.

7

Integrative Behavioral and Family Therapy for Adolescent Substance Abuse

HOLLY BARRETT WALDRON, JANET L. BRODY,
and NATASHA SLESNICK

The integrative behavioral and family therapy (IBFT) model is a multi-systemic intervention model combining two common treatment approaches for adolescent substance abuse: family systems therapy and individual cognitive–behavioral therapy. The model is designed to be effective for adolescents presenting for treatment within the broad spectrum of substance abuse and dependence diagnoses and related problem behaviors (see also Myers, Brown, Tate, Abrantes, & Tomlinson, Chapter 9, this volume). The IBFT model is conceptualized as a moderate intensity, predominantly office-based, relatively brief outpatient intervention that can be conducted in 10 to 16 sessions. In general, family therapy is a treatment of choice for many problem behaviors in adolescence (Alexander, Holtzworth-Munroe, & Jameson, 1994) and has considerable support for the treatment of adolescent substance use disorders (Stanton & Shadish, 1997; Waldron, 1997). The rationale for combining family therapy with individually based interventions into an integrated model derives from empirical findings that lend support to both treatment approaches and from the distinct theoretical formulations concerning the etiology of substance abuse of these two treatment modalities.

Cognitive–behavioral models are based on the assumption that drinking and drug use are largely learned and are best understood in the context of the antecedents and consequences surrounding the behavior, one aspect of which involves the social context of the family. In family systems models, on the other hand, alcohol and drug abuse and dependence are viewed as behaviors that occur in response to problems with existing family relationships and that have a specific meaning in the context of the family. Each approach has some empirical support, suggesting that both approaches may be important in remediating substance abuse and related problem behaviors. Yet these models are frequently adopted in treatment and research settings with little regard as to whether resources for intervening with adolescents who abuse alcohol or other substances should focus on the adolescent only, on the entire family, or both (Kumpfer & Alvarado, 1996). The IBFT model was developed in response to the concern that implementing one model over the other may ignore critical components necessary for establishing and maintaining change in drinking and drug use among adolescents. The strength of the IBFT model is that treatment can both alter the dysfunctional family interactions that fostered the development and maintenance of substance abuse and dependence and address the concern that alcohol and drugs have unique features (e.g., reinforcing properties of the substance itself) that operate independently of the family and must be taken into account in the context of treatment. This chapter provides an overview of the behavioral, family systems, and ecological theories on which the IBFT model is based, describes the core components of intervention, and presents empirical support for such a multidimensional approach. Special issues and challenges in the implementation of IBFT with families of adolescents who abuse alcohol and other drugs are also discussed.

THEORETICAL BACKGROUND AND RATIONALE

Cognitive–Behavioral Perspectives

Many cognitive–behavioral models for the treatment of addictive behaviors include elements derived from classical and operant learning principles established within experimental psychology. For example, much research has examined the classically conditioned acquisition of preferences for and aversions to alcohol and drugs, tolerance, and urges and cravings and has shown that some aspects of substance use behaviors, such as urges to use in the context of a particular time or place, appear to be under stimulus control (Sherman, Jorenby, & Baker, 1988; Stewart & Grupp, 1986). Such studies suggest that interventions that help clients anticipate and avoid high-risk situations will facilitate sobriety (Dimeff & Marlatt, 1995; Monti, Rohsenow, Colby, & Abrams, 1995). Other research has examined substance use from the operant-conditioning perspective that alcohol and drug use behaviors develop and are maintained in the context of the antecedents and consequences surrounding the behavior. Both animal studies

(Balster, 1991; Carroll, Carmona, & May, 1991) and human studies (Bickel, Hughes, DeGrandpre, Higgins, & Rizzuto, 1992; Hursh, 1991) amply demonstrate the responsiveness of drug-taking behavior to reinforcement contingencies. Moreover, therapeutic strategies derived from an operant model have already shown promise in treating drug problems for adults (Higgins et al., 1995; Stitzer, Bigelow, & Liebson, 1979; Stitzer & Kirby, 1991) and for adolescents (Gilchrist & Schinke, 1985).

The social learning model incorporates classical and operant learning principles, acknowledging the influence of environmental events on the acquisition of behavior but also recognizing the role of cognitive processes (e.g., how environmental influences are perceived and appraised) in determining behavior (Bandura, 1977). Cognitively mediated learning through observation and imitation of models, social reinforcement, the anticipated effects of the substance, the direct experience of alcohol's effects as rewarding or punishing, the self-efficacy to refrain from use, and physical dependence all influence the acquisition and maintenance of drinking and drug use behaviors (Abrams & Niaura, 1987). Many cognitive–behavioral interventions that were developed using social learning theory as a base involve multiple components of intervention. Avoidance of stimulus cues, altering reinforcement contingencies, training in coping skills to manage and resist urges to use, and other skills-focused interventions to promote sobriety are often integrated into treatment programs (Marlatt & Gordon, 1985; Monti, Abrams, Kadden, & Cooney, 1989; Monti et al., 1993).

Family Therapy Perspectives

Family systems perspectives view the family as a basic unit or system subject to the same properties as other systems. According to such perspectives, all families tend to establish an equilibrium along a continuum of adaptive and dysfunctional behavior, characterized by observable and repeated patterns of family interaction. Moreover, the behaviors of family members are viewed as reciprocally determined, such that the behavior of each member influences and, in turn, is influenced by the behavior of every other member. The family system is characterized holistically, taking into account the mutual interdependence among family members, together with the processes (e.g., rules for behaving, roles, repeated sequences of behaviors, communication interactions) in which the families engage. The essential core and distinguishing feature of systems models, then, is that the locus of problem behavior is systemic, transcending the individual, and therefore the focus of treatment should be relational.

Alcohol and substance abuse are conceptualized as maladaptive behaviors expressed by one or more family members but reflecting dysfunction in the system as a whole (Stanton & Todd, 1982). The goal of family systems therapy is to correct faulty family interaction patterns and other aspects of family functioning. Family systems interventions are designed to effect change in a number of substance use risk and protective factors, including parent and sibling drug use, ineffective supervision and discipline (monitoring), negative parent–child relationships, and family conflict. In general, however, changing family interactions and improving relationship functioning is key to reducing adolescents' involvement with alcohol and other drugs.

Integrative Behavioral and Family Therapy

The IBFT model is a multisystemic, multidimensional treatment approach that is based on the recognition that substance use and other related problem behaviors derive from many sources of influence and occur in the context of multiple systems (Henggeler et al., 1991; Liddle et al., 1995). Consistent with Bronfenbrenner's theory of social ecology, the individual is viewed as being nested within a complex array of interconnected systems that encompass the individual, family, and extrafamilial (e.g., peer, school, neighborhood) factors (Bronfenbrenner, 1979). In this integrative model, treatment is directed toward assessing these multiple influences and intervening so that change is supported throughout a number of systems that affect the problem behavior, including the intrapersonal system of the individual adolescent, the interpersonal systems of the family and peers, and the extrapersonal systems of the school and the community. The combination of cognitive–behavioral therapy and family therapy in the IBFT model targets change in adolescent substance use at the level of the individual, while also placing heavy emphasis on the various substance use risk and protective factors directly associated with the family. This integration of the two modalities is necessary to successfully address the multiple systems of influence associated with the complexities of adolescent substance abuse.

Overview of the Model

Like other multisystemic intervention programs, our model includes sessions or parts of sessions held conjointly with the adolescent and other family members but also includes individual sessions with the adolescent that target coping, decision making, emotion regulation, or other intrapersonal factors or processes that may be influencing substance use (see Table 7.1). Actual techniques implemented during treatment are generally drawn from family and cognitive–behavioral models within the substance abuse and family intervention literatures. The family-based sessions within the IBFT model have been adapted from functional family therapy (FFT), a behavioral-systems family therapy approach developed for high-risk youths and

TABLE 7.1. IBFT Treatment Phases and Session Topics

Session number	Treatment modality	Session topic
Phase I: Motivation for change and initial skill building		
Session 1	Family therapy	Engagement and motivation
Session 2	Family therapy	Motivation and assessment
Session 3	Individual therapy	Functional analysis
Session 4	Individual therapy	Skill building
Session 5	Individual therapy	Skill building
Phase II: Implementation of individual and family behavior change		
Session 6	Individual therapy (15 minutes)	Monitor skill progress
	Family therapy (45 minutes)	Behavior change
Session 7	Individual therapy (15 minutes)	Monitor skill progress
	Family therapy (45 minutes)	Behavior change
Session 8	Individual therapy (15 minutes)	Monitor skill progress
	Family therapy (45 minutes)	Behavior change
Session 9	Individual therapy (15 minutes)	Monitor skill progress
	Family therapy (45 minutes)	Behavior change
Session 10	Individual therapy (15 minutes)	Monitor skill progress
	Family therapy (45 minutes)	Behavior change
Phase III: Generalization of behavior change and relapse prevention		
Session 11	Individual therapy	Problem solving
Session 12	Individual therapy	Problem solving
Session 13	Individual therapy	Relapse prevention
Session 14	Family therapy	Generalization and termination

their families (Alexander & Parsons, 1982; Barton & Alexander, 1981). The individually focused elements of the IBFT model involve multiple treatment components adapted from several cognitive–behavioral intervention programs (Kadden et al., 1992; Meyers & Smith, 1995; Monti et al., 1989).

The basic objectives of the IBFT intervention for families of substance-abusing members are twofold: (1) to reduce or eliminate substance use and other problem behaviors, and (2) to improve.family relationships. These objectives are met within the three phases of the IBFT model. The first phase focuses on both the family and the individual. The initial family sessions concentrate on engaging the family in treatment, enhancing the family's motivation for change, and assessing aspects of the family relationship to be targeted for change. The initial individual session with the adolescent involves conducting a functional analysis of behavior and then using the functional analysis to guide the identification of targets for skills training. At this early juncture, a menu of treatment options is discussed with the adolescent, and intervention components are selected and incorporated into the treatment plan, tailored to the individual adolescents' needs and treatment goals. The middle phase of therapy focuses primarily on establishing behavioral changes in the family but is designed so that portions of each session are spent with the adolescent to reinforce implementation of newly acquired skills. The last phase of therapy focuses on generalization of new family and individual behaviors to the natural environment, with an emphasis on independent problem solving within the family and substance abuse relapse prevention. The implementation of the three phases of the IBFT model are described in the following sections.

PHASE I: MOTIVATION FOR CHANGE AND INITIAL SKILL BUILDING

Family Therapy Sessions

The family-based component of the IBFT approach begins with two sessions that focus on treatment engagement, motivation, and family relationship assessment. By initiating the therapeutic process with family sessions, the therapist can begin to develop a therapeutic alliance with all family members and discuss the overall treatment plan with the entire family. In addition, the therapist can identify and begin to resolve any resistance to the therapeutic process and observe family interactions that may provide important assessment information for subsequent individual sessions with the youth and for guiding the implementation of behavior change strategies with the family.

Treatment Engagement

The importance of engaging families in treatment is underscored by the reality that families who fail to appear for their first session or who attend only one or two sessions probably do not benefit from treatment. The process of engaging families relies primarily on creating positive expectations for therapy. A host of variables can influence treatment expectancies, including characteristics of the service delivery system (e.g., reputation, location, friendliness of staff), family attitudes and beliefs, and therapist characteristics (e.g., age, gender, ethnicity, cultural sensitivity, education level, experience, interpersonal warmth). In this relatively transitory period, the family members' perceptions that the therapist can help them are more important than any specific technique the therapist could employ. Although high therapist credibility initially may not determine positive outcome, poorer outcome is sure if the family finds the therapist unconvincing as a change agent (Alexander, Waldron, Newberry, & Liddle, 1988). From the first contact with the therapist, families are attuned to aspects of therapy that are important to them, such as the therapist's confidence that their problems can be solved, his or her ability to listen and validate their feelings, and his or her use of humor. Therapists can make some adjustments to maximize credibility (e.g., such as adopting the language system used by the family) but can also anticipate challenges to credibility and respond to them directly.

Enhancing Motivation

Families with substance use problems frequently enter treatment with an established pattern of conflictual exchanges characterized by intense negative affect and malevolent attributions (Alexander, Waldron, Barton, & Mas, 1989). The presenting complaints tend to be viewed as internal properties or traits of the substance-abusing family member (e.g., "self-involved," "irresponsible," or "sick"). The recipient of the complaints, in turn, frequently responds defensively and appears disinclined to cooperate. Often, therapy is not expected to help, as the family has given up on finding solutions. These patterns and behaviors represent a major impediment to change at the onset of treatment. Therapists' direct requests to change are rarely effective, as they are perceived as confrontational by the referred individual and as irrelevant by family members, who typically do not have an appreciation for their role in the problem.

The purpose of inducing motivation is to offer family members an alternative, less negative, relationship-based definition of the problem that will predispose families to accept systemic change. Two main strategies for motivating families include relabeling or reframing and focusing on the relational aspects of family members' behaviors. The therapist's use of warmth, empathy, and humor in responding contingently and nonconfrontationally to family members in implementing these strategies is vital to the success of motivational enhancement with families. It is the explicit goal of motivationally focused sessions with families that each member should experience feeling cared for and sided with by the therapist, while also examining their contribution to and share of responsibility for the family's problems, all in the safety of the therapeutic environment.

Relabeling problem behavior is considered a core technique in many family therapy models (and other motivation-focused treatments; Miller & Rollnick, 1991) to effect a shift in the family's perspective about their problems. Relabeling a person, behavior, situation, or event is designed to change the meaning and value of a negative behavior by casting it in a more benign, or even benevolent, light. Morris, Alexander, and Waldron (1988) proposed that relabeling may operate by: (1) suspending the automatic negative thinking and response patterns in families, (2) requiring them to search for new explanations of family behavior, and (3) offering a cognitive perspective that opens the door to more effective communication and expression of feelings and reconnects families with their underlying love and caring for each other. If family members can be helped to consider that their own and others' behaviors are motivated and maintained by variables other than individual malevolence (e.g., that anger reflects underlying hurt or worry), they are more likely to see change as possible and become more motivated.

MOTHER: His behavior shows us that he doesn't care about us at all.

THERAPIST: I wonder if his getting in trouble all the time is his way of letting you know he still needs you to be very involved in his life.

ADOLESCENT: My mother nags me all the time, she's always after me. The only time she talks to me is when she wants me to do something.

THERAPIST: My guess is that the reason your mom nags you so much is because of how much she loves you. It's your mom's job to make sure that you grow up okay, and she takes that responsibility very seriously. Unfortunately, a lot of times with families that love and caring comes out wrong and the real message gets lost in the nag.

In this example, the mother interprets the adolescent's acting out behavior as a message about his lack of caring for the family. The therapist offers a more positive interpretation, reframing the behavior as a request for attention. The therapist also reframes the mother's nagging as a sign of her love. In both cases, the reframes provide alternative explanations for behaviors and are designed to enhance positive connections between the family members.

Another important motivational tool for family therapy involves emphasizing the relational nature of behavior. In disturbed families, individuals do not usually see their behavior as contributing to their current difficulties in a contingent or interdependent fashion. Rather, they view their own behavior as a necessary reaction to the misbehavior of other members. Part of the therapist's task is to make observations or comments and ask questions that highlight the interactions between family members and the interrelatedness of their actions so that they become aware of how they affect each other and how undesirable behaviors have emerged in a relational context. The therapist can facilitate a relationship focus by identifying sequences of behavior that highlight the relational impact of family behaviors, thoughts, and feelings and can guide the family away from discussions of substance use and related problem behaviors that cast these behaviors as a reflection of the adolescent's individual disturbance. For example, if during a family session a mother were complaining about her daughter's behavior, the therapist might turn to another family member and ask where he or she was during the episode under discussion. By shifting the focus away from the complaint about the daughter and onto the interaction patterns between family members, the therapist "takes the heat off" the referred adolescent, lowers defensiveness and the likelihood of hostile exchanges ensuing or escalating during the session, and facilitates the consideration of changes that may be needed throughout the family system.

THERAPIST: (*To father*) What would you like to get from this treatment?

FATHER: Frankly I don't see why I need to be here, she's the one with the drug problem.

THERAPIST: Tell me about how things are at home.

FATHER: Right now it's terrible, we fight all the time, she always has this attitude and I'm fed up.

THERAPIST: So one thing that would make treatment worthwhile is if you and your daughter were able to talk about things differently?

FATHER: Yeah, I guess so.

THERAPIST: (*To daughter*) What about you, are you as concerned about getting along with your dad as he is, would you like to see it get better?

DAUGHTER: Yes. We used to do lots of fun things together and now all we do is fight.

MOTHER: We are both having trouble communicating with her.

THERAPIST: (*To daughter*) Sounds like one thing that's going on in this family is that you've been in the hot seat for quite a while and are having trouble getting your folks to understand you. One goal we can have for the whole family, then, is to help you understand each other better so you aren't at each other's throats all the time. Maybe we can even figure out some ways that you and your dad can have some fun together again.

In this example, the therapist redirects the father's focus from the daughter's substance use to an examination of the interactions at home. The therapist broadens the father's narrow view of the problem and helps redefine the concerns as belonging to all members of the family, not just the daughter. In this instance, it also helps provide a rationale for the father's participation in therapy and helps reduce resistance to family therapy. Focusing on relationships can be accomplished by asking about each family member's role in an important behavioral sequence ("So, Mom, where were you when Dad confronted John about coming home past his curfew?" or "When did you first hear that Mom had been called in to see the principal at John's school?") In these examples, the emphasis is on examining the behavioral relationships among family members rather than on the individual family member's thoughts and feelings about a particular event.

Enhancing motivation in families depends on the therapist's non-judgmental stance and use of relabeling, relationship focus, and other strategies to shift the focus off problem behavior. Therapists must also take care to avoid forming a coalition with one family member at the expense of another. Establishing a positive focus can also help to create a more collaborative tone in therapy. Inviting family members to reflect on aspects of family life that are working well for them or asking members to recall happier times, pleasant events, and rewarding family activities can emphasize strengths, raise expectations that family life can be better, and help motivate families to pursue more positive interactions.

Family Assessment

A final task of the therapist in the first two sessions is to begin the process of assessing family functions. Assessment takes place at two levels: (1) what change is needed (i.e., the behavioral targets of change), such as drug use, nonproductive use of time, or family conflict; and (2) how the behavior change has to occur in order to maintain the functions served by the behavior within the family. Using both sets of information, the therapist can devise a unique plan for each family that takes into account the characteristics and needs of each individual, as well as the fit between individuals' characteristics at the relationship level.

Family therapists often observe that families cling tenaciously to their interaction patterns, even when they can articulate that their behavior (e.g., parents lecturing and sending teenagers to their rooms) is not having the effect they intended and the youth continues to engage in the same misbehavior again and again. The concept of the interpersonal or relationship function of behavior helps the therapist understand some of the resistance to change encountered when working with families by examining the ways in which each family member attempts to regulate relationships within the family and the interpersonal outcome or payoff that the maladaptive behaviors and patterns achieve. Analyzing interpersonal functions also reveals aspects of the relationships that family members may be unable to tell the therapist. Family assessment in this model, then, requires the therapist to look beyond the apparent problem and refocus on all relationships and the interpersonal impact of repetitive or problematic behavioral sequences.

According to the model, all behaviors can be viewed in terms of the interpersonal relatedness or interdependency they allow each family member to achieve with each other (Alexander & Parsons, 1982; Alexander et al., 1988). The essence of understanding the interpersonal function of behaviors that characterize the relationship between family members is in the outcome of the behavior. If a behavior is associated with repeated interaction patterns in families that result in family members experiencing significant physical or psychological separation from one another, then the outcome (i.e., function) of the behavior is distance. By contrast, if the outcome of behavior is that family members experience greater connection or interdependency, then the function of the behavior is closeness. In some relationships family members consistently exhibit elements of both separation and closeness. One example is the couple that spends a lot of time together but only in the context of group activities. This blending of closeness and distance is referred to as midpointing (Alexander & Parsons, 1982).

Although the functional states of closeness and distance are often seen as opposite ends of a continuum, they are considered here as separate dimensions, with the magnitude of each dimension varying from little to large amounts. Although certain behaviors more commonly produce certain functions (e.g., the state of drunkenness produces distance), a particular behavior must never be assumed to create a specific function. For example, an adolescent's drug use could create considerable distance in that the youth spends the majority of free time with other drug-abusing peers. Alternatively, drug use may initiate a repeated behavioral sequence in the family that routinely results in increased closeness when mother and father rally around the adolescent in a renewed effort to support him or her. Or drug use could involve a mix of both closeness and distance (i.e., midpointing) when the youth alternates messages that cry for help with messages that reject parental attempts to help. Thus an entire behavioral sequence must be examined and the final result determined so that an accurate functional assessment can be inferred for each family member. The identification of the functions for each dyad in the family allows the therapist to develop a change plan that will target maladaptive behaviors while preserving each family members' functions with others and in so doing increase the likelihood that behavioral changes will be more readily instituted and maintained.

MOTHER: One thing that infuriates me is that they are always fighting with each other. I don't understand why they can't get along better as brothers.

THERAPIST: Sounds like this happens a lot. Let's look at this a little more closely. (To mother) What are you doing when they start fighting?

MOTHER: I work from home and spend a lot of time at my computer. Usually they start fighting as soon as I sit down to work. I end up yelling at them to stop over and over again. I usually have to get up and go in there before they pay attention.

SON: We never fight when you're not around.

THERAPIST: It looks like one reason they may fight so much is that they have figured out it's one good way to get your attention.

In this example, the therapist explains to the family that fighting is one method used by the brothers to get attention from their mother (a contact function). However, it is not necessary to explain the concept of functions to family members. Rather, the therapist uses the information concerning functions to develop a treatment plan that involves substituting adaptive behaviors for maladaptive ones. In this example, the therapist would attempt to find positive ways of increasing the mother's contact time with the boys in order to lessen their need for attention when she is attempting to work.

Concurrent Individual Therapy Sessions

In order to maximize the momentum of adolescents' motivation and engagement into the therapy process, individual therapy sessions may be held concurrently with the family sessions in the first 3 weeks of therapy. In this instance, a 1-hour individual session with the adolescent and a 1-hour session with the entire family would be held each week. The individual skill-building sessions focus on initiating behavior change, using the adolescent's functional analysis of behavior to determine which skills are most needed early in treatment to establish a momentum for change. Together, the therapist and youth will choose from a menu of skill-building topics those that will be implemented in the upcoming sessions. In this way, the intervention is tailored to the individual strengths and weaknesses of each client.

Functional Analysis

The first individual therapy session with the youth focuses on developing a functional analysis of substance use behavior. A functional analysis is a structured interview that examines the antecedents and consequences of a specific behavior, such as drinking or using drugs (Meyers & Smith, 1995). This information is integral to identifying stimulus cues associated with higher risk for substance use and to identifying the positive and negative consequences the adolescent experiences with respect to substance use and restraint from use. A unique advantage of this integrative model is that the therapist has the opportunity to observe the adolescent in the family system and, as a result, may be able to assist the youth in identifying triggers or cues for using alcohol or drugs associated with family interaction. The functional analysis may be useful in a number of other ways as well. For example, the assessment may be used to identify goals that are appropriate and attainable with the individual client. In addition, the functional analysis may be used to explore positive, prosocial behaviors that would help the adolescent in establishing a healthier life style. In general, developing alternative methods of coping with high-risk situations without using alcohol or drugs involves learning specific skills and strategies. Once the situations and problems that contribute to the individual's use are known, the coping strategies and other skills needed to manage those situations can be identified and skills training can begin.

As part of the functional analysis, the therapist might ask questions about the kinds of situations in which the adolescent uses; the typical triggers for use, such as when, where, and with whom; thoughts and feelings associated with use; what the adolescent dislikes about using; and what some of the positive results of use might be (Meyers & Smith, 1995). The therapist may then ask the client to complete a self-monitoring record and may demonstrate its use for the adolescent by recording on it the responses to the questions just asked. The therapist should summarize for the client the apparent determinants of substance use and confirm these determinants by asking for other examples. Upon completion of the functional analysis, the content of the next two individual sessions is chosen from the following menu of skill-building topics, depending on the problem areas in need of most immediate attention to facilitate sobriety.

Coping with Cravings and Urges to Use

Upon abstaining from the use of alcohol or drugs, youths may experience cravings, or urges to use, and skills must be presented early in treatment so that they may learn to cope with them. Urges to use can be triggered by environmental, physical, and psychological signs, sometimes without the youth even realizing it. However, cravings and urges usually last only a short time, often only 3–5 minutes, and will become less frequent and less intense as the youth learns how to cope with them.

One important coping strategy is for adolescents to learn to recognize triggers in order to reduce exposure to them or avoid them completely. A self-monitoring record may be assigned so that triggers can be identified. When a craving cannot be avoided, it is necessary to find an alternative method for managing it, such as getting involved in a distracting activity, talking it through with friends or family members, and challenging or changing thoughts (through reminders of the benefits of not using and the negative consequences of using). Some urges are too strong to ignore, and when this happens, the client may be instructed to focus on the urge to use systematically until it passes, using a technique called "urge surfing"

(Kadden et al., 1992). Using this procedure, urges are likened to ocean waves that start small, grow in size, and then break up and dissipate. Urge surfing, then, involves having the client imagine him- or herself as a surfer who will ride the wave as it grows, peaks, and crashes.

Communication and Problem-Solving Skills

Good communication skills help individuals deal with problems more smoothly, calmly, and easily. That is, learning to use effective communication skills helps people to resolve future problems on their own and to feel more appreciated and understood. Moreover, people who are good at communicating can get their needs met, which is especially important when communicating with people who have power over youths, such as teachers, probation officers, and parents. Also, effective communication and problem-solving skills allow clients to cope with potentially problematic situations (Monti et al., 1989). Armed with these skills, youths are less likely to be vulnerable or at a loss when they need to use them.

In teaching communication skills to the adolescent, the therapist may demonstrate in an exaggerated fashion the ineffective implementation of nonverbal and verbal communication and ask the youth to make a better response. Posture, eye contact, facial expression, gestures, and voice quality are nonverbal communications that should be demonstrated. Verbal communication skills to be addressed include speaking in a confident tone of voice, using "I" instead of "you" messages, being specific and brief, checking to see that others are listening, asking questions when confused, and ending the communication when it is breaking down. Therapists may model patterns to be avoided (e.g., putdowns, blaming, denial, defensiveness) and again ask the client to engage in role play and try to exhibit more effective communication. Feedback and rehearsal are used to facilitate skill acquisition.

Problem solving requires recognizing that there is a problem, identifying what the problem is, considering various potential solutions, selecting the most promising approach, and implementing and evaluating the effectiveness of the selected approach (Monti et al., 1989). Again, role playing and behavioral rehearsal with feedback from the therapist may be used in the session to facilitate acquisition of the new skills. The therapist and client should reason through the process of weighing the alternatives in order to select the most promising ones. The therapist's task is to help the youth to prioritize the alternative solutions, to role play how to implement the best solution, and to determine whether the solution was effective in resolving the problem or whether another alternative solution must be identified.

Anger Awareness and Management

Anger awareness and management is a tool especially useful for substance-abusing youth. Conflict with parents, teachers, and the legal system commonly occur, and adolescents often struggle to communicate their angry feelings effectively. In some cases, anger expression and emotion regulation may not have been adequately modeled for the youth by parents who themselves struggle with emotional expression. Anger may be expressed through behaviors that have a negative impact on others (e.g., aggression) or on the client (e.g., self-mutilation). At the same time, however, anger can provide useful information about a situation. The goal of anger management is to help clients learn to recognize their own angry feelings and communicate them in a way that does not inflict injury on themselves or others (Monti et al., 1989).

The first step to managing anger is identifying the experience of anger before it proceeds unaddressed. This may be accomplished by helping the youth become aware of external situations that trigger anger and/or internal reactions to those situations (Monti et al., 1989). The therapist can help the adolescent record his or her list of triggers and reactions in much the same way as was done for the functional analysis. The therapist can also demonstrate for the adolescent an appropriate response to an anger-evoking situation, articulating self-statements for anger management aloud: calming down (e.g., counting to 10), thoughts about the situation (e.g., "Why am I upset?"), and thoughts about options. An alternative strategy is to demonstrate an assertive versus an aggressive response and have the adolescent role play a situation that they have found difficult. The youth should be instructed to "think out loud" using calming reminder phrases, positive thinking, and verbalizing aloud the consequences of overreacting.

Negative Moods and Depression

Given the high level of comorbid depression and other negative moods that occur in adolescents who abuse alcohol and other substances (cf. Aseltine, Gore, & Colten, 1998; Chassin, Pitts, DeLucia, & Todd, 1999; Whitmore et al., 1997), coping skills learned in the context of substance abuse treatment can be applied to alleviate and prevent relapse to depression. In particular, communication and problem-solving skills and anger management skills provide a foundation for coping with other negative emotions. As with anger, adolescents can learn to recognize thought patterns associated with depression and other negative moods and can learn to intervene to control the negative emotion through challenging their thought patterns and changing their behaviors in response to negative thoughts and moods.

As noted in Kadden and colleagues (1992), there are several approaches to helping youths deal with depression. These approaches include (1) thinking more positively about the world and oneself, (2) becoming aware of distorted, self-defeating thoughts, (3) responding to these thoughts with more realistic ones, and then (4) acting on the new thoughts. In particular, increasing the adolescent's involvement in positive activities and reducing involvement in negative ones can reduce depression and enhance mood.

Substance Refusal Skills

When working with adolescents, peer and other types of group pressure cannot be ignored, and adolescents need to be prepared to assert themselves in the face of such pressure. Individuals attempting to refrain from substance use often experience two forms of social or peer pressure: direct and indirect social pressure (Kadden et al., 1992). Direct pressure occurs when someone offers a substance to the client overtly. Indirect social pressure involves being immersed in situations or social contexts in which substance use occurs.

Avoidance of those situations and of people associated with drug use is the first recommended action. When avoidance is not possible, having the youth turn down an overt offer of an alcoholic beverage or drug requires the successful implementation of assertiveness, communication, and problem-solving skills. Practice in refusing substances will help clients to respond confidently and quickly when the actual situations occur (Monti et al., 1989). The more rapidly a person is able to say "no" to such requests, the less likely he or she is to relapse (Kadden et al., 1992). Nonverbal skills that can be addressed in the session include speaking firmly with direct eye contact. Verbal skills to focus on include suggesting an alternative, changing the subject, and avoiding the use of excuses and vague answers (Monti et al., 1989). The therapist may model responses to a high-risk situation, participate in a role play of a situation chosen by the adolescent, and provide feedback on the adolescent's responses.

Enhancing Social Support Networks

In general, it is difficult to maintain abstinence without seeking help from others and allowing others to provide support. An important aspect of sobriety, then, is developing social support in the environment. Although many youths may state that they can manage high-risk situations and difficulties on their own, the therapeutic experience and participation in the therapeutic relationship will provide a model for extending their trust and faith to others. The exploration of support networks through family, peers, and others will allow youths to experience the value and comfort of others in the management of their problems. Also, having a support network will have a positive impact on their confidence in their own ability to handle difficult situations and cope with feelings of distress.

The communication strategies rehearsed during therapy can be used to help build and maintain supportive relationships with others. As described by Monti and colleagues (1989), after the adolescent has decided on a problem with which he or she would like some help, he or she can take three basic steps to elicit the most effective support from others: (1) consider who might be helpful (e.g., school counselor, parent, sibling, etc.), (2) consider what types of support the client would like (e.g., moral support, information or resources, etc.), and (3) consider how the client can get the needed help (ask, give feedback, etc.). As in other skill-training sessions, the therapist may demonstrate ineffective and effective ways of asking someone to provide support, and the client may engage in a behavioral rehearsal with the therapist.

PHASE II: IMPLEMENTATION OF INDIVIDUAL AND FAMILY BEHAVIOR CHANGE

The next five sessions of therapy in the IBFT model consist of a combination of both family therapy and individual therapy. For the first 15 minutes of each weekly session, the therapist meets individually with the youth. This time is devoted to monitoring the youth's progress in acquiring and practicing the cognitive behavioral skills discussed earlier, revising the functional analysis as the youth is able to recognize and disclose additional information, and planning for the acquisition of other skills in later sessions. An important and unique benefit of the IBFT approach is that these 15-minute sessions also enable the therapist to provide individual support and modeling for appropriate communication by the youth in the family session that immediately follows, thus facilitating parent–child communication about important topics that the youth might not otherwise address in therapy.

The primary goal of the family sessions in this phase is to establish new behaviors and patterns of interaction that will replace the old maladaptive patterns of behavior that were characteristic of the family prior to treatment, preventing maladaptive patterns from reappearing and producing long-term change in the family. During the treatment readiness phase, techniques are used to change the meaning of behavior, the attributions family members have about one another, and family members' motivations for change. Although such changes are important prerequisites to long-term change, by themselves those changes will not be maintained unless interaction patterns follow a specific plan.

In the family sessions, therapists draw from a menu of treatment strategies and behavior-change techniques, such as communication training, contingency management, negative mood regulation, and increasing rewarding shared activities, in order to achieve the objectives for change for each target behavior in the treatment plan. The particular selections of activities or techniques and how the techniques are applied in changing interaction patterns and behaviors, however, depend on several considerations. An understanding of interpersonal functions is key; intervention attempts can lead either to rapid change or to resistance, depending on how well the intervention strategy fits with each family member's interpersonal function with each other family member. Even when the behavior-change strategy is technically correct and well developed, resistance will arise if the intervention implemented is inconsistent with one or more of family members' interpersonal functions. For example, a son who abuses marijuana and crack cocaine may achieve considerable distance from his parents while at the same time creating a context for his father's merging function with his mother. That is, the son's substance use allows the couple to draw closer, discussing their concerns and attempting to solve the problem of how best to help their son. Attempts to move the son into more interdependent and intimate interactions with his parents would be incompatible with the family's relational functions, and noncompliance with intervention would likely result.

An early goal in the family sessions in this second phase of treatment is to enhance the family's experience of positive change. The therapist strives to help the family initiate new and positive interactions and heightening their experience that such interactions are possible (Alexander & Parsons, 1982). Throughout the behavior-change phase, interactions are highly structured, and the therapist is active and directive. By maximizing the success experiences of families, the positive momentum and family motivation established in the treatment readiness phase will continue.

When change attempts do go awry, several sources of the problem should be considered. For example, the therapist may not have been sufficiently clear, directive, or otherwise informative for family members to understand and to be able to carry out the change plan. Another possibility is that the family's functions have not been met by the behavior-change plan. Or the therapist may need to cycle back to the treatment readiness phase to focus further on motivational enhancement. When compliance with change attempts does occur, the therapist should steadily decrease assistance as each behavior change technique is implemented and each target problem is addressed.

The specific techniques introduced by the therapist in the behavior-change phase can include any strategies or devices capable of changing behavior and accomplishing these goals. The model has not created a new set of techniques for changing behavior, as many excellent cognitive and behavioral treatment manuals are already available. The most commonly applied modules for changing families are communication-skills training, problem-solving and conflict resolution skills, strategies to increase pleasing behaviors and rewarding activities, parenting and contingency management skills, the use of technical aids to facilitate family process, and relapse prevention skills. Optional modules that can also be implemented with some families, depending on their particular needs, include emotional regulation (i.e., anger, depressed mood), relaxation training, self-esteem building, assertiveness training, contingency contracting, or methods of self-control. Detailed applications of these techniques are described by Alexander and Parsons (1982).

The emphasis of the model is on the application of techniques in the context of the assessment of functional payoffs in the family and is tailored to each set of family relationships. For example, the manner in which the therapist incorporates communication or problem-solving skills into family interactions may range from instituting nightly formal family meetings (high contact, low distance) to occasional informal "as needed" checkups between family members or even written notes used to convey messages and solve problems (low contact, high distance). Similarly, community-based approaches, such as Alcoholics Anonymous, could be incorporated into treatment. For example, a father and son who both have drinking problems could attend meetings together or attend different meetings on alternating nights of the week, again depending on their assessed relationship functions.

Families with addictive behavior problems also often have limited access to community resources that reduce the risk for alcohol abuse. Later in the behavior change phase, extrafamilial resources can be identified and contacts made to further support the treatment gains made in therapy. In addition, after the referred family member's substance use has decreased and family interactions have improved, other family problems that commonly occur may be addressed. Concerns about the marital relationship and parental drinking are common. The therapist should discuss these issues with the parents, and if they desire to continue treatment on these problems, the family therapist should continue treatment with the marital dyad alone.

PHASE III: GENERALIZATION OF BEHAVIOR CHANGE AND RELAPSE PREVENTION

As behavioral changes are established, the focus of treatment shifts toward generalization of the new behaviors across other contexts, establishing the family's independence from the therapist, and anticipating substance use relapse and other potential problems. The therapist encourages clients to take responsibility for solving problems on their own, bolstering their self-efficacy by reinforcing independent problem-solving behavior. In this phase, one session is typically held with the adolescent alone to plan for emergencies, review managing high-risk situations, and anticipate coping with substance use lapses. Another session is conducted conjointly with all family members to review treatment gains and to identify areas needing continued attention.

Individual Session: Planning for Emergencies and Coping with a Lapse

Following the conclusion of treatment, adolescents invariably will be confronted with situations that threaten sobriety. Relationships with peers and family and school or employment issues, positive or negative, can be sources of stress that increase the likelihood of a relapse. According to Kadden and colleagues (1992), a lapse or slip is likely to be accompanied by feelings of guilt or shame, which may be covered with an attitude of apathy. However, if these reactions to the slip, as well as the behaviors that led up to the lapse, are analyzed, the likelihood of further lapses may be reduced.

The therapist may ask the client to describe one or more situations (e.g., breaking up with a girlfriend or boyfriend) that could lead to craving for drugs or to a lapse. The adolescent may be asked to consider how these events might affect his or her behavior and interactions with others. The adolescent should be encouraged to draw on skills discussed in previous sessions and examine what specific strategies could be used to cope with high-risk situations. The therapist and adolescent should prepare a generic emergency plan for coping with any number of possible stressful situations that might arise unexpectedly. Strategies such as problem-solving skills, calling people for support, and cognitive coping methods should be identified for each anticipated situation. In the immediate aftermath of a substance use episode, the adolescent should be instructed to leave the situation, call someone for help, and get rid of the drugs. In the event of a longer term substance use episode, the adolescent should be encouraged to examine the slip with someone, analyzing possible triggers and considering expectations for use. The adolescent must beware of catastrophizing thoughts, for if allowed to proceed unchecked, these reactions can contribute to further substance use episodes.

Generalization of Family Changes and Treatment Termination

To develop the family's independence, the therapist gradually takes a less active role in the intrafamily process. As family members experience short-term changes, the therapist helps them to consider alternative ways to continue positive changes. In addition, issues that may involve systems external to the family are discussed. Many extrafamilial factors cannot be changed, such as neighborhood crime or institutional racism. However, other factors may be modifiable for a family, such as responsiveness of school personnel or employees. The therapist may interact directly with legal and educational systems on behalf of the family and help the families to interact independently and more effectively within these systems (Alexander, Barton, Waldron, & Mas, 1983). In addition, the therapist may help the family anticipate stressors and problems, exploring solutions to those future difficulties. Therapy moves toward termination when (1) drug and alcohol use and other problem behaviors are reduced or eliminated, (2) adaptive interaction patterns and problem- solving styles have been developed and are occurring independent of therapist's monitoring and prompting, and (3) the family appears to have the necessary motivation, skills, and resources to maintain a positive clinical trajectory without the support of ongoing services.

SPECIAL CONSIDERATIONS IN IMPLEMENTING THE INTEGRATIVE BEHAVIORAL AND FAMILY THERAPY MODEL

The IBFT model provides a multidimensional approach to treating adolescent substance abuse. However, a number of important issues must be considered when implementing this approach. These issues include considering the adolescent's social and cognitive development in relation to treatment, determining the appropriate target population and setting for treatment with the model, and maintaining confidentiality in the integrative context of the family and individual therapy modalities.

From a developmental perspective, the tasks of adolescence involve mastering the ability to move from concrete thinking to more abstract thought, identity development, and separation and individuation from the family unit. This process often necessitates that the adolescent struggle with competing sources of influence, such as parents' external limit setting and demands for conformity from both traditional and more deviant peer groups. The need for autonomy and the development of self-efficacy through this process become increasingly important for the adolescent. Understanding these concepts and the relative mastery that youths may display throughout the adolescent age span are important in the implementation of effective treatments for substance-abusing adolescents and may have implications for preventing premature termination from treatment and substance use relapse. For example, we have found that adolescents vary substantially in their ability to connect cause-and-effect events such as the relationship between violating a rule and being denied a future privilege

("You mean the reason you won't let me go out next Saturday is because I stayed out all night last Friday?"). They also tend to minimize the significance of problem behavior that occurred in the past ("That happened weeks ago and I'm not like that anymore") and to be overly optimistic about their ability to engage in new behaviors ("I'll fill out applications for 10 jobs this week"). By being sensitive to the developmental issues that underlie these kinds of behaviors, the therapist can help the adolescent develop a better appreciation of the connection between problem behavior and negative consequences, provide developmentally appropriate reinterpretations of behavior that reduce the tendency for the adolescent's behavior to be viewed as malevolent by parents, and reduce the likelihood that adolescents experience failure by establishing unrealistic goals.

A second important consideration relates to understanding the appropriate target population for treatment with the IBFT model. The model is designed to be effective for adolescents presenting for treatment within the broad spectrum of substance abuse and dependence diagnoses. However, ecologically based multisystemic treatments vary along a spectrum of intensity that can range from weekly sessions conducted with the individual and family to intensive in-home interventions that may also include extensive therapist involvement at school, with probation officers, and with other relevant systems. The IBFT model is conceptualized as a moderate-intensity, predominantly office-based outpatient intervention. It is anticipated that therapists using the model would intervene with relevant external systems such as schools and juvenile probation, but, as a relatively brief intervention that can be conducted in 10–16 sessions, the model is not designed for implementation at the intensity of a family-preservation model. As with any outpatient intervention, adolescents in need of more intensive intervention services such as inpatient detoxification or other residential treatment should be referred for appropriate services.

One challenge posed by the IBFT model relates to the critical issue of confidentiality. Because the therapist will be working with both the family and the youth individually, the therapist must exercise caution to protect disclosures made by the youth in the individual sessions. Establishing trust with the youth through nondisclosure of confidential information in family sessions is critical to therapeutic effectiveness. Moreover, the therapist must maintain neutrality in the family sessions while also maintaining a supportive relationship with the adolescent in the individual sessions. Some strategies that the therapist can employ to enhance this process include discussing with the adolescent in advance any plans the therapist may have to pursue particular issues with the family and encouraging the youth to initiate discussions of sensitive topics in the family sessions when appropriate.

EMPIRICAL FINDINGS

Research demonstrating the efficacy of cognitive–behavioral therapy approaches in reducing adult substance use is well established (cf. Miller et al., 1995; Miller & Heather, 1998). However, clinical trials to evaluate treatment efficacy for adolescent substance abusers, although increasing in number, are still limited. Cognitive–behavioral approaches have most often been applied in prevention settings, with outcome evaluations of such programs demonstrating significant delays in the onset of substance use and reductions in current use (Botvin & Botvin, 1992; Pentz, 1985). In a study examining cognitive–behavior therapy for adolescents treated for alcohol abuse or dependence, Myers and Brown (1990a, 1990b) found that adolescent alcohol abstainers and minor relapsers were more likely to utilize problem-solving coping strategies than were major relapsers. Further, coping factors have been identified as significant predictors of treatment outcome (Myers, Brown, & Mott, 1993).

In a controlled clinical trial, Turner, Liddle, and Dakof (1996) compared substance use outcomes for youths randomly assigned to one of three treatment conditions: cognitive–behavior therapy, multisystemic family therapy, or treatment as usual. Preliminary results indicated that both cognitive–behavioral therapy and family therapy produced greater reductions in substance use relative to treatment as usual. However, some findings suggested that although there were no differences between the two conditions through 6-month follow-up, the cognitive–behavioral treatment appeared more effective through a 12-month follow-up.

Reviews of formal clinical trials of family-based treatments have consistently found that more drug-abusing adolescents enter, engage in, and remain in family therapy than in other treatments and that family therapy produces significant reductions in substance use from pre- to posttreatment (Liddle & Dakof, 1995; Stanton & Shadish, 1997; Waldron, 1997). In seven of eight studies comparing family therapy to a non-family-based intervention, for example, adolescents receiving family therapy showed greater reductions in substance use than those receiving adolescent group therapy (Azrin et al., 1993; Joanning, Thomas, Quinn, & Mullen, 1992; Liddle et al., 1995), family education (Joanning et al., 1992; Liddle et al., 1995) and individual therapy, individual tracking through schools, or juvenile justice system intervention (Bry & Krinsley, 1992; Henggeler et al., 1991). In a study focusing specifically on adolescent alcohol abusers, Trepper, Piercy, Lewis, Volk, and Sprenkle (1993) found that both family and individual therapy approaches resulted in reductions in alcohol use, though no changes in use were observed from a drug education condition.

Findings from two recent studies highlight the potential benefit of a

treatment model such as IBFT, which combines family and individual cognitive–behavioral skills-training strategies. Brown, Myers, Mott, and Vik
(1994) found that decreased use was not necessarily associated with better
functioning in areas such as family relationships and suggested that individual skills-based treatment with adolescents had a "fluctuating" impact on
other life domains. In another study evaluating behavior therapy for drug
abusers, Azrin and colleagues (1993) noted that the adolescent participants
demonstrated significantly greater substance use reductions than adult participants. However, in discussing this finding, the authors attribute these results to active parental participation in the adolescents' treatment sessions.
Thus, for both theoretical and empirical reasons, combining family and
cognitive–behavioral skills treatment approaches may provide significant
advantages over either approach alone, as different risk factors are addressed in each treatment modality and combining treatments increases the
number of factors addressed.

To evaluate the efficacy of a combined intervention (i.e., family therapy and individual cognitive–behavioral therapy) for adolescent substance
abuse, we conducted a randomized clinical trial comparing adolescent substance use and family relationship outcomes for the combined intervention
with outcomes for three other treatment conditions: a stand-alone family
therapy condition, a stand-alone individual cognitive–behavioral therapy,
and a psychoeducational group intervention condition. The primary hypotheses were: (1) family therapy, individual cognitive–behavioral therapy,
and a combined family therapy and cognitive–behavioral therapy intervention would be superior to the psychoeducational group intervention, and
(2) the combined intervention would be superior to the other three interventions.

The study, funded by the National Institute on Drug Abuse, involved
120 families of adolescents referred for substance abuse treatment. Adolescents randomly assigned to family therapy, cognitive–behavioral therapy, or
group therapy received 12 sessions, and adolescents assigned to the combined condition received 12 sessions each of family therapy and cognitive–
behavioral therapy. Assessments were completed at intake and 4, 7, and 19
months after intake. Youth ranged in age from 13 to 17 years ($X = 15.54$),
with 23% of the sample female. They identified themselves as Hispanic
(35%), white (41%), Native American (6%), and mixed (15%).

Our preliminary findings revealed the strongest immediate benefits for
youth receiving family therapy but also provide support for combining
family and cognitive–behavioral interventions. Adolescents who received
family therapy or family therapy in combination with individual cognitive–
behavioral therapy showed significant reductions in substance use from
pretreatment to 4 months following the initiation of treatment, whereas no

pretreatment-to-4-month reductions in use were found for the individual cognitive–behavioral intervention alone or the psychoeducational-skills group intervention.

However, reductions in substance use from pretreatment to 7 months following the initiation of treatment were significant for both the combined intervention (family therapy and cognitive–behavioral therapy), and for the group condition, but not for the other two intervention conditions. This pattern of findings for the combined condition may have resulted from the additional therapy sessions adolescents received, but it does provide initial support for both the immediate and continuing benefit of integrating family and individual cognitive–behavioral therapy. To disentangle the effect of dose of treatment from the integrative effects of the intervention, we currently have another controlled trial underway that compares the IBFT model to family and individual interventions alone, as well as to our group intervention, equating amount of treatment received across the intervention conditions.

REFERENCES

Abrams, D. B., & Niaura, R. S. (1987). Social learning theory. In H. T. Blane & K. E. Leonard (Eds.), *Psychological theories of drinking and alcoholism* (pp. 131–178). New York: Guilford Press.

Alexander, J. F., Barton, C., Waldron, H. B., & Mas, C. H. (1983). *Beyond the technology of family therapy: The anatomy of intervention model.* New York: Brunner/Mazel.

Alexander, J. F., Holtzworth-Munroe, A., & Jameson, P. (1994). The process and outcome of marital and family therapy: Research review and evaluation. In S. L. Garfield & A. E. Bergin (Eds.), *Handbook of psychotherapy and behavior change* (4th ed., pp. 595–630). New York: Wiley.

Alexander, J. F., & Parsons, B.V. (1982). *Functional family therapy: Principles and procedures.* Carmel, CA: Brooks/Cole.

Alexander, J. F., Waldron, H. B., Barton, C., & Mas, C. H. (1989). Minimizing blaming attributions and behaviors in conflicted delinquent families. *Journal of Consulting and Clinical Psychology, 57*, 19–24.

Alexander, J. F., Waldron, H. B., Newberry, A.M., & Liddle, N. (1988). Family approaches to treating delinquents. In E. W. Nunnally & C. Chilman (Eds.), *Mental illness, delinquency, addictions, and neglect* (pp. 128–146). Newbury Park, CA: Sage.

Aseltine, R. H., Gore, S., & Colten, M. E. (1998). The co-occurrence of depression and substance abuse in late adolescence. *Development and Psychopathology, 10*, 549–570.

Azrin, N., McMahon, P., Donohue, V., Besalel, K., Lapinski, E., Kogan, R., Acierno, R. & Galloway, E. (1993). Behavior therapy for drug abuse: A controlled treatment outcome study. *Behavior Research and Therapy, 32*, 857–866.

Balster, R. L. (1991). Drug abuse potential evaluation in animals. *British Journal of addictions, 86,* 1549–1558.

Bandura, A. (1977). *Social learning theory.* Englewood Cliffs, NJ: Prentice-Hall.

Barton, C., & Alexander, J. F. (1981). Functional family therapy. In A. S. Gurman & D. P. Kniskern (Eds.), *Handbook of family therapy* (pp. 403–443). New York: Brunner/Mazel.

Bickel, W. K., Hughes, J. R., DeGrandpre, R. J., Higgins, S. T., & Rizzuto, P. (1992). Behavioral economics of drug self-administration. The effects of response requirement on the consumption of and interaction between concurrently available coffee and cigarettes. *Psychopharmacology, 107,* 211–216.

Botvin, G., & Botvin, E. (1992). Adolescent tobacco, alcohol and drug abuse: Prevention strategies, empirical findings, and assessment issues. *Journal of Developmental and Behavioral Pediatrics, 13,* 290–301.

Bronfenbrenner, U. (1979). *The ecology of human development: Experiments by nature and design.* Cambridge, MA: Harvard University Press.

Brown, S., Myers, M., Mott, M., & Vik, P. (1994). Correlates of success following treatment for adolescent substance abuse. *Applied and Preventive Psychology, 3,* 61–73.

Bry, B. H., & Krinsley, K. E. (1992). Booster sessions and long-term effects of behavioral family therapy on adolescent substance use and school performance. *Journal of Behavioral Therapy and Experimental Psychiatry, 23,* 183–189.

Carroll, M. E., Carmona, G. G., & May, S. A. (1991). Modifying drug reinforced behavior by altering the economic conditions of the drug and nondrug reinforcer. *Journal of the Experimental Analysis of Behavior, 56,* 361–376.

Chassin, L., Pitts, S. C., DeLucia, C., & Todd, M. (1999). A longitudinal study of children of alcoholics: Predicting young adult substance use disorders, anxiety, and depression. *Journal of Abnormal Psychology, 108,* 106–119.

Dimeff, L. A., & Marlatt, G. A. (1995). Relapse prevention. In R. K. Hester & W. R. Miller (Eds.), *Handbook of alcoholism treatment approaches: Effective alternatives* (pp. 176–194). Boston: Allyn & Bacon.

Gilchrist, L. D., & Schinke, S. P. (1985). Preventing substance abuse with children and adolescents. *Journal of Consulting and Clinical Psychology, 53,* 121–135.

Henggeler, S. W., Borduin, C. M., Melton, G. B., Mann, B. J., Smith, L. A., Cone, L., & Fucci, B. R. (1991). Effects of multisystemic therapy on drug use and abuse in serious juvenile offenders: A progress report from two outcome studies. *Family Dynamics of Addiction Quarterly, 1,* 40–51.

Higgins, S. T., Budney, A. J., Bickel, W. K., Badger, G. J., Foerg, F. E., & Ogden, D. (1995). Outpatient behavioral treatment for cocaine dependence: One-year outcome. *Experimental Clinical Psychopharmacology, 3,* 205–212.

Hursh, S. R. (1991). Behavioral economics of drug self-administration and drug policy. *Journal of Experimental Analysis of Behavior, 56,* 377–394.

Joanning, H., Thomas, F., Quinn, W., & Mullen, R. (1992). Treating adolescent drug abuse: A comparison of family systems therapy, group therapy, and family drug education. *Journal of Marital and Family Therapy, 18,* 345–356.

Kadden, R., Carroll, K., Donovan, D., Cooney, N., Monti, P., Abrams, D., Litt, M., &

Hester, R. (1992). *Cognitive–behavioral coping skills therapy manual* (Vol. 3). Rockville, MD: National Institute on Alcohol Abuse and Alcoholism.

Kumpfer, K. L., & Alvarado, R. (1995). Strengthening families to prevent drug use in multiethnic youth. In G. Botvin, S. Schinke, & M. Orlandi (Eds.), *Drug abuse prevention with multiethnic youth* (pp. 255–294). Newbury Park, CA: Sage.

Liddle, H. A., & Dakof, G. A. (1995). Family-based treatment for adolescent drug use: State of the science. In E. Rahdert & D. Czechowicz (Eds.), *Adolescent drug abuse: Clinical assessment and therapeutic interventions* (pp. 218–254). Rockville, MD: U. S. Department of Health and Human Services, Public Health Service, National Institutes of Health, National Institute on Drug Abuse, Division of Clinical and Services Research.

Liddle, H. A., Dakof, G. A., Parker, K., Barrett, K., Diamond, G. S., Garcia, R., & Palmer, R. (1995). *Multidimensional family therapy of adolescent substance abuse*. Unpublished manuscript.

Marlatt, G. A., & Gordon, J. R. (1985). *Relapse prevention: Maintenance strategies in the treatment of addictive behaviors*. New York: Guilford Press.

Meyers, R. J., & Smith, J. E. (1995). *Clinical guide to alcohol treatment: The community reinforcement approach*. New York: Guilford Press.

Miller, W. R., Brown, J. M., Simpson, T. L., Handmaker, N. S., Bien, T. H., Lorenzo, S. L., Montgomery, H. A., Hester, R. K., & Tonigan, J. S. (1995). What works? A methodological analysis of the alcohol treatment outcome literature. In R. K. Hester & W. R. Miller (Eds.), *Handbook of alcoholism treatment approaches: Effective alternatives* (2nd ed., pp. 12–45). New York: Allyn & Bacon.

Miller, W. R., & Heather, N. (Eds.) (1998). *Treating addictive behaviors: Processes of change*. New York: Plenum Press.

Miller, W. R., & Rollnick, S. (1991). *Motivational interviewing: Preparing people to change addictive behavior*. New York: Guilford Press.

Monti, P. M., Abrams, D. B., Kadden, R. M., & Cooney, N. L. (1989). *Treating alcohol dependence: A coping skills training guide*. New York: Guilford Press.

Monti, P. M., Rohsenow, D. J., Colby, S. M., & Abrams, D. B. (1995). Coping and social skills training. In R. K. Hester & W. R. Miller (Eds.), *Handbook of alcoholism treatment approaches: Effective alternatives* (2nd ed., pp. 221–241). New York: Allyn & Bacon.

Monti, P. M., Rohsenow, D. J., Rubonis, A. V., Niaura, R. S., Sirota, A. D., Colby, S. M., Goddard, P., & Abrams, D. B. (1993). Cue exposure with coping skills treatment for male alcoholics: A preliminary investigation. *Journal of Consulting and Clinical Psychology, 61*, 1011–1019.

Morris, S. B., Alexander, J. F., & Waldron, H. (1988). Functional family therapy. In I. R. H. Falloon (Ed.), *Handbook of behavioral family therapy* (pp. 107–127). New York: Guilford Press.

Myers, M., & Brown, S. (1990a). Coping and appraisal in potential relapse situations among adolescent substance abusers following treatment. *Journal of Adolescent Chemical Dependency, 1*, 95–115.

Myers, M., & Brown, S. (1990b). Coping responses and relapse among adolescent substance abusers. *Journal of Substance Abuse, 2*, 177–189.

Myers, M., Brown, S., & Mott, M. (1993). Coping as a predictor of adolescent substance abuse treatment outcome. *Journal of Substance Abuse, 5*, 15–29.

Pentz, M. A. (1985). Social competence skills and self-efficacy as determinants of substance use in adolescents. In S. Shiffman & T. A. Wills (Ed.), *Coping and substance use* (pp. 117–142). New York: Academic Press.

Sherman, J. E., Jorenby, D. E., & Baker, T. B. (1988). Classical conditioning with alcohol: Acquired preferences and aversions, tolerance, and urges/cravings. In C. D. Chaudron & D. A. Wilkinson (Eds.), *Theories on alcoholism* (pp. 173–287). Toronto, Ontario, Canada: Addiction Research Foundation.

Stanton, M. D., & Shadish, W. R. (1997). Outcome, attrition, and family/couples treatment for drug abuse: A review of the controlled, comparative studies. *Psychological Bulletin, 122,* 170–191.

Stanton, M.D., & Todd, T.C., and Associates. (1982). *The family therapy of drug abuse and addiction.* New York: Guilford Press.

Stewart, R. B., & Grupp, L. A. (1986). Conditioned place aversion mediated by orally self-administered ethanol in the rat. *Pharmacology, Biochemistry and Behavior, 24,* 1369–1375.

Stitzer, M. L., Bigelow, G. E., & Liebson, I. (1979). *Reinforcement of drug abstinence: A behavioral approach to drug abuse treatment.* Rockville, MD: National Institute on Drug Abuse.

Stitzer, M. L., & Kirby, K. C. (1991). Reducing illicit drug use among methadone patients. In R. W. Pickens, C. G. Leukefeld, & C. R. Schuster (Eds.), *Improving drug abuse treatment* (pp. 178–203). Rockville, MD: U.S. Department of Health and Human Services, Public Health Service, Alcohol, Drug Abuse, and Mental Health Administration, National Institute on Drug Abuse.

Trepper, T. S., Piercy, F. P., Lewis, R. A., Volk, R. J., & Sprenkle, D. H. (1993). Family therapy for adolescent alcohol abuse. In T. J. O'Farrell (Ed.), *Treating alcohol problems: Marital and family interventions* (pp. 261–278). New York: Guilford Press.

Turner, R. M., Liddle, H., & Dakof, G. (1996, November). *Experimental evaluation of cognitive–behavior therapy for adolescent substance abuse.* Paper presented at the annual meeting of the Association for Advancement of Behavior Therapy, New York.

Waldron, H. B. (1997). Adolescent substance abuse and family therapy outcome: A review of randomized trials. In T. H. Ollendick & R. J. Prinz (Eds.), *Advances in clinical child psychology* (Vol. 19, pp. 199–234). New York: Plenum Press.

Whitmore, E. A., Mikulich, S. K., Thompson, L. L., Riggs, P. D., Aarons, G. A., & Crowley, T. J. (1997). Influences on adolescent substance dependence: Conduct disorder, depression, attention deficit hyperactivity disorder, and gender. *Drug and Alcohol Dependence, 47,* 87–97.

8

Motivational Interviewing and the Prevention of HIV among Adolescents

LARRY K. BROWN and KEVIN J. LOURIE

Adolescent sexual risk behavior and substance use are related to the majority of adolescent morbidity and mortality (Kann et al., 1998; Tubman, Windle, & Windle, 1996). Cross-sectional and longitudinal data from nationally representative samples show that adolescent substance use is a key risk factor for the early onset of sexual behaviors (Mott & Haurin, 1988; Zabin, Hardy, Smith, & Hirsch, 1986). For both female and male adolescents, early initiation of sexual intercourse predicts early use of alcohol and drugs compared with older cohorts and vice versa (Warren et al., 1997). Early intercourse experiences are in turn associated with higher levels of substance abuse, externalizing childhood behavior problems, and antisocial behaviors (Tubman et al, 1996). Adolescents who initiate sexual activity at earlier ages are more likely to experience unprotected intercourse and to expose themselves to STDs and other risks (Haignere, Gold & McDanel, 1999). Cross-sectional analysis of the 1991 Centers for Disease Control (CDC) Youth Risk Behavior Survey found that those who initiated sexual activity early had greater numbers of partners, were 50% less likely to use condoms regularly, and were two to seven times more likely to have been pregnant or have caused a pregnancy (Coker et al., 1994).

Adolescents are thus at risk for acquiring HIV because of sexual and drug behaviors that are commonly initiated during this developmental period. Illustrating this risk is the fact that one fourth of all new HIV infections occur among those under the age of 22 and that more than one half occur among those under the age of 26 (Office of National AIDS Policy, 1996). In the United States, HIV infection rates are increasing most rapidly among women and youth, particularly those who are in racial and ethnic minorities (National Institutes of Health [NIH], 2000). Prevention efforts therefore must utilize models and techniques appropriate to adolescents and minority communities. Unfortunately, no single theoretical model adequately encompasses adolescent risk behavior (Brown, DiClemente, & Reynolds, 1991). Models such as the theory of reasoned action (Fishbein, 1990), the health belief model (Petosa & Jackson, 1991), the transtheoretical model (Prochaska, 1989), and Bandura's model of self-efficacy (1994) have been useful for designing interventions. However, because each model has definite limits, most effective programs have used combinations of these approaches (Kim, Stanton, Li, Dickersin, & Galbraith, 1997). Furthermore, adolescent-specific factors such as cognitive immaturity, impulsiveness, and exploratory learning behavior need to be incorporated in any such model (Irwin & Millstein, 1997). The prevention of sexual risk behavior in minority communities is similarly limited by the absence of a "gold standard" for a conceptual framework or intervention design (Stanton, Kim, Galbraith, & Parrott, 1996).

The lack of a single most efficacious or best approach to changing sexual risk behavior underscores the need for alternative techniques. Therapeutic models are often used in other areas of behavior change to guide treatment, even if our understanding of the origins of disease is incomplete. The motivational approach is one such strategy for influencing behavior that may be useful across a wide spectrum of conditions. Many of the commonly used HIV prevention programs are lengthy, stand-alone interventions (National Institute of Mental Health [NIMH] Multisite HIV Prevention Trial Group, 1998). In contrast, the motivational method may be effective in brief contact and integrated into the larger context of clinical care. In this chapter, we review program elements that are routinely utilized by HIV prevention interventions in order to highlight their similarities with and differences from motivational interviewing. Clinical case studies are used during brief clinical encounters with adolescents to illustrate the application of motivational techniques in order to encourage safer sexual behavior. In addition, the processes of change that stimulate motivation to change, as developed by Prochaska (1989), are illustrated in case vignettes. Last, we discuss specific issues concerning adolescent development, culture, psychological impairment, and intervention format as they relate to motivational techniques for adolescent sexual behavior change.

ADOLESCENT SEXUAL RISK BEHAVIOR CHANGE TECHNIQUES

HIV prevention programs for adolescents have commonly used several techniques based on a variety of theories. Effective interventions have attempted to increase perceived susceptibility to HIV, to enhance favorable attitudes toward condoms, to build social skills, to improve self-efficacy, and to create peer norms supportive of safer sex (Kalichman, Carey, & Johnson, 1996; Kim et al., 1997; Wren, Janz, Corovano, Zimmerman, & Washenko, 1997). Each of these frequently targeted factors will be considered in turn.

Increasing Perceived Susceptibility

Recent intervention studies have shown that an important prerequisite for change is personal concern about HIV (Ellen, Boyer, Tschann, & Shafer, 1996). Most adolescents possess knowledge about HIV, but knowledge has to be personalized in order for an individual to perceive HIV as a relevant health threat (Kalichman, Adair, Samlai, & Weir, 1995). Therefore, risk assessment exercises in adolescent groups are tailored to increase self-awareness. In general, a greater sense of vulnerability has been correlated with AIDS-preventive behaviors (Pleck, Sonenstein, & Ku, 1993). For example, a study of 1,953 noninjecting female sexual partners of injection drug users in the United States found that an intervention to raise awareness about HIV risk resulted in significant changes in risky sexual behaviors of participants (Ashery, Wild, Zhao, Rosenshine, & Young, 1997). Six months after the intervention, the number of the women's sexual partners decreased by more than one fourth; the number of sexual partners with history of intravenous drug use declined by almost one half; and the frequency of engaging in unprotected vaginal sex decreased by over 15%.

Changing Attitudes toward Condoms

Some adolescents perceive condoms as not pleasurable, too much trouble, or too costly. These "hedonistic" attitudes are associated with inconsistent condom use (Jemmott, Jemmott, & Fong, 1992; Pleck et al., 1993). Early in the AIDS epidemic, behavior change among gay males in San Francisco focused on eroticization of safer sex and condom use, with a reduction in sexual risk behavior as indicated by a dramatic decrease in rates of sexually transmitted diseases (STDs) (Catania et al., 1989; McKusick, Coates, Morin, Pollack, & Hoff, 1990). Interventions for adolescents have improved consistent condom use in part by challenging negative attitudes about condoms through teaching erotic and sexy attitudes that may be associated with condoms (Tanner, 1988). Explicitly erotic material has not been used in public school settings, which limits the ability of large programs to alter hedonistic attitudes. The availability of condoms in schools does, at least, portray condoms as acceptable to society and probably increases their use (Schuster, Bell, Berry, & Kanouse, 1998). Despite earlier fears that condom availability in schools would result in increased rates of sexual intercourse by adolescents, there is now compelling evidence that sexual activity is not increased overall (Guttmacher et al., 1997).

Building Social Skills

Effective interventions for adolescents and young adults usually emphasize training in cognitive–behavioral skills, particularly the teaching of assertive sexual negotiation skills (DiClemente & Wingood, 1995). One study specifically tailored a curriculum for multiethnic urban high school students in order to teach the sexual decision-making and negotiation skills needed for condom use (Walter & Vaughan, 1993). It caused modest improvements in students' self-efficacy and risk behavior scores. Jemmott, Jemmott, and Fong (1992) found similar results with a program tailored for inner-city African American adolescent males in community settings. Likewise, in an STD clinic setting, a project for adolescent females that targeted condom negotiation skills found an increased use of condoms at 6 months after the intervention (Orr, Langefeld, Katz, & Caine, 1996). Despite the report of increased condom use, 30% of participants still reported that they "never" used condoms, and, compared with a nonintervention sample, the incidence of STD infection did not decline significantly. Although programs to improve social skills do influence sexual behavior in the short run, risk behaviors appear to resume. Therefore, many researchers feel that booster sessions or ongoing programs are needed to reinforce and sustain behavior change (Kim et al., 1997; Levy et al., 1995).

Improving Self-Efficacy

In general, health-promoting behaviors have been found to be associated with self-efficacy for those behaviors (Bandura, 1986; O'Leary, 1985). Adolescents must feel confident that they can initiate discussions with a partner about safer sex or resist pressures to engage in high-risk sex if they are to assertively set limits in real sexual encounters (Bandura, 1994; St. Lawrence, 1993). For example, in a study of 116 low-income African American adolescents in San Francisco, DiClemente and colleagues (1996) found that self-efficacy regarding the use of condoms predicted the self-report of consistent condom use over a 6-month interval. An information-motivation-behavioral intervention by Fisher, Fisher, Misovich, Kimble, and Malloy (1996) for 521 college students, consisting of three 2-hour sessions, significantly increased participants' perceptions of the effectiveness and ease with which they would be able to use condoms in "real life" situations. Two months following the intervention there was an increase in the self-report of the purchase and use of condoms.

Changing Perceived Peer Norms

Peer norms about sexuality can either reinforce risky behavior or encourage the emergence of safer sex practices (Marin, Gomez, & Hearst, 1993; NIH, 1997). Recent research suggests that subjective peer group norms are one of the strongest predictors of whether or not a person will practice safer sex (DiClemente et al., 1992; Fishbein et al., 1995; Fisher, Misovich, & Fisher, 1992; Lagana & Hayes, 1993; Walter & Vaughan, 1993). One study found that adolescents who perceived peer support for condom use were more than three times more likely to intend to use condoms than their peers (Brown, DiClemente, & Park, 1992). Another project found that improving peer norms for HIV risk-reduction behaviors among college students resulted in a significant increase in safer sex (Fisher et al., 1996). Other projects have successfully targeted peer norms in other ways. A randomized, controlled trial of a community-based intervention delivered in eight weekly sessions involved 76 naturally formed peer groups consisting of 383 African American youths 9 to 15 years of age. Rates of self-reported condom use were significantly higher among intervention than control youths at the 6-month follow-up. Unfortunately, by 12 months postintervention, significant differences no longer appeared between the groups (Stanton et al., 1996). The AIDS Risk Reduction Education and Skills Training (ARREST) program, which trained inner-city African American and Latino adolescents to resist peer pressure, also found an increase in self-reported condom use (Kipke, Boyer, & Hein, 1993).

Peer norms are also a significant influence among those who are HIV infected. A 12-month motivational-skills-based intervention for adolescents living with hemophilia and HIV was designed to improve safer sexual behaviors (Schultz, Brown, & Butler, 1996). The intervention comprised two individual sessions, a peer group activity and an extensive peer group retreat. Condom use and safer, nonpenetrative sexual behaviors increased significantly over the intervention year, as did reports of self-efficacy for safer sexual behaviors (Schultz et al., 1996). Moreover, participants who maintained or improved safer sex behaviors were significantly more likely than their peers to have improvements in their perception of the support of peers for safer sex (odds ratio = 5.4) and to have attended the first peer group activity (odds ratio = 4.7).

Other Considerations

A variety of other factors moderate sexual behavior and are sometimes targeted by programs or influence how the interventions are delivered. These factors include impulsivity, distress, and adverse life experiences (Brooks-Gunn, Boyer, & Hein, 1988; Emans, Brown, Davis, Felice, & Hein, 1991). Impulsivity increases vulnerability to transient and coercive relationships and, coupled with a lack of judgment, may lead to inappropriate risk assessment (Epstein, 1991). Adolescents who experience high levels of psychological distress may lack the confidence needed to use the assertiveness skills required in real-life situations. A reduction of distress may thus be a prerequisite for behavior change. Studies on the behavioral sequelae of abuse and poverty indicate that adverse life experiences are of great importance to HIV prevention efforts, because adolescents in such circumstances are less capable of engaging in protective behaviors and are more prone to engage in sex with multiple partners in unsafe conditions (Allers, Benjack, White, & Rousey, 1993; Brown, Kessel, Lourie, Ford, & Lipsitt, 1997; Lodico & DiClemente, 1994; Zierler et al., 1991).

In summary, group interventions for HIV prevention generally use skill-building techniques and address factors such as adolescents' perceived susceptibility to HIV, attitudes toward condoms, safer sex self-efficacy, and peer norms. The application of motivational interviewing methods to adolescent programs is an important opportunity to further refine prevention efforts. This application requires the integration of motivational techniques that have been used commonly with adults in an individual format with techniques for adolescents in a group setting. Motivational techniques in the group setting may stimulate adolescents to alter their attitudes about condoms or modify their perceptions of peer support for safer behavior. For example, videotaped role playing that is critiqued by the group is a way to address common barriers to protective behaviors (e.g., fear of partner rejection) and to improve adolescents' sense of control in relationships (e.g., improved assertiveness). These alterations may, in turn, be associated with movement from lack of awareness of sexual risk behaviors to practicing safer sexual behaviors. The implications of motivational interviewing in HIV prevention for adolescents are described in the next section.

WHAT MOTIVATIONAL METHODS CAN CONTRIBUTE TO HIV PREVENTION STRATEGIES?

Motivational interviewing methods have been mostly used for substance abuse treatment but also have many techniques and foci in common with sexual behavior change programs for adolescents. The few descriptions of the application of motivational interviewing to HIV prevention research reveal several similarities to and differences from standard HIV prevention models (Prochaska, Redding, Harlow, Rossi, & Velicer, 1994). Motivational interviewing techniques attempt to increase the individual's perception of the risks associated with a particular behavior problem, such as smoking or drinking or drug use, just as HIV prevention programs try to increase participants' perceptions of the risks associated with unsafe sexual behaviors, such as unprotected intercourse. No matter which risk behavior is targeted, the barriers to behavior change (i.e., lack of awareness of a problem, perceived invulnerability, and hedonistic attitudes) must be overcome through a process of self-motivated change. The processes of change arise from the transtheoretical model of behavior change and are associated with progressive movement toward greater action and maintenance of safer behaviors (Prochaska, 1989). These processes are well explicated in the literature dealing with motivational techniques and can be successfully applied to the HIV prevention effort among adolescents (Tober, 1991).

Applications of Motivational Interviewing to Sexual Risk Reduction

The motivation to change a problematic behavior is a significant predictor of protective health behaviors and can be an important factor for choosing and changing sexual risk behaviors (Bell, 1996). Motivations, in turn, are influenced by many factors. For example, the motivations to use condoms consistently are linked to emotions and inclinations concerning sexuality. Consider one study of 559 Dutch men who visit prostitutes that found that certain emotional patterns (such as "the need for sexual variation") were correlated with inconsistent condom use, whereas greater consistency of condom use was correlated with less compulsive attitudes toward visiting prostitutes (De Graaf, Van Zessen, Vanwesenbeeck, Straver, & Visser, 1997). This literature suggests that people engage in sexual behavior according to their own motives and perceived needs, despite the "objective" risks. Indeed, sometimes perceived benefits are more predictive of sexual behavioral change than perceived risks (Parsons, Siegel, & Cousins, 1997; Prochaska, Velicer, et al., 1994).

With adults, the motivational approach has already been particularly useful for changing multiple problematic behavior patterns (e.g., related to drinking, eating, smoking, domestic violence, and sexual risks). Among those at highest risk, behavior patterns often overlap, as is the case of patients with both psychiatric and substance abuse disorders (Smyth, 1996). Because it is nonconfrontational and engaging, the motivational approach is particularly useful for higher risk individuals who may have multiple behavioral problems and who are unprepared to change (Miller, 1998; Smyth, 1996). For example, this approach has been shown to be an effective alternative to the standard behavioral skill training approach in problem drinkers (Heather, Rollnick, Bell, & Richmond, 1996). It has been successfully used by Baker and Dixon (1991) to reduce risky sexual behavior among adult injection drug users and combined with relapse prevention techniques among adult sexual offenders by several researchers (Garland & Dougher, 1991; Kear-Colwell & Pollock, 1997; Marshall & Pithers, 1994; Wormith & Hanson, 1992). Although the application of motivational interviewing to HIV prevention among adolescents has not been reported in the literature, examples from our pilot research are described in the following section on clinical applications.

Collaborative Techniques

There appears to be a natural progression in the process of behavior change. Individuals do not change health-related behaviors in a single act but, rather, go through a series of predictable stages of behavior change that can result in the long-term maintenance of the newly acquired behavior. According to the transtheoretical model, individuals move from being unaware of or unwilling to do anything about the problem (precontemplation) to awareness of the problem (contemplation) to making a commitment to change (preparation) to actually making behavior change (action) and to sustaining the new behavior change for more than 6 months (maintenance) (Prochaska, 1989). An approach that matches the intervention to the individual's readiness for change makes the application of motivational techniques to sexual behavior change in adolescents particularly relevant (Schultz, Brown, & Butler, 1996). Methods that are nonconfrontational may work best to change sexual behaviors of adolescents. A lecturing approach may "turn off" the teenager and may have "many potentially serious consequences for clients at risk for HIV and their significant others" (Baker & Dixon, 1991, p. 294). Didactic approaches have also been found to be of limited effectiveness for sexual behavior change in adolescents. Since 1988, studies have shown that increasing knowledge seldom results in an increase in intention to employ safer sexual behavior, just as teaching abstinence seldom results in decreased sexual behavior (Kirby et al., 1994). In fact, the goal of a motivational approach among sexually active adolescents is not sexual abstinence but rather, taking a harm reduction approach to reduce unprotected sex (Baker & Dixon, 1991).

Brief Delivery

HIV prevention programs that have been shown to be moderately effective have been lengthy group sessions with multiple contacts over many weeks (NIMH Multisite HIV Prevention Trial Group, 1998). Until recently, interventions have shown little impact in fewer than four 1-hour sessions

(Rotheram-Borus, Koopman, Haignere, & Davies, 1991). Briefer programs for adolescents have generally been didactic and limited in skill building, with little evidence of behavioral impact (Kirby et al., 1994). There is, however, some recent evidence that brief, focused interventions may be effective (Boekeloo et al., 1999). Project RESPECT (Kamb et al., 1998) used a short, two-session approach to individualized HIV counseling and demonstrated safer sex behavior change in adolescents by 6 months after the intervention. Such programs are ideal for teens who are only briefly involved in treatment or educational programs outside of the context of school (Tober, 1991). Adolescents often lack access to transportation and other resources for participating in community-wide scheduled events and might not be motivated to attend the multiple health education sessions required by lengthy, "in-depth" interventions.

Brief interventions are well-suited for clinical settings. The collaborative relationship that is needed for a motivational intervention has already been established in the "client–provider" relationship in the primary care medical office (Rollnick & Bell, 1991). Recent research on the development of office-based sexual risk reduction programs for young adolescents indicates that a single brief session may be effective in reducing reported inconsistent condom use at 3-month follow-up (Boekeloo et al., 1999). Although evidence for the efficacy of the motivational approach to HIV prevention among teens is lacking, studies suggest that this approach is useful in busy medical settings for nonsexual behavior problems. For example, at 3-month follow-up, 100 adolescents enrolled in a motivational alcohol reduction study reported less frequent alcohol consumption than their peers who received standard care (Monti et al., 1996; see Monti, Barnett, O'Leary, & Colby, Chapter 5, this volume, for additional details).

CLINICAL APPLICATIONS: STRATEGIES AND CASE STUDIES

Motivational Methods to Increase Perceived Susceptibility

Personalizing the risks of sexual behavior increases contemplation of the possibilities of behavior change and begins the process of such change (Baker & Dixon, 1991). The application of motivational techniques to increasing perceived susceptibility is based foremost on the use of empathic, nonconfrontational techniques, as the following case study illustrates:

> Andy, a 15-year-old white male at an inner-city primary health care clinic, at first refused to talk about sexual experience, but he did want to discuss his family situation. "My mother told me that I don't have

to talk about sex if I don't want to." The interviewer allowed Andy to formulate and voice his own concerns in the context of topics he deemed to be meaningful, and open-ended questions about his family (such as, "What is your relationship with your mom like?") eventually led to discussion of a failed relationship with a girlfriend. Affirming questions about the difficulties concerning his former girlfriend soon led to a discussion of his sexual frustration, experimentation experiences, and fears about having sexual intercourse for the first time. "I wanted to get tested [for HIV], because I wanted to have sex with my girlfriend, but that was last year. . . . " The interviewer: "It sounds like you're still pretty worried about sex."

An empathetic approach sets the groundwork for increasing perceived susceptibility by illustrating the incongruence between the individual's stated desire for safety and actual risky actions. Specific techniques assist clients in reflecting on adverse consequences of sexual risk behavior in order to entertain plans for change. As described in the following, techniques for increasing perceived susceptibility include (1) open-ended questions, (2) affirming language, (3) reframing, and (4) a menu of strategies.

Ask Open-Ended Questions That Cannot Be Answered by a Simple "Yes" or "No"

Open-ended questions allow adolescents to begin talking about the good things in sex and the difficult or worrisome aspects of sex. Such questions also help the interviewer to evaluate the adolescent's motivational stage. For example,

> "Tell me, when did you first start dating?"
> "What can you tell me about your relationship with your boyfriend?"
> "What sexual experiences have you had?"
> "What do you think about condoms, anyway?"

Open-ended questions are also a good strategy for eliciting the discrepancy between stated goals and actual behaviors. For example, Latisha, a 16-year-old African American female patient at a residential psychiatric treatment facility, agreed with the group facilitator that it would be wise to consider using condoms based on her goals for her own life:

IINTERVIEWER: It sounds like the two of you are very close. . . . What do you do to protect yourself?

LATISHA: I'm on the pill . . . and we're careful . . . because I can't get pregnant again. I got too much I want to do. . . .

INTERVIEWER: But there are probably other things you want to protect yourself from. What about getting HIV or another STD? What do you two do to protect yourselves from getting infected?

LATISHA: Nothin', I guess, not any more. . . . In the beginning we used a jimmy, but not lately, 'cause I'm just tryin' to forget about all that. But probably we should use one. . . .

Open-ended questions can prompt the teenager to discuss personal topics and feelings relevant to sexual risk without a sense of failure or fear of giving the wrong answer or a defiant answer. If they are probing yet nonconfrontational, such questions help adolescents better realize the nature of their own contradictions, including both the source of the problem and potential solutions.

Use Affirming Language

An expression of empathy toward the client helps to counteract the self-criticism and stigma often associated with unhealthy behaviors, as illustrated in the following interview. Maria is an 18-year-old Latina woman who was interviewed in a primary care clinic. She discussed her attitudes concerning her boyfriend's casual sexual relationships with other women and its impact on her vulnerability to HIV infection:

MARIA: He used to go around with other girls, but he don't no more. . . .

INTERVIEWER: That must have been really hard to deal with. I can see how you would be worried when he stays out late with his friends.

MARIA: Yeah, he stays out, but he says he don't go around no more. He says he don't.

INTERVIEWER: It sounds like you trust him.

MARIA: Well . . . sometimes I worry if he's safe, if we gonna be safe.

INTERVIEWER: How would you feel about going back to using condoms, just in case?

MARIA: But then he'd be like, I'm accusing him of cheating or like he ain't clean or somethin', like I don't trust him.

INTERVIEWER: You're right, it is really hard for most people to talk about some of this stuff with their partner. Is there a way you could start talking about condoms with Jose without causing a problem between you?

Despite Maria's initial denial of risk, affirmation of her feelings for her boyfriend and validation of her feelings concerning his other sexual relationships facilitated discussion of the barriers associated with the use of condoms.

Reframe Statements

Reframing statements sometimes helps to stimulate the participant's self-assessment and understanding of the problem behavior. Most behaviors have simultaneously healthy and unhealthy aspects. Acknowledging these different motivations and considerations is useful. Sometimes the unhealthy aspect can be highlighted, or *reframed*, in a paradoxical fashion. For example, instead of directly confronting an adolescent girl's minimization of a first risky sexual encounter, the interviewer might say, "It sounds like you can trust your partner a lot." The more the interviewer doubts whether the partner would have lied about his sexual history, the more the interviewer will elicit material concerning the inherent problems of trusting one's partner, his sexual history, and planning for safer sex in the future. Many of these principles are apparent in the following interview with Germaine, a 15-year-old African American male attending a psychiatric day treatment facility. He recently heard that a friend of his had been incarcerated and begins to talk of "risk" in his life:

GERMAINE: I got risk every which way, no matter what I do. Everything I do has risk, even if you go in a car.

INTERVIEWER: You're right. . . . But what are the most risky things that you do?

GERMAINE: I don't know, everything, I guess. Maybe drugs, fights, cops, goin' to [juvenile detention] again. . . . If I get caught, or get beat up . . . killed.

INTERVIEWER: That is a lot. What are some of the risky things you can control?

GERMAINE: I don't know . . . stop rippin' shit off, hanging out on the streets . . . stop doin' so much drugs. . . . That's why I ain't in a gang no more.

INTERVIEWER: That's good. Anything else?

GERMAINE: I dunno. . . .

INTERVIEWER: You were talking before about all your girlfriends. What about that?

GERMAINE: Naw, I ain't too worried about that. They safe. And they all love me.

INTERVIEWER: It doesn't sound like you are too worried about infection, HIV and STDs. I guess they are gonna keep you safe!

GERMAINE: Now we're talkin' about the virus? That ain't going to happen to me. . . . But my uncle's dyin' from the AIDS. And he quit shootin' up years ago! We don't know how he got it.

INTERVIEWER: What's that make you think about?

GERMAINE: What? "Safe sex"? Oh man, I ain't usin' condoms. You want me to use a condom? I mean, I can tell you, "yeah, I use 'em" but I got to really think about it at the moment . . . and I don't want to bother. But I know I should. . . .

INTERVIEWER: That's good to be thinking about it, at least, and to be aware of the problem. That's enough for right now. Maybe you'd like to take home some information. . . .

This conversation with Germaine illustrates the use of open-ended questions, affirming language, and reframing. The interviewer concludes with positive support for Germaine's having simply considered the possibility of change. Indeed, a shift from denial of the need for change to consideration of change is important progress. Too often interviewers reward only the maintenance of consistent safe actions and miss the process involved in changing intentions and inconsistent actions as presented in the transtheoretical model (Prochaska, 1989).

Use a Menu of Strategies

Increasing perceived susceptibility and motivational goal setting are based on the use of a "menu of strategies" or a "cluster of options" (Miller & Rollnick, 1991; Rollnick, Heather, & Bell, 1992). Motivational interviewing strategies are in many ways similar to the processes of change techniques suggested by the transtheoretical model of change (Prochaska, 1989). The two approaches are often combined in the research literature (Annis, Schober, & Kelley, 1996; Botelho & Novak, 1993; DiClemente, 1991; Miller & Rollnick, 1991; Rollnick, Heather, & Bell, 1992). The processes of change are methods used in the transtheoretical model to encourage the client or patient to contemplate a given problem and adopt suitable strategies to change this behavior based on the client's own intentions and behaviors (stage of change). Such processes can be applied to sex behavior change and include consciousness raising (increasing awareness of risky behaviors), dramatic relief (emotional expression about relevant behaviors), self-reevaluation (reappraising one's behavior and oneself in light of that behavior), counterconditioning (substituting adaptive and positive behaviors for maladaptive and problem ones), stimulus control (controlling the environment so that problem behaviors are encountered less often), and reinforcement management (reinforcing positive behaviors while extinguishing negative ones). These processes are described in more detail in the following paragraphs. In general, processes such as consciousness raising and self-reevaluation increase perceived susceptibility and are appropriate for clients not yet considering a change in behavior (the precontemplation stage). In contrast, processes of change such as stimulus control and reinforcement are more useful for those who begin to enact the safe behavior, as described in the following case vignettes.

Dawn, a 16-year-old white mother, was interviewed in the primary care setting. During an earlier discussion, Dawn had expressed no awareness of risk for HIV. However, contrasting HIV risk with her hopes for a long life as a mother and her desire to maintain the health of her new baby helped to stimulate contemplation of sexual risk:

INTERVIEWER: You've worked so hard to give your baby everything. He's so big!

DAWN: I do everything for him, first, before anyone, even me.

INTERVIEWER: But if you take better care of yourself, he's gonna benefit too, because you'll be around longer to take care of him and watch him grow up. I mean if you get AIDS from having unprotected sex, who will take care of him?

DAWN: Oh no! I'm the *only* one he's got. I'll always be here for him. I'll make sure of that!

The discussion with Dawn is an example of the use of dramatic relief, providing the opportunity for her to express emotions about her behaviors and personal situation. Using dramatic relief, such as asking Dawn how she would feel if she could no longer care for her baby or transmitted HIV to a future child, is likely to increase perceived susceptibility to the consequences of HIV infection. Environmental reevaluation is a process that facilitates re-appraisal of the impact of one's behavior on others, as illustrated in this brief interaction. This dialogue helped Dawn to express and identify the emotions related to her sexual risk behavior and to assess the potential impact on her child. The brief opportunity to express the need to care for her baby and to avoid situations that could imperil her family was an important stimulus to the initiation of behavior change. Other processes of change that may be appropriate for individuals in denial or precontemplation about risk behaviors include consciousness raising (e.g., "What can happen to people who have sex that isn't safe?"), and self-reevaluation (e.g., "How would you feel about yourself if you were HIV-infected?"). Some individuals who are not yet contemplating a change in risk behavior find it useful to examine the advantages of safer behavior. The perceived disadvantages of safer sex ("condoms are a hassle to remember to have around") are also useful to explore as individuals become prepared to begin to enact safe behaviors. In this interview with Amanda, a Hispanic teenage mother in the STD clinic, self-reevaluation and the affirmation of prior success are employed in order to increase perceived self-efficacy for condom negotiation:

INTERVIEWER: How do you feel about using condoms?

AMANDA: I don't need to, because I'm on the pill anyway. . . .

INTERVIEWER: But you already said that you knew that the pill won't protect you from HIV and getting AIDS. What do you think about protecting yourself with condoms?

AMANDA: I used to use them all the time, actually, but I stopped once I went on the pill, almost a year ago.

INTERVIEWER: How do you feel about yourself, that you are not using condoms?

AMANDA: I know I should use 'em, though, especially with my boyfriend now. I hate to admit it, but you never know where he's been. I mean he loves me, but he's a player. He used to be a player.

INTERVIEWER: So he was a player?

AMANDA: I do worry. I try not to, but I know it happens.

INTERVIEWER: Well, do you think you could use a condom with him, if you wanted to?

AMANDA: Yeah, I know I could. I'm just out of practice. It's been a while.

INTERVIEWER: Okay, no problem. That's great that you've used them before. It will make it a lot easier to use them again. Tell me how you were able to do it before. . . .

Goal Setting

Improved self-esteem and self-efficacy can occur in the context of motivational interviewing programs for adolescents (Tober, 1991). "A general goal of motivational interviewing is to increase the client's perceptions of his or her capability to cope with obstacles and to succeed in change" (Miller & Rollnick, 1991, p. 61). Once motivation is increased (the preparation stage), then collaborative goal setting assists in making the process of change real. The objectives in goal setting are to (1) help to identify and remove barriers to change, (2) elicit a decisional balance of perceived costs and rewards of change, (3) increase perceived choices, and (4) set realistic and attainable goals. Some of the techniques that are used to achieve these objectives include reviewing of one's personal risk assessment, discussing discrepancies between stated goals and actions, tailoring strategies of change for the individual or group, and rewarding any positive change.

Review Personal Risk Assessment

The process of sexual behavior change using motivational methods begins with reviewing the client's concerns about risk. This information is used to segue to options and strategies for change. The interviewer may have already asked about the individual's general health, lifestyle, and stresses and discussed common risks (e.g., diet, smoking, and alcohol and drug use) with the client. The purpose of reviewing the client's risk assessment is thus to ask about previously stated concerns, to provide additional information as needed, and to provide the opportunity to voice new concerns in order to rethink strategies for change. Often individuals perceive that behaviors other than risky sexual behaviors are also in need of change and may recognize the relationships between these target behaviors. For example, adolescents are commonly aware that they have more unprotected sex during alcohol and drug use or that they smoke more cigarettes when they are drinking alcohol. Thus reviewing the context of risk behavior is an important aspect of the assessment of personal risk. The interviewer may then summarize the client's current situation until both the client and interviewer are satisfied with the summary.

Identify Discrepancy

Discrepancy may be identified to increase perceived susceptibility to a problem, as discussed previously, but may also be useful to help set goals and reevaluate strategies for changing the problem. Intentions for subsequent safe behavior may be increased by encouraging the adolescent to recognize the discrepancy between the stated goals and ongoing risk behaviors (e.g., refraining from drug use but at the same time engaging in unprotected intercourse). For example, the interviewer might say, "Your girlfriend means a lot to you. On the one hand, you've stopped getting high and drinking, but, on the other hand, you haven't been using condoms." Explication of the contradictory behaviors is a natural prompt for discussing the facilitators and barriers of safer sexual behavior in order to devise a better plan for positive change. This technique has been applied to interventions among adolescent mothers who have used condoms consistently but then stopped using condoms in order to get pregnant: "What were some of the reasons you used condoms before you wanted to get pregnant?" "Now that you don't want to get pregnant, what's stopping you from using condoms, if you know that it's a lot more risky without them?"

Tailor Change Strategies

Use the processes of change that are appropriate for those ready to begin or to maintain actions of safe behavior. Examples of strategies that encourage action and help to maintain positive behavior change include stimulus control, counterconditioning, helping relationships, reinforcement management, and social liberation. In the case of each strategy, however, the plan for change must be acceptable to the client (Miller & Rollnick, 1991). The following role play with Amanda is an example of self-liberation to facilitate movement from the preparation stage to the action stage. It demonstrates the importance of tailoring behavior change strategies to the needs of individual clients:

INTERVIEWER: What's going to happen when you try to use condoms next time you have sex with your boyfriend?

AMANDA: I don't know, because my boyfriend hates condoms. He thinks that it's too much trouble to use them anyway, especially if I'm on the pill.

INTERVIEWER: When did you start with your boyfriend again, 3 months ago?

AMANDA: Yeah. . . . I know that it's probably risky. He'd probably use them if I brought one out, 'cause he knows that I know that he's been with other girls. . . . I tried once, with another boy, and it wasn't a big deal.

INTERVIEWER: How did you make it not such a big deal?

AMANDA: He was just different. He didn't have a problem with condoms.

INTERVIEWER: Let's try to pretend you're talking to your boyfriend now and telling him that you want to use a condom. How could you make it fun, you know, "sexy"?

AMANDA: Oh, you mean like those flavored ones, all kinds of colors?

INTERVIEWER: As long as they're made from latex.

AMANDA: I could say, "Baby, you know how much I want to be with you. But this time I got a little surprise. . . . It might tickle a bit, but I think you're gonna like it!"

INTERVIEWER: But your boyfriend might say, "What you got a condom for?"

AMANDA: "I just want to be extra careful about not being risky, and it's gonna make you last even longer, just for me. . . . C'mon now. . . . "

INTERVIEWER: Great role play! You made yourself clear but also had a lot of fun.

It is important that the processes of change employed by the interviewer can be realistically applied within the life of the client. The purpose of the interaction with Amanda was to promote "self-liberation," her own belief in her ability to change and in her commitment to follow through with her goals. By reaffirming prior successes and small positive changes, the interviewer helps to increase the client's self-efficacy for condom negotiation and use. At the same time, some clients who feel committed to changing their behaviors may continue to encounter barriers to change and appear to lack such small positive changes. For them, "stimulus control" (so that stimuli leading to the problem are less likely) and "reinforcement management" (to promote positive behaviors and discourage negative actions) may be more important processes of change.

Reward Positive Change

Another important aspect of goal setting is to give personal feedback in a way that expresses optimism about any current changes in the client's life. Positive change, no matter how small, should be encouraged and reinforced, as illustrated in the following interview with Dan, an adolescent who only 2 years ago arrived to the United States with his parents from the Cape Verde Islands:

DAN: It's not that big a deal in my family, anyway. We don't talk about girls and sex, or condoms.

INTERVIEWER: How did you learn about condoms then?

DAN: They talk about it at school, in health class, some of the guys.

INTERVIEWER: Where did you learn the most?

DAN: School taught me a lot . . . but it sounded weird.

INTERVIEWER: You had some HIV education in health class at school?

DAN: Yeah, "only use latex, lubricated latex condoms."

INTERVIEWER: I'm impressed that you remember what they said!

DAN: They even passed one around to touch. Gross. I don't think I'd use one, even if I was having sex.

INTERVIEWER: At least you've touched one. A lot of kids have never even seen a condom.

DAN: They made us put them on these things, you know like the guy, like a banana. . . . It was so stupid, but I did it anyway. . . . I had to go through the whole thing for the whole class. But I won some race and got a prize.

INTERVIEWER: That's not bad. So you actually know how to use a condom. You're way ahead . . . for when you do start having sex.

The accomplishments of the individual can be affirmed while at the same time facilitating discussion of the next step toward behavior change, as illustrated in the following interview. Latisha was open about having unprotected intercourse with multiple partners but denied that there were any alternatives: "Boys don't want to have sex with a condom. They'll just get somebody else." The interviewer affirmed her need for intimacy and the importance of having a boyfriend but also emphasized the importance of being safe and using a condom:

INTERVIEWER: You also said that you're afraid of getting HIV, and that you want to start using condoms.

LATISHA: Yeah, I know that I should, but it ain't that easy.

INTERVIEWER: I know that your boyfriend is very important to you. I just wonder if there is a way to get him to use a condom.

LATISHA: He's used them before, when he got 'em.

INTERVIEWER: So if you had them around, would you be able to use them with him?

LATISHA: If I really wanted him to. He'd probably use it.

INTERVIEWER: All you'd have to do is ask him to use a condom, and he'd do it?

LATISHA: Well, I'd have to be nice about it, so he don't think I'm sayin' he's dirty or go around anymore. I'd have to be nice.

INTERVIEWER: It sounds like you know what he would be sensitive about. What could you say to make it sound nice?

By examining motivation for behavior change, the interviewer is able to focus on a strategy that matches the client's degree of readiness for change. In summary, strategies that elicit reappraisal of motivation and increase perceived susceptibility through examination of the discrepancies between goals and behaviors are useful with clients who are less ready for change. For those who express desire to initiate behavioral change or who have already attempted change, examination of the roadblocks to change and practicing specific techniques (i.e., role playing, assertiveness training, etc.) are the more useful strategies.

STRENGTHS AND LIMITATIONS OF THE MOTIVATIONAL APPROACH TO SEXUAL BEHAVIOR CHANGE

As applied to changing adolescent sexual behavior, motivational interviewing offers discrete intervention strategies that are appropriate for teenagers from different backgrounds and that may be useful in various settings. Motivational interviewing has generally been described with adults (Kadden, 1995) and usually occurs individually, in contrast to HIV prevention with teens, which usually occurs in groups (NIMH Multisite HIV Prevention Trial Group, 1998). Thus some motivational interviewing strategies may need to be adapted for groups. In addition, as described subsequently, specific developmental, cultural, and psychological considerations must also be taken into account in order to adapt motivational approaches to clinical care.

The Group Format

Motivational interviewing has been successful when used in individual interviews. A one-on-one format allows the interviewer to take an in-depth personal approach to the barriers and processes of change of the client. However, adolescent sexual risk prevention programs are largely delivered in the peer group setting (Wren et al., 1997). Therefore, adaptations of motivational methods for the group setting need to be further designed and tested. Motivational techniques have been used in combination with cognitive–behavioral skills training in groups for problem behaviors such as adolescent eating disorders and adult alcohol abuse (Kadden, 1995; Long & Hollin, 1995). However, additional data concerning the use of motivational interviewing methods in the group setting are needed. Among adolescents, the group context may be an important factor in the application of motivational interviewing techniques. Adolescents may be more motivated to change when they hear others discussing a personal behavior plan. In addition, a public review of their plans may be a precipitator of change. For example, role playing and skill building are important components of the application of motivational models and are particularly well suited to groups. It is thought that a group format can increase self-efficacy as a result of exposure to examples of successful change by other peers and by using peer modeling of preventive behaviors (Miller & Rollnick, 1991). The best composition of groups for sexual behavior change is unclear, but small, same-sex groups of closely knit ethnic affiliation have been found to be one effective format for delivery of HIV prevention programs in the inner city (Stanton, Li, et al., 1996).

The utility of motivational interviewing methods as compared with social learning theory in the adolescent group context is unknown. Standard

HIV prevention groups generally attempt to teach knowledge about HIV, to increase perceived susceptibility to HIV, and to provide a context for practicing new social skills among peers. However, these groups have shown only limited success in personalizing this information and these skills in order to increase motivation toward positive behavior change (Lagana & Hayes, 1993). Motivational techniques for matching intervention strategies to clients' needs may increase perceived susceptibility and intentions to change. Moreover, a culturally relevant group format that incorporates developmental and psychological concerns may provide an optimal context for HIV prevention.

Developmental Considerations

HIV/AIDS information and activities need to be developmentally appropriate if they are to be effective (Osborne, Kistner, & Helgemo, 1993; Siegel, 1993). For example, some adolescents will lack basic factual information or understanding of the common terminology for risk behaviors, symptomatology, and testing (Flaskerud & Uman, 1993; Obeidallah et al., 1993). Other adolescents may lack personal awareness of vulnerability to HIV or relevant sexual experience. Generally, adolescents are less personally aware of the consequences of their risk behaviors due to the short history of their behavior (Tober, 1991; Trigwell, Grant, & House, 1997). Teenagers' understanding of the concepts relevant to HIV is a reflection of their general conceptual abilities, but it may be overwhelmed by anxiety about sexuality (Brown, DiClemente, & Beausoleil, 1992; Schonfeld, Johnson, Perrin, O'Hare, Cicchetti, 1993). One of the advantages of the application of motivational techniques to HIV prevention programs for adolescents is that intervention materials may be tailored to all age levels, specifically according to the appropriate developmental and conceptual levels. At the same time, this flexibility requires a wide range of motivational materials, scripted probes, and behavior change strategies that are applicable to adolescents across the developmental spectrum.

The use of developmentally appropriate materials for HIV prevention programs without a specific motivational component has been found to be effective. For example, one longitudinal study of 383 African American adolescents by Stanton, Li, and colleagues (1996) found that using developmentally appropriate activities that tailored group discussions, videos, games, role playing, storytelling, and arts and crafts according to the ages and ethnic orientations of participants increased the use of oral contraceptives and condoms by 30%. There are numerous reports of the efficacy of developmentally and culturally tailored interventions that target a change in sexual risk behavior or promote abstinence (Kim et al., 1997; Stanton, Kim, et al., 1996). Few intervention projects, however, examine the precursors of safer sex behaviors. Among younger, not yet sexually active, adolescents, it may be advantageous to target high-risk situations rather than condom use and sexual intercourse alone (Paikoff, 1995). Motivation to be safe in other domains may then carry over to affect condom self-efficacy when that behavior is relevant. Also, the motivators for learning to use condoms may be different if the adolescent is sexually naive rather than experienced with unprotected intercourse, just as motivators are different for prevention of smoking rather than smoking cessation. Motivators may also differ at each developmental stage. For example, younger adolescents are more influenced by their families, as opposed to older teens, who are more influenced by their peers (Resnick et al., 1997).

In summary, among adolescents who may lack sexual experience and do not perceive any threat of sexual risk behaviors or vulnerability to HIV infection, prevention strategies must be adapted to include developmentally appropriate themes and situations. One of the strengths of the motivational interviewing model, in both the individual and group formats, is that it provides the opportunity to tailor educational information, role playing, and standard skill-building exercises according to the unique needs of specific clients and their developmental abilities and issues.

Cultural Considerations

Another important predictor of HIV prevention effectiveness is the cultural relevance of the intervention (DiClemente & Wingood, 1995; Janz et al., 1996; NIH, 2000). Adolescents' own personal experience of sexuality (including, for example, perceptions of privacy, gender roles and sexual orientation, and use of alcohol and drugs during sex), as well as the involvement of families and peers, must be taken into account in order to make intervention content culturally sensitive (Lagana & Hayes, 1993; Rotheram-Borus et al., 1991; Weeks, Schensul, Williams, Singer, & Grier, 1995). For example, in some urban Latino populations in the United States, the woman's expression of submissiveness during sexual negotiation and decision making is a validation of femininity and of the man's masculinity, which may undermine these women's abilities to engage in HIV-preventive behaviors (Amaro, 1995; Cochran & Mays, 1989; Sobo, 1993). Another example is that white youths tend to have greater exposure to information about AIDS and condoms, whereas Latino youths receive more information about intravenous drug use as a route of transmission (Hofstetter et al., 1995). In order to increase Latino youths' perceived sense of susceptibility to HIV from sexual behaviors, more emphasis must be placed on delivery of culturally relevant information about HIV transmission among young heterosexuals. In addition, further information on intravenous drug use may also be appropriate for white youths.

Although ethnic culture may determine some factors, it may not be the major factor in shaping attitudes for all adolescents. For some teens, the context of a "minority, inner-city" culture is a more significant determinant of attitudes than their specific ethnic background. Conditions stemming from poverty may underlie high-risk behaviors such as sex for money, cocaine addiction, and intravenous drug use (Connors, 1992). These contextual situations, rather than ethnic affiliation, cut across urban culture groups and may shape risk behavior (Koniak-Griffin, Nyamathi, Vasquez, & Russo, 1994). By incorporating social and cultural considerations into the design and delivery of behavior change programs, the culturally sensitive motivational intervention provides a model that can offer, in the words of Resnicow, Royce, Vaughan, Orlandi, and Smith (1997), "strategies that appeal to a range of individual needs and preferences" (p. 380).

Psychological Factors

In addition to the influence of developmental and cultural factors, sexual motivation is shaped by psychological factors (Hill & Preston, 1996). For example, in a cross-sectional, longitudinal study of 1,167 10th- and 11th-grade students from suburban high schools, Tubman, Windle, and Windle (1996) found that repeated unprotected intercourse with multiple partners was associated with higher levels of childhood behavior problems, earlier onset of antisocial behaviors, and substance use. Findings such as these suggest that sexual risk behavior may sometimes be related to earlier trauma, depression, and conduct problems (Brown, Danovsky, Lourie, DiClemente, & Ponton, 1997). Psychological distress and dysfunction may increase sexual risk behaviors due to a lack of regard for safety, greater impulsivity, and peer norms that reinforce risk. These factors have been illustrated most clearly among adolescents in intensive psychiatric treatment, among whom rates of sexual risk behaviors are far greater than among adolescents who attend public schools (Brown, Kessel, et al., 1997; DiClemente & Ponton, 1993; Stiffman, Dore, Earls, & Cunningham, 1992).

Those at greatest risk for exposure to HIV are those with the greatest levels of distress and the least social support, education, socioeconomic opportunity, and access to health care services (Rotheram-Borus et al., 1991). Therefore, simply "giving people information and changing their perception of the seriousness of their risk may not be a particularly effective intervention. . . . Interventions do not appear to be effective if there is no change in the underlying causes that move people to engage in the risk in the first place" (Bell, 1996, p. 52). The motivational approach may not target depression and impulsivity, although it does challenge the maladaptive attitudes and cognitions often associated with psychological distress. For example, processes of change such as self-liberation, helping relationships, and stimulus control are specifically directed at improving one's confidence in one's ability to make positive changes, at increasing support from others for behavior change, and at influencing the environment so that negative stimuli are decreased. One program found that interventions that successfully induced changes in the psychosocial domains of emotional well-being and cognitive functioning among 454 chronic drug users showed the greatest promise to produce changes in AIDS risk behaviors (Bell, 1996).

A study of HIV-infected adolescents with hemophilia underscores the important relationship between distress and sexual risk behavior (Brown, Schultz, & Gragg, 1995). The intervention aimed to increase motivation for and participation in safer sexual behaviors. It found that increasing emotional distress (unrelated to physical illness) over the year-long project period was associated with greater sexual risk behavior. In summary, there is ample evidence to suggest that psychological distress and dysfunction are important influences on sexual behavior. It is clear that motivational interviewing methods can address the attitudes and motivators of individual clients and thus may target each person's unique concerns, even if they are based on maladaptive and distorted cognitive processes. It has yet to be shown whether motivational interviewing methods can improve sex risk behaviors among adolescents with rigid or fixed emotional disturbances, such as mood, anxiety, and personality disorders.

SUMMARY

HIV prevention programs for adolescents based on social learning theory have shown moderate efficacy for changing high-risk sexual behaviors by focusing on HIV-related personalized knowledge, attitudes, peer norms, condom self-efficacy, and communication skills. Most of the published data, however, are based on multisession, intensive group programs that require considerable time commitments from both interviewers and participants. Recently, a few studies that have used brief, individualized interview methods in adolescent HIV prevention have also shown efficacy in changing HIV-related attitudes and behaviors. Motivational interviewing techniques are currently used in various risk behavior programs for both adolescents and adults and present valuable tools for application to adolescent HIV prevention efforts, in both individual and group settings. However, both the advantages and limitations of integrating motivational methods and the social learning approach must be delineated and tested in order to pursue this new direction for HIV prevention research.

Considerations for applying motivational methods to sexual risk behavior change in adolescents include developmental and cultural differences, psychological factors, group versus individual format, and issues specifically related to adolescent sexuality. Case studies of interviews and role plays with teenagers in the primary care, STD clinic, and psychiatric facilities illustrate the application of motivational techniques and the use of discrete processes of change to motivate progress along the stages of sexual behavior change. These case studies reveal a repertoire of strategies for applying motivational methods to sexual behavior change for adolescents from diverse cultural backgrounds. These strategies should be useful for both clinicians and researchers attempting to integrate individual and group methods in settings of brief contact with adolescents in an effort to reduce sexual risk behavior and the transmission of HIV.

REFERENCES

Allers, C., Benjack, K., White, J., & Rousey, J. (1993). HIV vulnerability and the adult survivor of childhood sexual abuse. *Child Abuse and Neglect, 17*, 291–298.

Amaro, H. (1995). Love, sex, and power: Considering women's realities in HIV prevention. *American Psychologist, 50*, 437–447.

Annis, H., Schober, R., & Kelley, E. (1996). Matching addiction outpatient counseling to client readiness for change: The role of structured relapse prevention counseling. *Experimental and Clinical Psychopharmacology, 4*, 37–45.

Ashery, R., Wild, J., Zhao, Z., Rosenshine, N., & Young, P. (1997). The wheel project: Women helping to empower and enhance lives. *Journal of Substance Abuse Treatment, 14*, 113–121.

Baker, A., & Dixon, J. (1991). Motivational interviewing for HIV risk reduction. In W. R. Miller & S. Rollnick (Eds.), *Motivational interviewing: Preparing people to change addictive behavior* (pp. 293–302). New York: Guilford Press.

Bandura, A. (1986). *Social foundations of thought and action: A social cognitive theory.* Englewood Cliffs, NJ: Prentice-Hall.

Bandura, A. (1994). Social cognitive theory and exercise of control over HIV infection. In R. J. DiClemente (Ed.), *Preventing AIDS: Theories and methods of behavioral interventions. AIDS Prevention and Mental Health* (pp. 25–59). New York: Plenum Press.

Bell, D. (1996). The effect of psychosocial domains on AIDS risk behaviors. *Drugs and Society, 9*, 37–55.

Boekeloo, B. O., Schamus, L. A., Simmens, S. J., Cheng, T. L., O'Connor, K., & D'Angelo, L. J. (1999). A STD/HIV prevention trial among adolescents in managed care. *Pediatrics, 103*, 107–115.

Botelho, R., & Novak, S. (1993). Dealing with substance misuse, abuse, and dependency. *Primary Care, 20*, 51–70.

Brooks-Gunn, J., Boyer, C., & Hein, K. (1988). Preventing HIV infection and AIDS in children and adolescents: Behavioral research and intervention strategies. *American Psychologist, 43*, 958–964.

Brown, L., Danovsky, M., Lourie, K., DiClemente, R., & Ponton, L. (1997). Adolescents with psychiatric disorders and risk of HIV: A review of the literature. *Journal of the American Academy of Child and Adolescent Psychiatry, 36*, 1609–1617.

Brown, L., DiClemente, R., & Beausoleil, N. (1992). Comparison of HIV-related knowledge, attitudes, intentions and behaviors among sexually active and abstinent young adolescents. *Journal of Adolescent Health, 13,* 140–145.

Brown, L., DiClemente, R., & Park, T. (1992). Predictors of condom use in sexually active adolescents. *Journal of Adolescent Health, 13,* 651–657.

Brown, L., DiClemente, R., & Reynolds, L. (1991). HIV prevention for adolescents: Utility of the health belief model. *AIDS Education and Prevention, 3,* 50–59.

Brown, L., Kessel, S., Lourie, K., Ford, H., & Lipsitt, L. (1997). The influence of sexual abuse on AIDS-related attitudes and behaviors in psychiatrically hospitalized adolescents. *Journal of the American Academy of Child and Adolescent Psychiatry, 36,* 316–322.

Brown, L. K., Schultz, J., & Gragg, R. (1995). HIV-infected adolescents with hemophilia: Adaptation and coping. *Pediatrics, 96,* 459–463.

Catania, J., Coates, T., Kegeles, S., Ekstrand, M., Guydish, J., & Bye, L. (1989). Implications of the AIDS risk-reduction model for the gay community: The importance of perceived sexual enjoyment and help-seeking behaviors. In V. Mays (Ed.), *Primary prevention of AIDS: Psychological approaches* (pp. 242–261). Newbury Park, CA: Sage.

Cochran, S. D., & Mays, V. M. (1989). Women and AIDS-related concerns: Roles for psychologists in helping the worried well. *American Psychologist, 44,* 529–535.

Coker, A. L., Richter, D. L., Valois, R. F., McKeown, R. E., Garrison, C. Z., & Vincent, M. L. (1994). Correlates and consequences of early initiation of sexual intercourse. *Journal of School Health, 64,* 372–377.

Connors, M. (1992). Risk perception, risk taking and risk management among intravenous drug users: Implications for AIDS prevention. *Social Science and Medicine, 34,* 591–601.

De Graaf, R., Van Zessen, G., Vanwesenbeeck, I., Straver, C., & Visser, J. (1997). Condom use by Dutch men with commercial heterosexual contacts: Determinants and considerations. *AIDS Education and Prevention, 9,* 411–423.

DiClemente, C. C. (1991). Motivational interviewing and the stages of change. In W. R. Miller & S. Rollnick (Eds.), *Motivational interviewing: Preparing people to change addictive behavior* (pp. 191–202). New York: Guilford Press.

DiClemente, R., Durbin, M., Siegel, D., Krasnovsky, F., Lazarus, N., & Comacho, T. (1992). Determinants of condom use among junior high school students in a minority, inner-city school district. *Pediatrics, 89,* 197–202.

DiClemente, R., Lodico, M., Grinstead, O., Harper, G., Rickman, R., Evans, P., & Coates, T. (1996). African-American adolescents residing in high-risk urban environments do use condoms: Correlates and predictors of condom use among adolescents in public housing developments. *Pediatrics, 98,* 269–278.

DiClemente, R. J., & Ponton, L. E. (1993). HIV-related risk behaviors among psychiatrically hospitalized adolescents and school-based adolescents. *American Journal of Psychiatry, 150,* 324–325.

DiClemente, R., & Wingood, G. (1995). A randomized controlled trial of an HIV sexual risk-reduction intervention for young African-American women. *Journal of the American Medical Association, 274,* 1271–1276.

Ellen, J., Boyer, C., Tschann, J., & Shafer, M. (1996). Adolescents' perceived risk for STDs and HIV infection. *Journal of Adolescent Health, 18,* 177–181.

Emans, S. J., Brown, R. T., Davis, A., Felice, M., & Hein, K. (1991). Society for adolescent medicine position paper on reproductive health care for adolescents. *Journal of Adolescent Health, 12,* 649–661.

Epstein, S. (1991). Impulse control and self-destructive behavior. In L. P. Lipsitt & L. L. Mitnick (Eds.), *Self-regulatory behavior and risk taking: Causes and consequences* (pp. 273–284). Norwood, NJ: Ablex.

Fishbein, M. (1990). AIDS and behavior change: An analysis based on the theory of reasoned action. *Interamerican Journal of Psychology, 24,* 37–56.

Fishbein, M., Trafimow, D., Middlestadt, S., Helquist, M., Frances, C., & Eustice, M. (1995). Using an AIDS KABP survey to identify determinants of condom use among sexually active adults from St. Vincent and the Grenadines. *Journal of Applied Social Psychology, 25,* 1–20.

Fisher, J., Fisher, W., Misovich, S., Kimble, D., & Malloy, T. (1996). Changing AIDS risk behavior: Effects of an intervention emphasizing AIDS risk reduction information, motivation, and behavioral skills in a college student population. *Health Psychology, 15,* 114–123.

Fisher, J., Misovich, S., & Fisher, W. (1992). Impact of perceived social norms on adolescents' AIDS-risk behavior and prevention. In R. J. DiClemente (Ed.), *Adolescents and AIDS: A generation in jeopardy* (pp. 117–136). Newbury Park, CA: Sage.

Flaskerud, J., & Uman, G. (1993). Directions for AIDS education for Hispanic women based on analyses of survey findings. *Public Health Reports, 108*(3), 298–304.

Garland, R. J., & Dougher, M. J. (1991). Motivational intervention in the treatment of sex offenders. In W. R. Miller & S. Rollnick *Motivational interviewing: Preparing people to change addictive behavior* (pp. 303–313). New York: Guilford Press.

Guttmacher, S., Lieberman, L., Ward, D., Freudenberg, N., Radosh, A., & Des Jarlais, D. (1997). Condom availability in New York City public high schools: Relationships to condom use and sexual behavior. *American Journal of Public Health, 87,* 1427–1433.

Haignere, C. S., Gold, R., & McDanel, H. J. (1999). Adolescent abstinence and condom use: Are we sure we are really teaching what is safe? *Health Education and Behavior, 26,* 43–54.

Heather, N., Rollnick, S., Bell, A., & Richmond, R. (1996). Effects of brief counseling among male heavy drinkers identified on general hospital wards. *Drug and Alcohol Review, 15,* 29–38.

Hill, C., & Preston, L. (1996). Individual differences in the experience of sexual motivation: Theory and measurement of dispositional sexual motives. *Journal of Sex Research, 33,* 27–45.

Hofstetter, C., Hovell, M., Myers, C., Blumberg, E., Sipan, C., Yuasa, T., & Kreitner, S. (1995). Patterns of communication about AIDS among Hispanic and Anglo adolescents. *American Journal of Preventive Medicine, 11,* 231–237.

Irwin, C. E., & Millstein, S. (1997). Risk-taking behavior in adolescents: The paradigm. *Annals of the New York Academy of Sciences, 28,* 1–35.

Janz, N. K., Zimmerman, M. A., Wren, P. A., Israel, B. A., Freudenberg, N., & Carter, R. J. (1996). Evaluation of 37 AIDS prevention projects: Successful approaches and barriers to program effectiveness. *Health Education Quarterly, 23,* 80–97.

Jemmott, J., Jemmott, L., & Fong, G. (1992). Reductions in HIV risk-associated sexual behaviors among black male adolescents: Effects of an AIDS prevention intervention. *American Journal of Public Health, 82,* 372–377.

Kadden, R. (1995). Cognitive-behavioral approaches to alcoholism treatment. *Alcohol Health and Research World, 18,* 279–286.

Kalichman, S., Adair, V., Samlai, A., & Weir, S. (1995). The perceived social context of AIDS: A study of inner-city sexually transmitted disease patients. *Journal of AIDS Education and Prevention, 7,* 298–307.

Kalichman, S., Carey, M., & Johnson, B. (1996). Prevention of sexually transmitted HIV infection: A meta-analytic review of the behavioral outcome literature. *Annals of Behavioral Medicine, 18,* 6–15.

Kamb, M., Fishbein, M., Douglas, J., Rhodes, F., Rogers, J., Bolan, G., Zenilman, J., Hoxworth, T., Malotte, K., Iatesta, M., Kent, C., Lentz, A., Graziano, S., Byers, R., & Peterman, T. (1998). Efficacy of risk-reduction counseling to prevent human immunodeficiency virus and sexually transmitted diseases. *Journal of the American Medical Association, 280,* 161–167.

Kann, L., Kinchen, S. A., Williams, B. I., Ross, J. G., Lowry, R., Hill, C. V., Grunbaum, J. A., Blumson, P. S., Collins, J. L., & Kolbe, L. J. (1998). Youth Risk Behavior Surveillance—United States, 1997. *Journal of School Health, 68,* 355–369.

Kear-Colwell, J., & Pollock, P. (1997). Motivation or confrontation: Which approach to the child sex offender? *Criminal Justice and Behavior, 24,* 20–33.

Kim, N., Stanton, B., Li, X., Dickersin, K., & Galbraith, J. (1997). Effectiveness of the 40 adolescent AIDS-risk reduction intervention: A quantitative review. *Journal of Adolescent Health, 20,* 204–215.

Kipke, M., Boyer, C., & Hein, K. (1993). An evaluation of an AIDS risk reduction education and skills training (ARREST) program. *Journal of Adolescent Health, 14,* 533–539.

Kirby, D., Short, L., Collins, J., Rugg, D., Kolbe, L., Howard, M., Miller, B., Sonenstein, F., & Zabin, L. (1994). School-based programs to reduce sexual risk behaviors: A review of effectiveness. *Public Health Reports, 109,* 334–360.

Koniak-Griffin, D., Nyamathi, A., Vasquez, R., & Russo, A. (1994). Risk-taking behaviors and AIDS knowledge: Experiences and beliefs of minority adolescent mothers. *Health Education Research, 9,* 449–463.

Lagana, L., & Hayes, D. (1993). Contraceptive health programs for adolescents: A critical review. *Adolescence, 28,* 348–359.

Levy, S. R., Perhats, C., Weeks, K., Handler, A. S., Zhu, C., & Flay, B. R. (1995). Impact of a school-based AIDS prevention program on risk and protective behavior for newly sexually active students. *Journal of School Health, 65,* 145–151.

Lodico, M., & DiClemente, R. (1994). The association between childhood sexual abuse and prevalence of HIV-related risk behaviors. *Clinical Pediatrics, 35,* 498–502.

Long, C., & Hollin, C. (1995). Assessment and management of eating disordered patients who overexercise: A four-year follow-up of six single case studies. *Journal of Mental Health (UK), 4,* 309–316.

Marin, B., Gomez, C., & Hearst, N. (1993). Multiple heterosexual partners and condom use among Hispanics and non-Hispanic whites. *Family Planning Perspectives, 25,* 170–174.

Marshall, W., & Pithers, W. (1994). A reconsideration of treatment outcome with sex offenders. *Criminal Justice and Behavior, 21*, 10–27.

McKusick, L., Coates, T., Morin, S., Pollack, L., & Hoff, C. (1990). Longitudinal predictors of reductions in unprotected anal intercourse among gay men in San Francisco: The AIDS Behavioral Research Project. *American Journal of Public Health, 80*, 978–983.

Miller, W. (1998). Enhancing motivation for change. In W. Miller & N. Heather (Eds.), *Treating addictive behaviors: Applied clinical psychology* (2nd ed., pp. 121–132). New York: Plenum Press.

Miller, W. R., & Rollnick, S. (1991). *Motivational interviewing: Preparing people to change addictive behavior.* New York: Guilford Press.

Monti, P., Colby, S., Spirito, A., Myers, M., Rohsenow, D., Woolard, R., & Lewander, W. (1996, September). *Motivational interviewing for adolescent drinking: Preliminary results from an emergency department intervention study.* Paper presented at the Addictions Conference, Hilton Head Island, SC.

Mott, F., & Haurin, R. (1988). Linkages between sexual activity and alcohol and drug use among American adolescents. *Family Planning Perspectives, 20*, 128–136.

National Institute of Mental Health Multisite HIV Prevention Trial Group. (1998). The NIMH Multisite Prevention Trial: Reducing HIV sexual risk behavior. *Science, 19*, 1889–1894.

National Institutes of Health. (2000, September). Interventions to prevent HIV risk behaviors. *AIDS, 14*(Suppl. 2), S85–S96.

Obeidallah, D., Turner, P., Jannotti, R., O'Brien, R., Haynie, D., & Galper, D. (1993). Investigating children's knowledge and understanding of AIDS. *Journal of School Health, 63*, 125–129.

Office of National AIDS Policy. (1996). *Youth and HIV/AIDS: An American agenda: A report to the president.* Washington, DC: The White House.

O'Leary, A. (1985). Self-efficacy and health. *Behaviour Research and Therapy, 23*, 437–451.

Orr, D., Langefeld, C., Katz, B., & Caine, V. (1996). Behavioral intervention to increase condom use among high-risk female adolescents. *Journal of Pediatrics, 128*, 288–295.

Osborne, M., Kistner, J., & Helgemo, B. (1993). Developmental progression in children's knowledge of AIDS: Implication for education and attitudinal change. *Journal of Pediatric Psychology, 18*, 177–192.

Paikoff, R. (1995). Early heterosexual debut: Situations of sexual possibility during the transition to adolescence. *American Journal of Orthopsychiatry, 65*, 389–401.

Parsons, J., Siegel, A., & Cousins, J. (1997). Late adolescent risk taking: Effects of perceived benefits and perceived risks on behavioral intentions and behavioral change. *Journal of Adolescents, 20*, 381–392.

Petosa, R., & Jackson, K. (1991). Using the health belief model to predict safer sex intentions among adolescents. *Health Education Quarterly, 18*, 463–476.

Pleck, J., Sonenstein, F., & Ku, L. (1993). Changes in adolescent males' use of and attitudes toward condoms: 1988–1991. *Family Planning Perspectives, 25*, 106–109, 117.

Prochaska, J. (1989). What causes people to change from unhealthy to health enhancing behavior? In C. Cuming & J. Floyd (Eds.), *Human behavior and cancer risk reduction* (pp. 30–34). Atlanta, GA: American Cancer Society.

Prochaska, J., Redding, C., Harlow, L., Rossi, J., & Velicer, W. (1994). The transtheoretical model of change and HIV prevention: A review. *Health Education Quarterly, 21,* 471–486.

Prochaska, J., Velicer, W., Rossi, J., Goldstein, M., Marcus, B., Rakowsky, W., Fiore, C., Harlow, L., Redding, C., Rosenbloom, D., & Rossi, S. (1994). Stages of change and decisional balance for 12 problem behaviors. *Health Psychology, 19,* 39–46.

Resnick, M. D., Bearman, P. S., Blum, R. W., Bauman, K. E., Harris, K. M., Jones, J., Tabor, J., Beuhring, T., Sieving, R. E., Shew, M., Ireland, M., Bearinger, L. H., & Udry, J. R. (1997). Protecting adolescents from harm: Findings from the National Longitudinal Study on Adolescent Health. *Journal of the American Medical Association, 278*(10), 823–832.

Resnicow, K., Royce, J., Vaughan, R., Orlandi, M. A., & Smith, M. (1997). Analysis of a multicomponent smoking cessation project: What worked and why. *Preventive Medicine, 26,* 373–381.

Rollnick, S., & Bell, A. (1991). Brief motivational interviewing for use by the nonspecialist. In W. R. Miller & S. Rollnick, *Motivational interviewing: Preparing people to change addictive behavior* (pp. 203–213). New York: Guilford Press.

Rollnick, S., Heather, N., & Bell, A. (1992). Negotiating behaviour change in medical settings: The development of brief motivational interviewing. *Journal of Mental Health (UK), 1,* 25–37.

Rollnick, S., Heather, N., Gold, R., & Hall, W. (1992). Development of a short "readiness to change" questionnaire for use in brief, opportunistic interventions among excessive drinkers. *British Journal of Addiction, 87,* 743–754.

Rotheram-Borus, M. J., Koopman, C., Haignere, C., & Davies, M. (1991). Reducing HIV sexual risk behaviors among runaway adolescents. *Journal of the American Medical Association, 266,* 1237–1241.

Schonfeld, D. J., Johnson, S. R., Perrin, E. C., O'Hare, L. L., & Cicchetti, D. V. (1993). Understanding of acquired immunodeficiency syndrome by elementary school children: A developmental survey. *Pediatrics, 92,* 389–395.

Schultz, J., Brown, L., & Butler, R. (1996, November). *Promoting safer sex among HIV-positive youth.* Abstract presented at the International Conference on AIDS Education, Atlanta, GA.

Schuster, M. A., Bell, R. M., Berry, S. H., & Kanouse, D. E. (1998). Impact of a high school condom availability program on sexual attitudes and behaviors. *Family Planning Perspectives, 30,* 67–72, 88.

Siegel, L. (1993). Children's understanding of AIDS: Implications for preventive interventions. *Journal of Pediatric Psychology, 18,* 173–176.

Smyth, N. (1996). Motivating persons with dual disorders: A stage approach. *Families in Society: The Journal of Contemporary Human Services, 77,* 605–614.

Sobo, E. J. (1993). Inner-city women and AIDS: The psycho-social benefits of unsafe sex. *Culture, Medicine and Psychiatry, 17,* 455–485.

Stanton, B., Kim, N., Galbraith, J., & Parrott, M. (1996). Design issues addressed in published evaluations of adolescent HIV-risk reduction interventions: A review. *Journal of Adolescent Health, 18,* 387–396.

Stanton, B., Li, X., Ricardo, I., Galbraith, J., Feigelman, S., & Kaljee, L. (1996). A randomized, controlled effectiveness trial of an AIDS prevention program for low-income African-American youths. *Archives of Pediatric and Adolescent Medicine, 150,* 363–372.

Stiffman, A., Dore, P., Earls, F., & Cunningham, R. (1992). The influence of mental health problems on AIDS-related risk behaviors in young adults. *Journal of Nervous and Mental Disease, 180,* 314–320.

St. Lawrence, J. (1993). African-American adolescents' knowledge, health-related attitudes, sexual behaviors and contraceptive decisions: Implications for the prevention of adolescent HIV infection. *Journal of Consulting and Clinical Psychology, 61,* 104–112.

Tanner, W. (1988). The effect of condom use and erotic instructions on attitudes toward condoms. *Journal of Sex Research, 25,* 537–541.

Tober, G. (1991). Motivational interviewing with young people. In W. R. Miller & S. Rollnick, *Motivational interviewing: Preparing people to change addictive behavior* (pp. 248–259). New York: Guilford Press.

Trigwell, P., Grant, P., & House, A. (1997). Motivation and glycemic control in diabetes mellitus. *Journal of Psychosomatic Research, 43,* 307–315.

Tubman, J. G., Windle, M., & Windle, R. C. (1996). Cumulative sexual intercourse patterns among middle adolescents: Problem behavior precursors and concurrent health risk behaviors. *Journal of Adolescent Health, 18,* 181–191.

Walter, H., & Vaughan, R. (1993). AIDS risk reduction among a multiethnic sample of urban high school students. *Journal of the American Medical Association, 270,* 725–730.

Warren, C. W., Kann, L., Small, M. L., Santelli, J. S., Collins, J. L., & Kolbe, L. J. (1997). Age of initiating selected health-risk behaviors among high school students in the United States. *Journal of Adolescent Health, 21,* 225–231.

Weeks, M., Schensul, J., Williams, S., Singer, M., & Grier, M. (1995). AIDS prevention for African American and Latina women: Building culturally and gender-appropriate intervention. *AIDS Education and Prevention, 7,* 251–263.

Wormith, J., & Hanson, R. (1992). The treatment of sexual offenders in Canada: An update. *Canadian Psychology, 33,* 180–198.

Wren, P., Janz, N., Corovano, K., Zimmerman, M., & Washenko, K. (1997). Preventing the spread of AIDS in youth: Principles of practice from 11 diverse projects. *Journal of Adolescent Health, 21,* 309–317.

Zabin, L. S., Hardy, J. B., Smith, E. A., & Hirsch, M. B. (1986). Substance use and its relation to sexual activity among inner-city adolescents. *Journal of Adolescent Health Care, 7,* 320–331.

Zierler, S., Feingold, L., Laufer, D., Velentgas, P., Kantrowitz-Gordon, I., & Mayer, K. (1991). Adult survivors of childhood sexual abuse and subsequent risk of HIV infection. *American Journal of Public Health, 81,* 572–575.

9

Toward Brief Interventions for Adolescents with Substance Abuse and Comorbid Psychiatric Problems

MARK G. MYERS, SANDRA A. BROWN, SUSAN TATE,
ANA ABRANTES, and KRISTIN TOMLINSON

This chapter represents an initial effort to outline the potential utility of brief interventions for substance-abusing adolescents with comorbid psychiatric problems. Youths with alcohol and other drug use problems frequently suffer from concomitant psychiatric disorders (Lewinsohn, Rhode, & Seeley, 1995). Unfortunately, substance abuse problems among adolescents presenting for psychiatric treatment in various settings are often not adequately assessed or addressed despite the deleterious influence of substance use on concomitant psychopathology. More generally, the availability of mental health services for adolescents is limited, and adequate assessment is frequently lacking. Brief intervention approaches represent a flexible and potentially cost-effective means for addressing substance use problems, and they can be implemented in a diversity of settings. Such approaches can provide initial assessment and serve as a bridge to more intensive intervention, if needed.

Brief interventions may also help to overcome the reluctance of mental health care providers (and other professionals who work with adolescents) to raise or address issues related to substance abuse. Despite the substantial overlap between psychopathology and substance use problems, many clinicians feel ill prepared to assess and manage substance abuse (Miller & Brown, 1997). Brief interventions that can be applied by specialists and nonspecialists alike can draw increased attention to substance use problems in settings that serve youths. The primary focus of this chapter examines efforts aimed at youths who experience substance use problems that have not been identified and/or treated. As conceptualized herein, the potential utility of brief interventions lies in identifying substance use problems, motivating adolescents in various settings to attend to their substance use behaviors, and facilitating behavior change.

PREVALENCE

Although comorbidity of substance use disorders and psychopathology in adolescents has not been studied as extensively as it has in adults, the past decade has shown increased awareness of this issue in youth. Recent studies have shown high prevalence rates of psychiatric disorders among substance-abusing adolescents across many different settings. The most commonly described studies in the literature, and those for which prevalence rates will be reported, include community, inpatient, and outpatient mental health and juvenile justice settings.

Rates of psychopathology in substance-abusing adolescents from community samples are similar to rates found in adult community samples (Rieger et al., 1990). Lewinsohn, Rhode, and Seeley (1995) examined lifetime comorbid psychiatric disorders in a community sample of adolescents aged 14 to 18 years. They found that 66% of adolescents who met criteria for a substance use disorder as defined by the *Diagnostic and Statistical Manual of Mental Disorders* (*DSM-III-R*; American Psychiatric Association, 1987) also met criteria for at least one other Axis I disorder (e.g., depressive disorders, disruptive behavior disorders). The Methods for the Epidemiology of Child and Adolescent Mental Disorders (MECA) study obtained similar rates with a community sample of 1,285 children and adolescents aged 9 to 18 years (Kandel et al., 1997). They found that 66% of weekly drinkers also met diagnostic criteria for a psychiatric disorder. Of those who used illicit drugs three or more times in the past year, 85% of females and 56% of males met criteria for at least one psychiatric disorder.

As expected, rates of psychiatric disorders in inpatient substance-abusing adolescents tend to be higher than those among community samples. Stowell and Estroff (1992) reported that 82% of adolescents entering inpatient treatment for a substance use disorder also met *DSM-III-R* criteria for an Axis I disorder. Rates were also high in a sample of substance-abusing American Indian adolescents (Novins, Beals, Shore, & Manson, 1996), with 68% of these adolescents meeting criteria for a co-occurring psychiatric disorder.

Inpatient psychiatric facilities represent the most common setting in which adolescent comorbidity has been studied. Substance use disorders are relatively common among adolescent psychiatric inpatients. For example, Deas-Nesmith, Campbell, and Brady (1998) studied 100 consecutive admissions to an adolescent acute-care psychiatric inpatient unit and found that 33% met criteria for substance abuse or dependence. Another study found that 50% of consecutive admissions to an adolescent psychiatry unit met criteria for a substance use disorder. In addition, those with a substance use disorder were more likely to meet criteria for a Cluster B personality disorder (i.e., antisocial, borderline, histrionic, or narcissistic; Grilo et al., 1995). Similar rates of substance use disorders in psychiatrically hospitalized adolescents have been found elsewhere (Bukstein, Brent, & Kaminer, 1989; Greenbaum, Foster-Johnson, & Petrila, 1996; Piazza, 1996).

Relatively few studies have examined the rates of adolescent comorbidity in outpatient settings. One study conducted a systematic review of psychiatric diagnoses of adolescents aged 13 to 19 years who were referred for routine clinical care in a pediatric psychopharmacology unit (Wilens, Biederman, Abrantes, & Spencer, 1997). Rates of substance use disorders were found to be lower (11%) than rates reported in the studies reviewed previously.

Further research in these settings is necessary before conclusions and generalizations can be made. Given that inpatient psychiatric stays are becoming shorter as a consequence of managed care practices, outpatient services are becoming increasingly important in meeting the mental health needs of adolescents. This indicates the importance of future research in these settings.

The final setting considered is the juvenile justice system. In a study of 111 juvenile offenders referred by the court for psychiatric evaluation, 81% met *DSM-III-R* criteria for a substance use disorder (Neighbors, Kempton, & Forehand, 1992). Of these substance-abusing adolescents, 91% met criteria for conduct disorder, 68% for oppositional defiant disorder, and 58% for attention-deficit/hyperactivity disorder (ADHD). Similar rates of disruptive behavior disorders were found in a group of delinquent, substance-involved youths in a residential treatment program (Crowley, Mikulich, MacDonald, Young, & Zerbe, 1998). Clearly, comorbidity is prevalent among incarcerated youths, a group for which the availability of substance abuse or mental health interventions is typically limited.

Overall, the psychiatric disorders that are most often reported concomitant with substance abuse among adolescents include mood, anxiety, conduct, and attention-deficit/hyperactivity disorders (see, e.g., Lewinsohn et al., 1995). Yet the lack of a systematic approach in assessing psychiatric diagnoses in these individuals has made it difficult to determine precisely the rates of overlap for specific psychiatric disorders. In addition, rates of psychiatric disorders differ based on the type of population and setting studied. For example, there are higher rates of comorbidity of mood and anxiety disorders with substance abuse in inpatient psychiatric settings, whereas in juvenile detention settings conduct and other disruptive behavior disorders are most often concomitant with substance abuse.

Based on these findings, it is clear that a high concordance between substance use and other psychiatric disorders exists in adolescents. This is an area of research that requires a great deal of further exploration. At this time, longitudinal studies that examine the clinical course of these adolescents are rare. Therefore, these types of studies will become increasingly more important in understanding the complexity of adolescent psychiatric and substance use disorder comorbidity. As information accrues regarding this phenomenon, better assessment, prevention, and intervention strategies can be designed to address the treatment needs of these adolescents.

WHY CONSIDER BRIEF INTERVENTIONS?

Brief interventions have proven efficacious in reducing alcohol consumption in adult problem drinkers in primary care settings (Fleming, Barry, Manwell, Johnson, & London, 1997) as well as in general hospital wards (Heather, Rollnick, Bell, & Richmond, 1996). In addition, encouraging preliminary findings have been reported with brief interventions for adolescent smoking (Colby et al., 1998) and drinking and driving (Monti et al., 1999). Yet brief interventions have thus far not been specifically applied to adolescents with comorbid psychiatric and substance use disorders.

There are several reasons to consider brief interventions as an option for youths with comorbid psychopathology and substance abuse. Brief interventions were initially designed to target adults who were problem alcohol users but who had not yet become physiologically dependent or experienced significant psychosocial problems. Because of their relatively shorter substance use histories, adolescents typically report lower rates of withdrawal symptoms and less severe problematic consequences than do adults with substance use disorders (see, e.g., Brown, 1993; Stewart & Brown, 1995). In addition, although brief interventions can be abstinence focused, they can also be goal oriented toward reducing problematic drinking. This approach might prove more appropriate for adolescents because moderate drinking or reducing drug use may appear to adolescents to be a more attainable initial goal than long-term abstinence. Therefore, adolescents are at a developmental stage at which brief interventions may prove particularly efficacious for curtailing harmful or risky alcohol and other drug involvement, deterring progression to more severe substance use and related problems.

Another reason for considering the utility of brief interventions derives from the availability of health care for adolescents. In general, concern exists as to whether children and adolescents receive adequate care for their emotional and mental health needs (Philips, 1990). Adolescents with comorbid substance use and psychiatric disorders often come from families that also have high rates of psychopathology (Miles et al., 1998). Given the limited availability of mental health services for youth, brief interventions may present a cost-effective means of increasing treatment availability. A significant advantage of brief interventions is that they can be incorporated within diverse settings, an approach that would increase the likelihood that adolescents in need would be attended to and have their needs addressed. For example, brief interventions could be developed for school systems, primary care settings, inpatient and outpatient psychiatric facilities, and juvenile detention centers.

In addition to the problem of insufficient treatment services for youth, evidence indicates that assessment procedures typically employed in mental health settings geared toward youth are often inadequate for generating useful treatment plans. In a recent study, researchers examined rates of substance use disorders in adolescents admitted to an inpatient psychiatric facility (Deas-Nesmith et al., 1998). Although none of the study participants had been identified as substance abusers during their hospitalization, diagnostic interviews conducted as part of the study revealed that 33% of the adolescents met diagnostic criteria for a substance use disorder. Therefore, it seems likely that adolescents may be underassessed with respect to substance use disorders and consequently be less likely to receive intervention for alcohol and other drug abuse. Brief interventions could thus be utilized to serve both as assessment and therapeutic tools for substance use disorders in contexts in which an adolescent may be receiving treatment (outpatient or inpatient) for an emotional or psychiatric disorder.

Last, the implementation of brief substance-focused interventions in varied settings may result in decreased psychiatric symptomatology for adolescent substance abusers. The relationship between substance abuse and psychopathology is quite complex. However, decreases in substance involvement have been associated with subsequent improvement in psychiatric symptoms (see, e.g., Brown & Schuckit, 1988). Therefore, brief interventions can serve a dual purpose in both treating the substance use disorder and aiding the goals of intervention for other mental health problems. This dual impact is especially important in such a difficult-to-treat population (Bukstein et al., 1989).

The high prevalence of comorbidity and frequent underidentification of substance use among comorbid adolescent populations clearly indicate the need for interventions developed specifically for these youths. Although brief interventions have received significant research attention, at this time no empirical studies with comorbid adolescents are available. Thus we extrapolate from related research findings and developmental considerations in suggesting intervention strategies.

UTILITY OF BRIEF INTERVENTIONS

Given the challenging nature of intervening with adolescents and the complexity associated with comorbidity, how might a brief therapeutic contact with these youths be of benefit? As noted, brief interventions may aid in the identification of substance involvement and problems. Brief interventions can also be utilized to heighten motivation to consider and engage in treatment. Resistance to intervention efforts and low internal motivation represent significant impediments to behavioral change for comorbid adolescents. Because adolescents seldom initiate treatment requests and are commonly referred by adults (e.g., parents, teachers, legal authorities), personal motivation may be lower than among other clients seen by counselors or therapists. Normal development in adolescent years includes movement toward independence and autonomy, a process that may lead adolescents to resist perceived adult efforts to control or curb personal freedom. Studies of clinical samples of substance-abusing youths reveal high rates of problems in school (e.g., truancy, deteriorating grades) and frequent negative sanctions in the form of suspension and expulsion (Brown, Mott, & Myers, 1990). Negative sanctions from school authority figures may serve to further increase resistance to adult intervention. Established motivational enhancement techniques, adjusted for adolescent populations (Tober, 1991) and clients who have been coerced into treatment (Miller & Rollnick, 1991), can be utilized to address motivational factors with comorbid youths. Brief interventions provide a supportive context within which these adolescents might explore personal ramifications of substance use and evaluate potential behavioral changes in a nonconfrontational setting.

Additionally, brief interventions may increase self-efficacy for behavior change. Low self-efficacy increases the difficulty of altering substance-related behaviors across populations and is associated with poorer outcomes for adolescents (Richter, Brown, & Mott, 1991). However, in addition to low-self esteem resulting from negative interactions with adult authority figures, as noted previously, adolescents may realistically feel limited in their ability to significantly alter their environments and may also experience barriers to accessing mental health services (e.g., transportation, financial/health insurance limitations, parental consent). As noted by one author, "Low self-esteem and low self-efficacy in young people will often be the results of a quite realistic perception that their views and desires are not taken into account in decisions that affect them. Rather than looking for examples of self-worth and mastery in their everyday lives, it may be more effective to create an opportunity for these feelings to be enhanced in the interview itself" (Tober, 1991, p. 248). Self-efficacy may also be enhanced through the exploration of treatment alternatives and problem solving related to personal barriers to engaging in such treatments (see Monti, Barnett, O'Leary, & Colby, Chapter 5, this volume).

As one example, adult comorbid substance abusers are less likely to participate in community support groups such as Alcoholics Anonymous, citing fear of crowds, difficulty sitting still through meetings, and difficulty meeting and relating to other people as reasons for not attending (Noordsy, Schwab, Fox, & Drake, 1996). Yet participation in alcohol- or drug-focused support groups is significantly correlated with improved adolescent substance abuse treatment outcomes. For example, several studies have demonstrated that more frequent attendance at 12-step meetings corresponds with lower rates of posttreatment substance involvement (Brown, 1993; Kelly & Myers, 1997). A recent study has demonstrated that 12-step meeting attendance may influence adolescent treatment outcome by serving to maintain motivation for abstinence (Kelly, Myers, & Brown, 2000). Additionally, adolescents who attended 12-step meetings composed primarily of adolescent participants had significantly less posttreatment substance use than those who attended meetings composed primarily of adults (Kelly & Myers, 1997). As found for adults, youth with comorbid psychopathology may experience barriers to participation in self-help groups. Such obstacles may arise as a consequence of social skill deficits or as a result of psychopathology (e.g., social anxiety, social withdrawal, etc.). As such, brief interventions can be employed to identify potential obstacles to participation and to assist with problem solving so as to minimize obstacles and facilitate involvement in such groups.

Finally, brief interventions can be used to provide personalized feedback and education tailored to specific substances and comorbid disorder characteristics, such as aggressive behaviors and symptoms of anxiety and depression. This type of focused information is seldom available to adolescents for several reasons. Alcohol and drug educational efforts for adolescent populations have predominantly focused on large-scale, school-wide prevention strategies, as opposed to individually tailored interventions aimed at students currently using substances. Additionally, physicians and counselors who as a matter of course counsel their adult patients on inter actions of alcohol and prescribed medications may not be uniformly addressing such issues with adolescents under legal drinking age. Finally, peer substance use is commonly overestimated by substance using populations. Personalized feedback on normative substance use (among similar age and gender youth), a common element in brief interventions, may decrease implicit pressure for comorbid youth to use substances in attempts to "fit in" with distorted perceptions of peer use. Education regarding reciprocal relationships between alcohol and drug effects, behavioral consequences, and psychiatric symptoms can be personally tailored to an adolescent's substance use patterns and comorbid disorder and discussed in a nonthreatening environment. For example, for an adolescent who drinks heavily and experiences significant depression, discussion would focus on the relationship between alcohol use and subsequent mood symptoms, along with an explanation of the depressogenic effects of alcohol. This type of discussion can be employed to clarify the reciprocal relationship whereby depression may motivate drinking; the drinking may result in increased depressive symptoms, which may then lead to further drinking for symptom relief; and so on, in a vicious cycle.

Thus brief interventions can be utilized to heighten motivation, enhance self-efficacy, and provide education and feedback to comorbid youths. By addressing potential impediments, adolescents may become receptive to collaborative goal setting aimed at altering substance use behaviors.

GOALS

Collaborative goals formulated in the brief therapeutic context may be directed toward engagement in professional substance abuse interventions. Adolescents referred through non-mental health settings (e.g., juvenile justice system, education system) may be directed toward use of professional health care settings to address the comorbid disorder, in addition to substance use. Discussing treatment options (inpatient versus outpatient, adult versus adolescent specific programs, individual versus group therapy) may help to engage the adolescent in the decision-making process.

Alternatively, brief intervention goals may include facilitating involvement in community resource support groups such as Alcoholics Anonymous, Narcotics Anonymous, or Rational Recovery. Ideally, those who provide brief interventions should be familiar with the resources available in the local area to increase the likelihood of referral to optimal groups (e.g., those with predominantly adolescent participants, those that make transportation accessible to the adolescent).

Generally, abstinence-focused interventions are advisable for comorbid substance abusers due to the potential for prescribed psychotropic medication interactions with substances of abuse and for decreased treatment compliance in the context of ongoing substance use and due to the illegality of substance involvement. However, those who provide brief intervention services should be prepared to discuss harm reduction techniques with adolescents who resist recommendations for immediate or lifetime abstinence from substance use. The interested reader is referred to Miller, Turner, and Marlatt (Chapter 2, this volume) for further consideration of harm reduction techniques with adolescents.

Important intervention areas to address with adolescents include the effects of substance use on anxiety and depressive symptoms, academic performance, violent or aggressive behaviors associated with substance use, driving while under the influence, and risky sexual behaviors. For assessed areas in which the adolescent has experienced consequences that appear related to substance use, the therapist can provide comparisons with frequency and rates of these consequences and behaviors in a normative sample (e.g., same age and gender students from a local school). For example, if an adolescent reports driving under the influence multiple times in the past year, this report can be compared with data on overall percentage of youth of the same age and gender who engaged in this behavior.

Although far less prevalent, intravenous drug use represents a danger for a small minority of youth. Brief intervention contact may also provide the therapist with the opportunity to raise the topic of teratogenic effects of alcohol and drug use on fetal development with sexually active substance abusers; more extensive information can be provided if the adolescent expresses interest. Ideally, harm reduction interventions are best delivered in settings easily accessible to youths, so the therapist should ensure that additional information or intervention contact is available on demand in the event circumstances or motivation change.

RECOMMENDATIONS

General Recommendations

General motivational principles described in the motivational enhancement literature are also applicable to interventions with comorbid adolescents. Thus empathic, nonconfrontational interactions that support self-efficacy and develop discrepancy are important components of brief interventions with youth. The reader is referred to the excellent literature on this topic for a general introduction to motivational and brief intervention strategies (see, e.g., Miller & Rollnick, 1991) and to the applied chapters in this volume (see, e.g., Monti et al., Chapter 5). We describe additional general recommendations that are useful in working with comorbid adolescents, followed by setting-specific recommendations.

First, because of the transitory nature of motivation among youth and the fluctuating, cyclical nature of many comorbid disorders, brief interventions should be made available "on demand," with little or no delay between the time a problem is identified and the time treatment is offered. Treatment should be easily accessible at "teachable moments" when motivation is high or difficulties are salient to the adolescent. Providing brief intervention in a timely fashion will also facilitate follow-up contact, if the adolescent desires it. Noordsy and colleagues (1996) advise meeting with dually diagnosed adults following initial attendance at 12-step meetings to answer questions, resolve misunderstandings, and solve any difficulties encountered as a means of enhancing the likelihood of future participation. Adolescents will likely benefit from premeeting discussions and similar follow-up assistance in managing unanticipated experiences in their attempts to alter substance use behaviors. Brief assistance in managing other life stressors (such as family or peer conflict, legal difficulties, academic problems) that may function to derail initial substance use changes may also improve the likelihood of positive treatment outcomes. Such assistance would be limited by design and might focus on helping the adolescent manage negative emotions related to these events by providing support and using strategies such as cognitive restructuring.

Second, a therapist should avoid labeling. In brief interventions, diagnostic labels offer little benefit and have the potential for generating negative reactions. The natural recovery literature has identified undesirable labeling, embarrassment, and stigma as reasons people give for not seeking treatment (Tucker, Vuchinich, & Gladsjo, 1994). Adolescents in particular are sensitive to self-identity issues, making labels even more troublesome (Chassin, Presson, Young, & Light, 1981). This suggests that adolescents may be resistant to stereotypical images associated with labels such as "alcoholic" or "addict." For comorbid youths, confusion and resentment may already exist based on prior labels associated with comorbid disorders (i.e., conduct disorder, ADHD). In discussing substance-use-related issues, along with avoiding labels, the therapist should focus on the problems experienced by the adolescent rather than on substance use per se (e.g., discuss the consequences of a DWI citation rather than the drinking behavior). By emphasizing areas of difficulty rather than specifics of substance use behavior, the treatment provider avoids a judgmental stance and functions as an ally of the adolescent in examining possible ways to reduce negative experiences. For example, discussion of the role of alcohol in exacerbating depressive symptoms for a depressed youth can link the issue of alcohol use with the primary identified problem and can serve to shift the focus from substance use per se to substance-related and psychiatric problems.

Third, in working with comorbid youth, a therapist should offer realistic and practical choices. Adolescents vary significantly in psychiatric symptomatology, as well as in their developmental stages and their functional abilities to access various services. All of these factors influence an adolescent's ability to participate in and benefit from treatment services. The process of selecting treatment alternatives also serves to engage the adolescent in the planning process, increasing a sense of personal responsibility and self-determination. If clinicians providing brief interventions align with a single treatment option, the adolescent may reject the provider in the process of rejecting a single intervention alternative, thereby closing opportunities for future intervention contact. As discussed previously, a range of treatment goals (abstinence, reduced consumption, harm reduction) may increase the likelihood that an adolescent will engage in some form of substance use behavior change.

Finally, general motivational techniques commonly encourage clients to access existing skills and resources. However, work with comorbid youths may require intervention to ameliorate skills deficits or decrease psychiatric symptoms associated with comorbidity in order to enhance an adolescent's ability to utilize resources. For example, brief social skills training can be incorporated to enhance communication with adult authority figures and treatment providers, to develop and practice verbal substance-refusal efforts with peers, and to improve interpersonal skills that will help interactions in support groups. Referrals for medication evaluation or psychological treatment may be indicated to reduce anxiety and depressive symptoms, thereby improving ability to engage in treatment for substance-related behavior change.

Setting-Specific Recommendations

We now turn to unique considerations related to specific settings in which therapists frequently encounter adolescents with substance abuse and other mental health disorders. The settings addressed include mental health inpatient and outpatient settings, medical primary care settings, the juvenile justice system, and the educational system. See Table 9.1 for a list of major intervention goals by type of setting.

TABLE 9.1. Recommended Goals for Brief Interventions across Settings for Adolescents with Co-Occurring Psychiatric and Substance-Related Problems

Setting	Major goals of brief intervention
Inpatient	Assess for substance abuse; enhance motivation to change; refer for specialized treatment.
Outpatient	Identify problems; provide feedback; set goals for behavior change.
Primary care	Screen for substance abuse and psychopathology; identify problems; provide referrals; enhance motivation to follow through on recommendations.
Juvenile justice	Screen for substance abuse; refer for more intensive assessment; encourage participation in treatment or support groups following incarceration.
School	Screen for substance abuse and psychopathology; provide feedback; set goals for change; identify resources for referral.

Inpatient Mental Health Settings

As previously mentioned, adolescents with psychiatric disorders in inpatient mental health facilities have very high rates of substance use disorders. Due to changes in the health care system over the past decade, adolescents who enter inpatient treatment programs are the most severely emotionally disturbed (e.g., suicidal, homicidal, or psychotic). In addition, insurance companies and government-provided health benefits usually limit the duration of inpatient hospital care (often to no more than several days). As a result, an inpatient stay allows sufficient time only to address the most severe and threatening problems and disorders and to plan for more comprehensive treatment. Because substance use disorders are typically not the primary reason for adolescent psychiatric inpatient treatment admissions, these are often not assessed. Even when substance use disorders are assessed, clinicians are frequently unsure about the most effective methods of treatment (Roche, Parle, Stubbs, Hall, & Saunders, 1995).

Brief interventions can serve several purposes within an adolescent inpatient setting. Brief interventions can provide assessment information through administration of screening instruments to identify those adolescents who may have a substance abuse problem. Brief interventions can serve a therapeutic function by enhancing motivation to change through providing feedback and referral recommendations. When brief interventions were implemented in this manner with adult inpatients with comorbid psychiatric disorders, 35% of the patients went on to use addiction services after inpatient treatment (Dunn & Ries, 1997). Similarly, adolescents who receive a brief intervention during inpatient treatment may pursue other addiction services upon discharge. Therefore, brief intervention for substance use disorders represents an optimal format in an environment in which treatment is short and focused on more immediate emotional concerns and in which clinicians may lack experience in treating substance use disorders.

Implementation of brief interventions in an inpatient mental health setting may benefit from a focus on the most salient aspects of the situation. For example, when making referrals or recommendations to adolescents in inpatient settings, providing a menu of options may be especially important, as these adolescents may be there involuntarily and feel deprived of their autonomy. Providing the adolescent with a variety of choices and control over goal setting can contribute significantly to the efficacy of the brief intervention. In addition, because of the severity of emotional disturbance in inpatient settings, an understanding, empathic approach is crucial when conducting the brief intervention. A focus on the potential influence of substance use on psychiatric symptomatology is likely to be of particular importance in this type of setting. The latter approach also serves to remove substance use behaviors as the focal point, which may in turn reduce resistance and aid in engaging adolescents in the process of change.

Outpatient Mental Health Settings

Although rates of substance use disorders are lower in outpatient than in inpatient mental health settings, many of the issues are similar. Psychiatric outpatient sessions are often restricted in length and focus primarily on management of psychotropic medications. Counseling sessions often focus on either family system issues or on the identified psychiatric problem without addressing substance use behaviors. In these situations, clinicians may feel they do not possess the expertise to directly address substance use problems, a factor that may contribute to the frequent failure to assess adolescent substance use. Clinicians may also be primarily concerned with addressing the presenting problem before attending to other issues. In this type of setting, abstinence from alcohol or drugs may be particularly important in cases involving psychotropic medications, both for improving adherence to and effectiveness of medication regimens. A reasonable goal for brief intervention in outpatient settings may consist of providing assessment and referrals for substance use problems. A benefit of this approach is that the primary clinician is responsible for assessing substance abuse but not for providing treatment if the therapist lacks sufficient knowledge or expertise. Primary goals of brief interventions in outpatient mental health settings are thus to identify problems, to provide feedback, and to set goals for behavior change with a focus on appropriate referrals as indicated.

As with inpatient settings, providing adolescents with choices and a sense of control is critical to the success of a brief intervention. Because a therapist can provide more extended contact in outpatient settings, he or she can use brief interventions to increase adolescent self-efficacy for change. Adolescents can be encouraged as they pursue mutually agreed-upon goals toward behavior change and are reinforced for positive changes made over time.

Primary Care

In recent years primary care settings have been the focus for implementation of brief interventions across a variety of problem behaviors. Research has indicated that brief interventions for the treatment of substance use problems have been effective in nondependent substance-abusing adult populations. For example, among patients screened for problem drinking, those who received brief physician advice during a medical visit reduced average drinks per week, excessive drinking, and binge drinking by 20% at 1 year compared with patients who did not receive the intervention (Fleming et al., 1997). Similar findings were reported for a study of hospitalized male heavy drinkers. Patients who received brief counseling (skills-based counseling or brief motivational interviewing) showed decreased levels of weekly alcohol consumption at 6-month follow-up compared with control participants (Heather, Rollnick, Bell, & Richmond, 1996). The World Health Organization (WHO) evaluated the relative effects of simple advice and brief counseling with heavy drinkers identified in primary care settings in eight countries and found a significant effect of brief intervention on alcohol consumption across cultures (WHO, 1996). Thus support exists for the utility of primary care-based brief interventions in reducing drinking among adults.

Emerging evidence suggests that brief interventions implemented in health care settings with adolescents can also decrease substance use and related problems. In a recent study (Dimeff, 1998), undergraduate students seeking services at a student health center who met criteria for heavy and hazardous drinking were provided either a brief intervention or treatment as usual. Participants with adequate exposure to the brief intervention (as opposed to students with minimal exposure) had fewer alcohol-related problems and fewer binge-drinking episodes at the 1-month follow-up than control participants and experimental participants without adequate exposure to the brief intervention. In another study, adolescents presenting at an emergency room following an alcohol-related event (e.g., injury, intoxication, etc.) received either a brief motivational intervention or standard care (Monti et al., 1999). Those who received a brief motivational intervention reported significantly lower rates of drinking and driving, traffic violations, alcohol-related injuries, and alcohol-related problems than those in the standard-care condition. Details of this brief intervention are presented in Monti and colleagues (Chapter 5, this volume).

These studies suggest that primary care settings may also be useful venues for addressing substance abuse problems in youths with psychiatric comorbidity. These types of settings present some advantages and challenges for intervening with this population. A major advantage of primary care facilities is that they serve a broad population of adolescents and thus provide an opportunity to reach youths who may not otherwise seek or receive treatment. The challenge lies in conducting screening and assessment to identify substance use and psychiatric problems. One approach is to focus on youths who present with either substance-related problems (e.g., who are injured in substance-related incidents) or psychiatric problems (e.g., who may receive treatment in emergency departments as a result of acute exacerbation of symptoms). Because of the nature of primary care settings, any interventions by necessity are minimal. In such cases, brief assessment of substance use or psychiatric symptoms (as appropriate) can be conducted, with the goal of identifying problems, providing appropriate follow-up referrals (for mental health and/or substance abuse treatment), and enhancing motivation to follow through on recommendations. Because of their role as primary contact with the adolescent, physicians and nurses are the appropriate providers of brief intervention in these settings. As in other settings, focusing on the influence of substance use on the presenting problem is likely to be most effective in motivating change efforts.

Juvenile Justice

Because of the social and economic impact of substance abuse on society, the juvenile justice system is a highly studied setting. Although alcohol and drug abuse is prevalent among adolescent offenders, substance-related treatment is not available in the majority of juvenile justice settings, and, when it is available, it tends to be episodic and short-lived (Dembo, 1995). This contrasts with research findings from the general population indicating that longer treatment is more effective for substance use disorders (Hubbard, Craddock, Flynn, Anderson, & Etheridge, 1997). The discrepancy between the high need for substance abuse interventions and the limited availability of services in the juvenile justice system increases the importance of brief intervention efforts as a means of screening to evaluate the need for more detailed assessment and treatment of mental health disorders, including substance use. Brief interventions should also be utilized to encourage long-term participation in substance-related treatment services or community support groups following involvement with the juvenile justice system. Research findings indicate that substance-related treatment reduces criminal behavior (Hubbard et al., 1997), and thus interventions aimed at engaging comorbid youths in alcohol- and drug-treatment services may represent the best means of reducing recidivism.

Brief interventions in juvenile justice settings would most likely initially be provided by personnel with limited training in mental health treatment, such as parole officers. Because of the punitive nature of the juvenile justice system, identifying alcohol and drug problems and then reducing adolescents' resistance and engaging them in behavior change efforts could represent a major challenge. Adolescents in these settings most often exhibit externalizing disorders, and resistance to change is exacerbated by psychiatric comorbidity (Neighbors et al., 1992). Drug testing is often mandated for juvenile offenders, with penalties imposed for positive tests. Thus a critical issue for brief intervention in these settings is instilling motivation for self-disclosure of substance use and change that is not solely predicated on consequences imposed by the juvenile justice system. Providing screening, assessment, and feedback regarding the negative consequences of drug use for life domains other than legal is imperative. Brief interventions in juvenile justice settings should also attend to enhancing self-efficacy and pro-viding positive reinforcement for setting goals and making efforts at behav-ior change.

Schools

School-based alcohol and drug programs primarily focus on education and prevention. These programs emphasize discouraging students from experi-menting with substances, and few have implemented strategies for interven-tion with students who currently use substances. There is some evidence from work with college students that screening and brief intervention for students at high risk for alcohol problems can effectively reduce negative consequences. In a recent study (Marlatt et al., 1998), students entering college as freshmen were identified as being at risk for heavy drinking prior to enrollment and were randomized to either an individualized motiva-tional brief intervention in their freshman year or to a no-treatment control condition. Follow-up assessments over 2 years indicated that the interven-tion group had greater reductions in drinking rates and harmful conse-quences than did to the control group.

This harm reduction approach provides a model that may be relevant to school settings. Although most such studies to date have been conducted with college students (see Miller, Kilmer, Kim, Weingardt, & Marlatt, Chapter 6, this volume), a recent study by D'Amico and Fromme (2000) provides initial support for the utility of a school-based brief intervention with high school students. In this study a single 50-minute session consist-ing of motivational techniques, feedback, and skills training was compared with an abbreviated version of the Drug Abuse Resistance Education (DARE) curriculum. At the postintervention assessment, students who par-ticipated in the brief intervention reported significantly greater reductions in frequency of heavy drinking and drug use than those who received the DARE program (D'Amico & Fromme, 2000). Brief interventions of this type seem relevant to youths with psychiatric comorbidity. Students exhib-iting academic, disciplinary, or interpersonal difficulties may be viewed as an "at risk" population and targeted within schools for assessment and brief intervention as appropriate. Because schools tend to have explicit pol-icies regarding substance use and problem behaviors, gaining the trust of students is likely to present a particular challenge. Thus implementation of assessment and intervention in a nonthreatening and nonjudgmental fash-ion would likely be critical for success. As in primary care settings that serve a broad cross-section of adolescents, assessment must address both substance use and psychopathology. In order to obtain valid assessment, students need to be reassured that the information they provide will be confidential (within the boundaries permitted) and that no adverse disciplinary actions will result. Personalized feedback from assessment could be provided with reference to the student body in each particular school, which may prove to be a powerful tool. Because schools typically have limited resources, the goals of brief intervention would consist of setting goals for change and identifying appropriate resources for referral. This type of brief intervention could be provided by school counselors or school psychologists.

LIMITATIONS

Brief interventions for adolescents with comorbid psychopathology and alcohol and drug problems is a new arena, both in terms of clinical services and research. Although such abbreviated therapeutic efforts are unlikely to replace more extensive interventions in cases of youths with co-occurring substance use disorders and mental health diagnoses, there does appear to be an important niche for such intervention activities. As noted throughout the chapter, brief interventions for comorbid youth populations are limited in scope and often have different objectives than traditional treatments. Brief interventions for adolescents with comorbid disorders have targeted goals of identifying problems, expanding motivation for resolution of substance involvement and problems, and facilitating engagement into specific treatments for substance use disorders. In some cases brief interventions may produce the desired behavioral change (i.e., abstinence); however, it is more likely that brief interventions will increase readiness to make changes in substance involvement.

Substance involvement and substance use disorders are inconsistently screened and assessed in public service settings in which youth with behavioral or health problems most commonly present. Further, few professionals outside of addiction specialists feel competent to assess these problems and typically do not feel well prepared to provide substance abuse treatment should problems be identified. The brief interventions outlined herein offer relatively straightforward means to fill this gap of assessment and transition to treatment.

Although brief interventions for youths are rapidly emerging, as of yet no standardized brief intervention package is available for use with adolescents who have mental health and substance problems. Empirical evidence of the effectiveness of these interventions for youth is sorely needed. Clearly, guidelines for professionals regarding assessment questions and facilitative procedures are necessary before staff from diverse settings can begin to implement these procedures.

An important limitation regarding brief interventions for substance involvement among youths with mental health disorders is the lack of a systematic approach to diagnosis in this population. Heretofore, little research has been available to guide the clinician in distinguishing between mental health disorders that may be substance induced and those that will likely persist despite abstinence. Such data are even more critical today, with the reduced duration of coverage of mental health inpatient and outpatient services. Without empirically based guidelines, it is difficult for a clinician to structure the normative feedback and advice that are central to brief interventions. Clearly, research is needed in this area to guide the development of brief interventions for youths presenting with both mental health and substance abuse symptoms.

Legal issues and their psychological impact may pose particular challenges for brief interventions with youths. Whereas alcohol and tobacco can be legally consumed by adults, any purchase or use by adolescents is illegal. Because of the illegality of use for adolescents, social systems seldom discriminate between experimentation, heavy use, or substance use disorders in their required actions. Consequently, youths at earlier stages of substance involvement may be as hesitant to seek help as those with substance use disorders.

A final social and professional issue regarding brief interventions for substance-abusing youths with mental disorders is the social zeitgeist of confrontation for substance-related problems. Most brief interventions are based on a motivational enhancement approach that is nonconfrontational by design. Confrontation represents an impediment to help seeking that may be particularly troublesome in populations of adolescents with mental health disorders such as depression or anxiety, in which low rates of help seeking are to be expected. Although much has been written about confrontational approaches as barriers to treatment (see, e.g., Tucker, 1999), little of this clinical research information has been disseminated into the predominately 12-step-oriented programs nationally, and even less has been implemented by way of new treatment engagement strategies.

A variety of social, legal, and political hurdles may greet attempts to disseminate brief interventions for such youths and incorporate them into practice. Professional and legal standards and procedures for the treatment of minors often inhibit utilization of available resources by youths. For example, once alcohol or drug problems are identified, parents often must be informed and approve intervention prior to implementation. Given the fluctuating motivation of youths and the common concerns of confidentiality (Windle, Miller-Tutzauer, Barnes, & Welte, 1991), "on demand" or immediate treatment of substance-related *problems*, as opposed to substance use *disorders*, would likely increase adolescent utilization rates for interventions.

SUMMARY

Brief interventions for adolescents with co-occurring substance use disorders and other mental health disorders is a particularly promising area. Such interventions offer a number of potential benefits for youths, including more reliable identification of problems, earlier engagement in treatment, curtailing the escalation and adverse consequences of substance abuse, and diminution in psychiatric symptoms secondary to substance involvement. Research on adult populations suggests that brief interventions may be valuable across a variety of settings in which individuals with co-occurring mental health and substance use disorders are commonly seen. Although such cross-system research with adolescents is lacking, the limited number of studies completed to date (see, e.g., Monti et al., 1999; Wagner, Brown, Monti, Myers, & Waldron, 1999) indicate that research for brief interventions for youths with comorbid mental health and substance use disorders is well merited.

The design of brief interventions for adolescents is in the developmental stage. However, it is expected that optimal approaches will vary markedly across settings, for each gender, and by age and cultural background. Consonant with the flexibility of the motivational enhancement model, brief interventions may be tailored to accommodate problems and issues that vary across types of psychopathology. Given the reduced help seeking of youths, brief, motivationally focused interventions may be the optimal approach to engage youths in efforts to attend to their substance-related problems and to serve as a useful bridge to more intensive substance-focused treatments when needed. Although it is unlikely that brief interventions will supplant more intensified intervention, their niche for identification, engagement, and transition to treatment is critical to provision of an optimal continuum of care.

REFERENCES

American Psychiatric Association. (1987). *Diagnostic and statistical manual of mental disorders*, (3rd ed., rev.). Washington, DC: Author.

Brown, S. A. (1993). Recovery patterns in adolescent substance abuse. In J. S. Baer, G. A. Marlatt, & R. J. McMahon (Eds.), *Addictive behaviors across the lifespan: Prevention, treatment, and policy issues* (pp. 161–183). Beverly Hills, CA: Sage.

Brown, S. A., Mott, M. A., & Myers, M. G. (1990). Adolescent drug and alcohol treatment outcome. In R. R. Watson (Ed.), *Prevention and treatment of drug and alcohol abuse* (pp. 373–403). Totowa, NJ: Humana Press.

Brown, S. A., & Schuckit, M. A. (1988). Changes in depression among abstinent alcoholics. *Journal of Studies on Alcohol, 49*, 412–417.

Bukstein, O. G., Brent, D. A., & Kaminer, Y. (1989). Comorbidity of substance abuse and other psychiatric disorders in adolescents. *American Journal of Psychiatry,* 146(9), 1131–1141.

Chassin, L., Presson, C. C., Young, R. D., & Light, R. (1981). Self-concepts of institutionalized adolescents: A framework for conceptualizing labeling effects. *Journal of Abnormal Psychology, 90,* 143–151.

Colby, S. M., Monti, P. M., Barnett, N. P., Rohsenow, D. J., Weissman, K., Spirito, A., Woolard, R. H., & Lewander, W. J. (1998). Brief motivational interviewing in a hospital setting for adolescent smoking: A preliminary study. *Journal of Consulting and Clinical Psychology, 66,* 574–578.

Crowley, T. J., Mikulich, S. K., MacDonald, M., Young, S. E., & Zerbe, G. O. (1998). Substance-dependent, conduct-disordered adolescent males: Severity of diagnosis predicts 2-year outcome. *Drug and Alcohol Dependence, 49,* 225–237.

D'Amico, E. J., & Fromme, K. (2000). Implementation of the Risk Skills Training Program: A brief intervention targeting adolescent participation in risk behaviors. *Cognitive and Behavioral Practice, 7*(1), 101–117.

Deas-Nesmith, D., Campbell, S., & Brady, K. T. (1998). Substance use disorders in adolescent inpatient psychiatric population. *Journal of the National Medical Association, 90,* 233–238.

Dembo, R. (1995). On the poignant need for substance misuse services among youths entering the juvenile justice system. *International Journal of the Addictions, 30,* 747–751.

Dimeff, L. A. (1998). Brief intervention for heavy and hazardous college drinkers in a student primary health care setting. *Dissertation Abstracts International, 58,* 6805B. (University Microfilms No. AAM9819231)

Dunn, C., & Ries, R. (1997). Linking substance abuse services with general medical care: Integrated, brief interventions with hospitalized patients. *American Journal of Drug and Alcohol Abuse, 23,* 1–13.

Fleming, M. F., Barry, K. L., Manwell, L. B., Johnson, K., & London, R. (1997). Brief physician advice for problem alcohol drinkers: A randomized controlled trial in community-based primary care practices. *Journal of the American Medical Association, 277,* 1039–1045.

Greenbaum, P. E., Foster-Johnson, L., & Petrila, A. (1996). Co-occurring addictive and mental disorders among adolescents: Prevalence research and future directions. *American Journal of Orthopsychiatry, 66,* 52–60.

Grilo, C. M., Becker, D. F., Walker, M. L., Levy, K. N., Edell, W. S., & McGlashan, T. H. (1995). Psychiatric comorbidity in adolescent inpatients with substance use disorder. *Journal of the American Academy of Child and Adolescent Psychiatry, 34*(8), 1085–1091.

Heather, N., Rollnick, S., Bell, A., & Richmond, R. (1996). Effects of brief counselling among male heavy drinkers identified on general hospital wards. *Drug and Alcohol Review, 15,* 29–38.

Hubbard, R. L., Craddock, S. G., Flynn, P. M., Anderson, J., & Etheridge, R. M. (1997). Overview of 1-year follow-up outcomes in the Drug Abuse Treatment Outcome Study (DATOS). *Psychology of Addictive Behaviors, 11*(4), 261–278.

Kandel, D. B., Johnson, J. G., Bird, H. R., Canino, G., Goodman, S. H., Lahey, B. B., Regier, D. A., & Schwab-Stone, M. (1997). Psychiatric disorders associated with substance use among children and adolescents: Findings from the methods for the epidemiology of child and adolescent mental disorders (MECA) study. *Journal of Abnormal Psychology, 25*(2), 121–132.

Kelly, J. F., & Myers, M. G. (1997). Adolescent treatment outcome in relation to 12-step group attendance [Abstract]. *Alcoholism: Clinical and Experimental Research, 21*, 27A.

Kelly, J. F., Myers, M. G., & Brown, S. A. (2000). The effects of adolescent 12-step group attendance on common processes of change following inpatient substance abuse treatment: Analysis of a mediational model. *Psychology of Addictive Behaviors, 14*(4), 376–389.

Lewinsohn, P. M., Rhode, P., & Seeley, J. R. (1995). Adolescent psychopathology: 3. The clinical consequences of comorbidity. *Journal of the American Academy of Child and Adolescent Psychiatry, 34*(4), 510–519.

Marlatt, G. A., Baer, J. S., Kivlahan, D. R., Dimeff, L. A., Larimer, M. E., Quigley, L. A., Somers, J. M., & Williams, E. (1998). Screening and brief intervention for high-risk college student drinkers: Results from a two-year follow-up assessment. *Journal of Consulting and Clinical Psychology, 66*(4), 604–615.

Miles, D. R., Stallings, M. C., Young, S. E., Hewitt, J. K., Crowley, T. J., & Fulker, D. W. (1998). A family history and direct interview study of the familial aggregation of substance abuse: The adolescent substance abuse study. *Drug and Alcohol Dependence, 49*(2), 105–114.

Miller, W. R., & Brown, S. A. (1997). Why psychologists should treat alcohol and drug problems. *American Psychologist, 52*, 1269–1279.

Miller, W. R., & Rollnick, S. (1991). *Motivational interviewing: Preparing people to change addictive behavior.* New York: Guilford Press.

Monti, P. M., Colby, S. M., Barnett, N. P., Spirito, A., Rohsenow, D. J., Myers, M. G., Woolard, R., & Lewander, L. (1999). Brief intervention for harm reduction with alcohol-positive older adolescents in a hospital emergency department. *Journal of Consulting and Clinical Psychology, 67*, 989–994.

Neighbors, B., Kempton, T., & Forehand, R. (1992). Co-occurrence of substance abuse with conduct, anxiety, and depression disorders in juvenile delinquents. *Addictive Behaviors, 17*, 379–386.

Noordsy, D. L., Schwab, B., Fox, L., Drake, R. E. (1996). The role of self-help programs in the rehabilitation of persons with severe mental illness and substance use disorders. *Community Mental Health Journal, 32*(1), 71–80.

Novins, D. K., Beals, J., Shore, J. H., & Manson, S. M. (1996). Substance abuse treatment of American Indian adolescents: Comorbid symptomatology, gender differences, and treatment patterns. *Journal of the American Academy of Child and Adolescent Psychiatry, 35*(12), 1593–1601.

Philips, I. (1990). Trends in the delivery of mental health services for children and adolescents. *Bulletin of the Menninger Clinic, 54*, 95–100.

Piazza, N. J. (1996). Dual diagnosis and adolescent psychiatric inpatients. *Substance Use and Misuse, 31*, 215–223.

Richter, S. S., Brown, S. A., & Mott, M. A. (1991). The impact of social support and self-esteem on adolescent substance abuse treatment outcome. *Journal of Substance Abuse, 3*, 371–385.

Rieger, D. A., Farmer, M. E., Rae, D. S., Locke, B. Z., Keith, S. J., Judd, L. L., & Goodwin, F. K. (1990). Comorbidity of mental disorders with alcohol and other drug abuse: Results from the epidemiologic catchment area (ECA) study. *Journal of the American Medical Association, 264,* 2511–2518.

Roche, A. M., Parle, M. D., Stubbs, J. M., Hall, W., & Saunders, J. B. (1995). Management and treatment efficacy of drug and alcohol problems: What do doctors believe? *Addiction, 90,* 1357–1366.

Stewart, D. G., & Brown, S. A. (1995). Withdrawal and dependency symptoms among adolescent alcohol and drug abusers. *Addiction, 90,* 627–635.

Stowell, R. J., & Estroff, T. W. (1992). Psychiatric disorders in substance-abusing adolescent inpatients: A pilot study. *Journal of the American Academy of Child and Adolescent Psychiatry, 31*(6), 1036–1040.

Tober, G. (1991). Motivational interviewing with young people. In W. R. Miller & S. Rollnick, *Motivational interviewing: Preparing people to change addictive behavior* (pp. 248–259). New York: Guilford Press.

Tucker, J. A. (1999). Changing addictive behavior: A historical and contemporary perspective. In J. A. Tucker, D. M. Donovan, & G. A. Marlatt (Eds.), *Changing addictive behavior: Bridging clinical and public health strategies* (pp. 3–44). New York: Guilford Press.

Tucker, J. A., Vuchinich, R. E., & Gladsjo, J. A. (1994). Environmental events surrounding natural recovery from alcohol-related problems. *Journal of Studies on Alcohol, 55,* 401–411.

Wagner, E. F., Brown, S. A., Monti, P. M., Myers, M. G., & Waldron, H. (1999). Innovations in adolescent substance abuse intervention. *Alcoholism: Clinical and Experimental Research, 23,* 236–249.

Wilens, T. E., Biederman, J., Abrantes, A. M., & Spencer, T. J. (1997). Clinical characteristics of psychiatrically referred adolescent outpatients with substance use disorder. *Journal of the American Academy of Child and Adolescent Psychiatry, 36*(7), 941–947.

Windle, M., Miller-Tutzauer, C., Barnes, G. M., & Welte, J. (1991). Adolescent perceptions of help-seeking resources for substance abuse. *Child Development, 62,* 179–189.

World Health Organization. (1996). A cross-national trial of brief interventions with heavy drinkers. *American Journal of Public Health, 86,* 948–955.

10

New Frontiers

Using the Internet to Engage Teens in Substance Abuse Prevention and Treatment

HARVEY SKINNER, OONAGH MALEY, LOUISE SMITH,
SHAWN CHIRREY, and MEG MORRISON

> Eighty percent of the technologies that we will still be using 20
> years from now have yet to be invented.
> —A PREDICTION MADE BY MANY FUTURISTS

Today's youths have access to more health information than ever in the
past. Yet health risk behaviors such as cigarette smoking, excessive drinking, and drug abuse have increased over the past 15 years. The major challenge is: How do we engage youth in health promotion? We live in a highly
media-oriented world. Music videos and computer games use a dynamic
approach that appeals to teens. The Internet, in particular, provides innovative opportunities for reaching youths, including those turned off by traditional health education approaches.

This chapter describes opportunities for using the Internet for substance abuse prevention and brief treatment with adolescents. The *seven
critical functions* model (Skinner, 2001) is presented as a framework that
practitioners can use for designing brief interventions. Practical examples
for alcohol, drug, and tobacco interventions are taken from the Web, as
well as from the TeenNet Website CyberIsle. A brief on-line intervention
for adolescent smoking prevention or cessation, called the Smoking Zine
(short for "magazine"), is used to illustrate how information can be presented in a nonjudgmental, fun environment through quizzes, simulations,
fact sheets, self-assessments, personalized feedback, and peer discussion
groups. A parallel Website called PractitionerNet provides a forum and
guidelines for practitioners in using the Internet for brief interventions with
young people.

297

THE CHALLENGE OF ENGAGING YOUTHS

We face a dilemma in substance abuse prevention in adolescence. This is the developmental stage at which potential health-risk behaviors (e.g., smoking, alcohol, and other drug use) may be initiated. On the other hand, the individual may pass successfully through this transition period into adulthood, when the likelihood of initiation decreases substantially.

During middle or high school, American and Canadian teenagers initiate use of alcohol, tobacco, and marijuana at a greater rate than at any other time. Indeed, with few exceptions, health-risk behaviors such as drug and alcohol use have remained steady or have increased among youths in America and Canada (Adlaf, Ivis, & Paglia, 1999; Johnston, Bachman, & O'Malley, 2000). For these reasons, adolescents are a primary target for prevention and health promotion initiatives. However, it is often difficult to engage teens in a serious examination of health consequences, because they believe negative consequences are too vague and far in the future to be concerned about.

The increasing availability of information technology creates an innovative channel for clinical prevention and health promotion with the ability to reach a large number of young people. Health promotion programs that are interactive and involve peer-led components have been shown to be the most effective (Botvin & Botvin, 1997; Dusenbury & Falco, 1997; Ellickson, 1995; Lynagh, Schofield, & Sanson-Fisher, 1997; Tobler & Stratton, 1997). The Web provides an ideal environment for this interactivity and peer-to-peer interaction.

HOW THE INTERNET CAN HELP PRACTITIONERS ENGAGE YOUTHS

Although computers have been heralded as a technological revolution, today we are at the doorstep of a much bigger transformation. The information technology revolution is having a profound impact on the way we live, learn, and educate. Driving this revolution is the explosive growth of the Internet, especially the World Wide Web. The Internet provides an environment that can be graphically appealing, anonymous, and nonjudgmental, that can incorporate mutual support and be accessible 24 hours a day, and is paced at the user's speed (Abbate, 1999; Abrams, 1998).

The Web provides an extremely powerful tool for health education and brief interventions regarding alcohol, drug, and tobacco use. Aspects that are particularly relevant for prevention and treatment programs with youths include:

1. Quick dissemination of information and ability to reach a large number of youths in all areas of a country (indeed, the world).
2. Vibrant graphics and innovative effects that youths find highly engaging.
3. Multiple pathways or means for youths to gain access to health information and brief interventions (e.g., from schools, local libraries, homes, community and health care settings).
4. Extensive linkages to related topics, such as discussion groups, lifestyle assessments and guided-change programs, specific health information, and interactive games related to health issues.
5. Information that can be readily updated and refreshed in order to provide a new look.
6. Connectivity (one-to-many) and mutual support, allowing users to assist others and to create an environment that stimulates collective action.

Young people have been the early adopters of this new technology. Teens go on the Web for numerous reasons: 83% for e-mail, 68% for specific information and research, 51% for games, and 40% for chat rooms (Pricewaterhouse Coopers, 2000). In Canada, over 50% of the adult population has general access to the Internet, but over 90% of adolescents have access. Similarly, in the United States, female "tweens" (girls 12 to 15 years old) are the fastest growing group on the Net (Teenage Research Unlimited, 2000): in 1996, 54% were on-line, and in 1999 that figure jumped to 87%. Thus most youths are already on the Internet. Our challenge is to provide relevant content and services regarding substance abuse.

Keeping on top of the rapid pace and diversity of information technology (IT) is a concern for busy practitioners. Some good sources to check out periodically include:

1. Benton Foundation (*www.benton.org*)
   • Organization that follows IT and community trends
2. Cyber Dialogue (*www.cyberdialogue.com*)
   • U.S. organization that tracks on-line health consumer trends
3. NUA (*www.nua.org* or *www.nua.ie*)
   • Irish organization that is the world leader in surveys of Net users
4. Slash Dot (*www.slashdot.org*)
   • Bible for all things open source (e.g., free software) and new technology
5. Wired (*www.wired.com*)
   • Good old standby on technology trends

6. Shift Magazine (*www.shift.com*)
   - Canada's answer to *Wired* (good IT coverage)
7. Cell phone technology and trends include:
   - Unwired News (*Wired* magazine) (*www.wired.com/news/wireless*)
   - Yahoo Mobile (*mobile.yahoo.com/wireless/home*)
   - W3C WAP Forum (*www.w3.org/TR/NOTE-WAP*)

SEVEN CRITICAL FUNCTIONS: A FRAMEWORK FOR BRIEF INTERVENTIONS

Already there are myriad Websites on the Internet that address elements of alcohol, drug, and tobacco use and abuse. Moreover, these sites are under continual evolution: Many will be substantially altered over the next months and years, and other links will become nonfunctional or extinct by the time this book appears. What is most needed is a framework or model that will be enduring and also help practitioners adapt these resources effectively for brief interventions. This is where the *seven critical functions* model (Skinner, 2001) can help.

The seven critical functions are essential components of substance abuse prevention for brief interventions. Both practitioners and adolescents (patients, clients, or students) need support if they are to be successful in changing health behavior related to alcohol, drug, and tobacco use. Each function encompasses a group of linked activities or processes directed at accomplishing a specific goal. For example, a computerized health-behavior assessment administered during clinical intake can automatically provide the practitioner with a patient's risk-factor profile regarding substance abuse in a timely fashion before the consultation begins. Integration of the functions in a dynamic system opens the window of opportunity for practitioners to use motivational interventions described in other chapters of this book and in key publications (Marlatt & Gordon, 1985; Miller & Rollnick, 1991; Prochaska, DiClemente, & Norcross, 1992; Rollnick, Mason, & Butler, 1999).

The seven critical functions are described in detail by Skinner (2001), along with an organizational assessment tool for conducting a critical functions analysis. The functions include:

1. Priming and prompting of patients, clients, and practitioners: to address prevention and substance abuse risk factors.
2. Identification of risk behaviors and related complications: using screening and case finding, both in clinical encounters and at the community population level.

3. Options for help: professional assistance, support groups that are professionally led, self-help groups, and community resources.
4. Continuing care: monitoring, reassessment, provision of additional care and follow-up.
5. Linkages and networks among services and resources: within and outside the specific health, community, or educational setting.
6. Information management: systems that support prevention and behavior-change initiatives, including timely feedback to patients and practitioners.
7. Personal and professional development in behavior change: individual (patient, practitioner) and organizational levels.

Each function encompasses a group of linked activities or processes that are directed at accomplishing a specific goal in behavior change. Their integration in a program of continuous improvement provides a fundamental approach to organizational renewal in supporting practitioners in prevention and brief interventions for adolescent substance abuse.

We have used the seven critical functions model as a framework for organizing Internet resources that can be adapted for different settings and needs. Table 10.1 contains resources for alcohol abuse interventions, Table 10.2 for drug abuse interventions, and Table 10.3 for smoking prevention and cessation. Internet links for the first four functions can be combined to create a prevention program or brief treatment intervention that is tailored to the practitioner's specific needs. The last three functions can provide background support for the interventions.

ALCOHOL INTERVENTIONS (TABLE 10.1)

A number of Web resources exist that encourage youths to look at the effects of alcohol, as well as at their attitudes and drinking behavior (*priming and prompting function*). The resources of the Alcohol Advisory Council of New Zealand take an interactive approach to engaging youths in thinking about alcohol. In FUEL (*www.alcohol.org.nz/fuel/index.html*), youths are invited to host a virtual party. During the party the youth pours the drinks and observes, the Website says there will be kissing, fighting, even vomiting. Once the party is over, the youth can host the party again to see how things could have been different. In HADENOUGH on the same Website, adolescents can explore their attitudes to alcohol and current drinking behavior through a number of self-assessments. Although aimed at youth, these resources can provide practitioners with a starting point for discussions with young clients. Additional Web resources provide practitioners

TABLE 10.1. Websites for Alcohol Use Interventions

Critical function	For teens	For practitioners
Priming and prompting	Alcohol Advisory Council (NZ) (*www.alcohol.org.nz*) Site includes FUEL (a game simulating drinking and partying scenarios and issues) and interactive quizzes to assess drinking habits and attitudes (HADENOUGH).	CyberIsle (*www.cyberisle.org*) Hot Talk discussion area shows practitioners what youth are talking about concerning alcohol use, interests, questions, and concerns.
	Addictions & More (*www.addictions.net/warning.htm*) Outlines warning signs of alcohol and drug abuse.	Alberta Alcohol and Drug Abuse Commission (*www.gov.ab.ca/aadac/addictions/abc/talking_to_teens_drugs.htm*) Links and tips for adults to talk with teens about drugs.
		Addictions & More (*www.addictions.net/warning.htm*) General addictions Website provides an outline of the warning signs of alcohol and drug abuse.
		CAMH—Youth & Alcohol Information (*www.arf.org/isd/infopak/youth.html*) Centre for Addictions and Mental Health's information package on youth and alcohol use (including identification and warning sign information).
Identification	University of Indiana, Alcohol and Drug Information Center (*http://campuslife.indiana.edu/~ADIC/checklist.html*) Provides a personal checklist about substance use.	
	Counseling Department at CalTech (*http://www.counseling.caltech.edu/drug/self/test/test1.html*) Drug and Alcohol Abuse Prevention program at Cal Tech provides an excellent alcohol self-test.	
	Mayo Clinic Drinking Quiz (*www.mayohealth.org/home?id=SC00010*) Mayo Clinic On-line, link to an on-line drinking quiz.	
Options for help	CyberIsle (*www.cyberisle.org*) Peer discussion and support groups, as well as links to on-line resources on alcohol.	National Clearinghouse for Alcohol and Drug Information (*www.health.org*) NCADI provides links, fact sheets, and linkages to

Kids Help Phone Discussion Groups (*http://kidshelp.sympatico.ca/talk#index.htm*)
Canadian phone help line for youth and children—linkages to phone base counseling and on-line peer-support discussion groups.

Action Steps for Youth (*www.ctclearinghouse.org/fdrugyout.htm*)

treatment resources.

Canadian Centre on Substance Abuse (*www.ccsa.ca*)
Includes a searchable database of treatment organizations in Canada.

Continuing care

CyberIsle (*www.cyberisle.org*)
Peer discussion and support groups, as well as links to on-line resources on drugs.

Support Groups (face-to-face and on-line) (*www.selfhelp.on.ca* or *http://mentalhelp.net/selfhelp*)
Links to on-line self-help clearinghouse and support groups in Canada and the United States.

American Medical Association: Adolescent Prevention Guidelines (*www.ama-assn.org/ama/publ/category/1980.htm*)
The AMA's set of recommendations that describe the content and delivery of comprehensive clinical preventive services for adolescents 11–21 years of age.

Linkages and networks

CyberIsle (*www.cyberisle.org*)
Peer discussion and support groups, as well as links to on-line resources on drugs.

Peer Help Approaches (Health Canada) (*www.hc-sc.gc.ca/hppb/alcohol-otherdrugs/pdf/peer_e.pdf*)
A research document from Health Canada emphasizing the use of peer support approaches in alcohol and drug treatment.

Brown University Center for Alcohol and Addiction Studies (*www.caas.brown.edu*)
Provides excellent resources and linkages on alcohol and addictions research and resources.

European Union Public Health Resources on Alcohol, Office of the Director of Alcohol Experts and Organizations (*www.sfsp-publichealth.org/europe.html*)
Excellent example of an EU policy and shared research model.

(continued)

TABLE 10.1. (*continued*)

Critical function	For teens	For practitioners
Linkages and networks (*continued*)	Canadian Health Network (*www.chn-rcs.ca*) Health Promotion Website that is a partnership between Health Canada and over 500 health organizations. Provides links and e-mail health information requests for individuals and practitioners. Health Finder (*www.healthfinder.com*) Developed by the U.S. Department of Health and Human Services, this Website provides access to consumer health and human services information.	Canadian Health Network (*www.chn-rcs.ca*) Health promotion Website that is a partnership between Health Canada and over 500 health organizations. Provides links and e-mail health information requests for both individuals and practitioners. National Institute on Alcohol Abuse and Alcoholism (*www.niaaa.nih.gov*) NIAAA provides up-to-date research, linkages, and resources for drug abuse, including an FAQ on alcohol abuse and alcoholism. Health Finder (*www.healthfinder.com*) Developed by the U.S. Department of Health and Human Services, this Website provides access to consumer health and human services information.
Information management	We were unable to find a comparable Website that addresses alcohol abuse in the comprehensive format in which CyberIsle (*www.cyberisle.org*) addresses tobacco prevention and cessation.	The whole CyberIsle (*www.cyberisle.org*) Website is a way of delivering seven critical functions, easily accessible 24 hours, paced at user speed, and allowing for interaction among practitioners.
Professional development		CEIDA (Australia) (*www.ceida.net.au*) Centre for Education and Information on Drugs and Alcohol (CEIDA) provides information and professional development resources for general practitioners. CAMH—Youth & Alcohol Information (*www.camh.net*) Centre for Addictions and Mental Health's information package on youth and alcohol use (including identification and warning sign information).

with tips for talking with adolescents (*www.gov.ab.ca/aadac/addictions/ abc/talking_to_teens_drugs.htm*), while youth discussion boards like Hot Talk on CyberIsle (*www.cyberisle.org*) can provide a window on how youths talk about alcohol in their own words (*professional development function*).

For youths who drink or are concerned about the drinking of someone they know, the Web provides access to a number of assessment resources (*identification function*), such as:

> *www.counseling.caltech.edu/drug/selftest/test1.html*
> *http://campuslife.indiana.edu/ADIC/checklist.html*

Adolescents can complete these assessments in private at any time of the day just by accessing the Web. Practitioners discussing potential alcohol problems with young clients can access the same assessments (*options for help function*).

When an adolescent identifies a drinking concern or problem, there are various "next steps" or interventions available (*options for help function*). The Internet provides environments to connect youths both to peer support, through discussion forums such as CyberIsle's Hot Talk (*www. cyberisle.org*), or to professional counseling through organizations such as Kids Help Phone (*http://kidshelp.sympatico.ca/talk/index.htm*). With the Internet, a youth does not have to wait for a clinic to open or make an appointment. Similarly, practitioners can use the Web to identify and access national and local resources. The National Clearinghouse for Alcohol and Drug Information (*www.health.org*) provides links to a searchable database of treatment facilities, as well as a list of referral hot line numbers.

For young people receiving treatment for alcohol abuse, relapse prevention is a major concern (*continuing care function*). As with identifying options for help, the Internet's 24/7 access (24 hours a days, 7 days a week) can provide critical support to a youth when a practitioner is not available. Support can be found on-line, as in CyberIsle's Hot Talk, or on-line resources can link youths to telephone support or to face-to-face support groups. In the United States, the American Self-Help Clearinghouse Website includes a searchable database of self-help groups (*http://mentalhelp. net/selfhelp*)

For practitioners who provide care to youths, having access to the most current treatment and care guidelines is essential (*professional development function*). The American Medical Association (AMA) Website provides access to the *Guidelines for Adolescent Preventive Services* (GAPS)— a set of guidelines for the delivery of clinical preventive services for adolescents: *www.ama-assn.org/ama/pub/category/1980.htm*.

In addition, a number of research and resource sites exist that practitioners can access for the latest findings, as well as up-to-date reviews and practice guidelines. Some recommended sites include:

(United States) Brown University, Center for Alcohol and Addiction Studies
www.caas.brown.edu
(United States) National Institute on Alcohol Abuse and Alcoholism
www.niaaa.nih.gov
(Canada) Centre for Addiction and Mental Health
www.camn.net
(Europe) European Union Public Health Resources on Alcohol
www.sfsp-publichealth.org/europe.html
(Australia) Centre for Education and Information on Drugs and Alcohol
www.ceida.net.au

DRUG ABUSE INTERVENTIONS (TABLE 10.2)

The Internet currently features fewer interactive resources for youths about drugs than about alcohol. However, youth and practitioners can access a wide range of approaches to drug education, from harm reduction to "just say no." Websites such as Dance Safe (*www.dancesafe.org*) and "D-2K" (*www.d-2k.co.uk*) outline the effects and risks of different drugs. These sites provide both youths and practitioners with starting points to explore various attitudes to drug use (*priming and prompting function*).

Very few resources provide youth with self-assessment tools to identify drug use problems (*identification function*). This most likely reflects the illegal nature of many recreational drugs and the fact that health education often focuses on preventing use. Clearly, there is a need to develop more resources, such as a Web-based version of the Drug Abuse Screening Test (DAST; Martino, Grilo, & Fehon, 2000; Skinner, 1982, 2000). For practitioners who treat adolescent clients, many of the same resources identified for alcohol (Table 10.1) provide linkages with drug treatment programs (*options for help function*) and professional or peer support (*continuing care function*). A few of the best resources include:

American Council for Drug Education: develops programs and materials, including those for health professionals and educators.
• www.acde.org/health

TABLE 10.2. Websites for Drug Use Interventions

Critical function	For teens	For practitioners
Priming and prompting	Drugs: The Facts (*http://hna.ffh.vic.gov.au/phb/hdev/drug/cover.html*) Information about drug use and abuse. Addictions & More (*www.addictions.net/warning.htm*) Outlines warning signs of alcohol and drug abuse. "D-2K" (*www.d-2k.co.uk*) This U.K. site provides information on a range of drugs, including effects, risks, and what to do in an emergency. Dance Safe (*www.dancesafe.org*) Provides harm reduction information on drugs used in the rave and dance communities.	CyberIsle (*www.cyberisle.org*) Hot Talk discussion area shows practitioners what youths are talking about concerning drug abuse, interests, questions, and concerns.
Identification	University of Indiana, Alcohol and Drug Information Center (*http://campuslife.indiana.edu/ADIC/checklist.html*) Provides a personal checklist about substance use. National Clearinghouse for Alcohol and Drug Information Straight Facts about Drugs and Alcohol (*www.health.org/govpubs/rpo884*) Includes signs of drug abuse for self or others	Addictions & More (*www.addictions.net/warning.htm*) General addictions Website provides an outline of the warning signs of alcohol and drug abuse.
Options for help	Dare World (*www.dare.com/index_3.htm*) Links and contact numbers for organizations targeting drug abuse.	Canadian Centre on Substance Abuse (*www.ccsa.ca*) Includes a searchable database of treatment organizations in Canada.

(continued)

307

TABLE 10.2. (continued)

Critical function	For teens	For practitioners
Options for help (continued)	CyberIsle (www.cyberisle.org) Peer discussion and support groups, as well as links to on-line resources on drugs. Kids Help Phone Discussion Groups (http://kidshelp.sympatico.ca/talk/index.htm) Canadian help phone line for youth and children—linkages to phone base counseling and online peer-support discussion groups.	National Clearinghouse for Alcohol and Drug Information (www.health.org) NCADI provides links, fact sheets, and linkages to treatment resources.
Continuing care	CyberIsle's Hot Talk (www.cyberisle.org) Peer discussion and support groups Kids Help Phone Discussion Groups (http://kidshelp.sympatico.ca/talk/index.htm) Canadian phone help line for youth and children—linkages to phone base counseling and on-line peer-support discussion groups.	American Medical Association: Adolescent Prevention Guidelines (www.ama-assn.org/ama/pub/catgory/1980.htm) The AMA's set of recommendations that describe the content and delivery of comprehensive clinical preventive services for adolescents 11–21 years of age.
Linkages and networks	CyberIsle (www.cyberisle.org) Peer discussion and support groups as well as links to on-line resources on drugs. Peer Help Approaches (Health Canada) (www.hc-sc.gc.ca/hppb/alcohol-otherdrugs/pdf/peer_e.pdf) A research document from Health Canada emphasizing the use of peer support approaches in alcohol and drug treatment.	National Institute on Drug Abuse (www.nida.nih.gov) NIDA provides up-to-date research, linkages, and resources for drug abuse, with some excellent resources on adolescent drug and alcohol abuse/use. Health Finder (www.healthfinder.com) Developed by the U.S. Department of Health and Human Services, this Website provides access to consumer health and human services information.

Linkages and networks (continued)	Canadian Health Network (www.chn-rcs.ca) Health promotion Website that is a partnership between Health Canada and over 500 health organizations. Provide links and e-mail health information requests for individuals and practitioners. Health Finder (www.healthfinder.gov) Developed by the U.S. Department of Health and Human Services, this Website provides access to consumer health and human services information.	TeenNet Websites (www.teennetproject.org) deliver the seven critical functions in a way that is easily accessible 24 hours, paced at user speed, and that allows for interaction among practitioners.
Information management	We were unable to find a comparable Website that addresses drug abuse in the comprehensive format in which CyberIsle addresses tobacco prevention and cessation.	
Professional development	Not applicable	CEIDA (Australia) (www.ceida.net.au) Centre for Education and Information on Drugs and Alcohol (CEIDA) provides information and professional development resources for general practitioners. American Council for Drug Education (www.acde.org/health) A substance abuse prevention and education agency that develops programs and materials. Also provides information and resources for health professionals and educators.

Note. Planet Know is an interactive antidrug site: http://www.planet-know.net/first.htm

National Institute on Drug Abuse: provides up-to-date research, linkages, and resources.
- www.nida.nih.gov/NIDAHome.html

Canadian Centre on Substance Abuse: includes searchable databases of treatment organizations in Canada.
- www.ccsa.ca

CyberIsle: peer discussion and support groups, plus links to on-line resources on drugs.
- www.cyberisle.org

Kids Help Phone Discussion Groups: Canadian help phone line for youth and children.
- http://kidshelp.sympatico.ca/talk/index.htm

SMOKING INTERVENTIONS (TABLE 10.3)

This section illustrates how TeenNet Websites can be used for smoking prevention and cessation programs. The overall goal of TeenNet (*www.teennetproject.org*) is to increase the number of teens engaged in health promotion activities, such as substance abuse prevention. The first Website, launched in 1997, was based on the concept of a teens-only "island" called CyberIsle (*www.cyberisle.org*). The main components of CyberIsle include:

1. *Home page:* Gateway to all components. A password is required in order to enter this teens-only island, which provides a means of gathering background information on users.
2. *Health information:* Interactive, multimedia information on a wide range of health, personal, and social issues.
3. *Self-assessment and guided change.* Assessment, individualized feedback, and guided self-change strategies that are matched to the individual's readiness for change.
4. *Hot Talk:* Chat rooms for ongoing discussion groups and special topic forums, such as drugs, parents, sex, and smoking,
5. *Hot Links:* Links to other relevant sites on the Internet. All links have been reviewed and approved by the TeenNet Quality Control Committee, consisting of parents, teachers, school board personnel, health workers, and teens.

Since the launch of CyberIsle, efforts have concentrated on developing a state-of-the-art Website for youth smoking prevention and cessation called the Smoking Zine, described in the next section, along with a comprehensive "e-Health" site called the Teen Clinic Online. Both are "located" on the main CyberIsle site. Also, a parallel site developed for practitioners (PractitionerNet) contains various resources and continuing education modules for adolescent health (*www.practitionernet.org*).

The TeenNet project is based on a person-centered health promotion model described by Skinner and Bercovitz (1997) that underscores the interconnection among self-care, mutual aid, and professional assistance. A highly participatory, community-based approach is taken in which teens and various community organizations are involved in all stages of project design, development, implementation, evaluation, and dissemination (Skinner et al., 1997). The project draws on concepts and methodologies from self-determination theory (Ryan & Deci, 2000), social learning theory (Bandura, 1997), the transtheoretical model of behavior change (Prochaska et al., 1992), harm reduction (Erikson, Riley, Cheung, & O'Hare, 1996), community mobilization (Minkler & Wallerstein, 1997) and action research (Argyris, Putnam, & Smith, 1985). Drawing on these theories and models, the development of TeenNet Websites is guided by five principles:

1. *Participatory*: key involvement (ownership) at all stages by teens.
2. *Relevant to teens*: focus on health, personal, and social issues identified by teens.
3. *Autonomy-supporting*: encourages individual choice and exploration of options regarding health behavior.
4. *Active learning and fun*: engaging, flexible and highly interactive, stimulates self-directed learning.
5. *Accessible*: designed and adapted to be accessible and relevant to diverse populations of adolescents (especially disadvantaged).

A WALK THROUGH THE SMOKING ZINE

The Smoking Zine is designed for both adolescent smokers and nonsmokers. Teens access the Zine from CyberIsle's navigation bar. The personalized password is the same as for CyberIsle. The Smoking Zine is organized according to five interactive stages, which can be completed by youths over a period of time. Adolescents are able to do this by taking advantage of the Zine's logout feature, which allows them to exit, then reenter the site. When youths log back in to the Zine, they are returned to the beginning of any incomplete stage.

Practitioners can use the Smoking Zine as a component of a prevention or clinical program (e.g., to link motivational counseling with feedback from the quizzes and decision balance) or can provide the Zine to

TABLE 10.3. TeenNet Websites for Smoking Interventions

Critical Function	CyberIsle's Smoking Zine (*www.cyberisle.org*)	PractitionerNet and Health Behavior Change (*www.practitionernet.org* and *www.healthbehaviorchange.org*)
Priming and prompting	• *It's My Life*—smoking assessment with personalized feedback (identifies youth as smoker, nonsmoker, or experimenter). • *Makin' Cents*—interactive game in which youth "go shopping with cigarette packages." Provides forum for consciousness raising by showing the cost of smoking. • *Tailored profiles*—Smoking Zine quizzes and assessments are tailored to youth's responses. At the end, youths are given a profile of their smoking behavior and attitudes. This profile can be printed for use by the youth alone or in consultation with a practitioner. • *Hot Talk* (CyberIsle's peer-to-peer discussion forum) provides practitioners with an opportunity to observe youth's smoking interests, questions, and concerns.	• *Tobacco HotTopic*—provides practitioners general and youth-specific information and resources. • Training module provides practitioners with an overview of the zine, including how to interpret results from *It's My Life* and exercises for using *Makin' Cents*. • *Smoking Zine Workbook* provides activities and prompts for using the Smoking Zine with youth.
Identification	• *It's My Life*—smoking assessment with personalized feedback (identifies youth as smoker, nonsmoker, or experimenter). • *To Change or Not to Change*—self-assessments to identify youth's readiness to change, including measures of the importance of change and self-confidence. • *It's My Life* and *To Change or Not to Change* can be used by youth alone or in consultation with practitioner.	• *Training module* provides practitioners with an overview of the zine, including how to interpret results from *It's My Life* and *To Change or Not to Change*. • *Smoking Zine Workbook* provides activities and prompts for using the Smoking Zine with youths.

Options for help	• *What Next*—the zine's interactive smoking cessation resource help youths set their goals, find out why they smoke, choose their quitting option, and identify rewards and supports. • On *CyberIsle*, youths can access on-line resources, including the Teen Clinic Online.	• *Training module* provides practitioners with tools for motivational counseling in conjunction with the Smoking Zine.
Continuing care	• *Zine Logout Feature*—enables youth to complete the stages of the zine when they are ready. Practitioners can encourage youths to complete the zine and to revisit the zine to see if their smoking behavior and attitudes have changed over time. • *Hot Talk*—provides youths with ongoing support (24/7).	• Clinical prevention practice guidelines. • *PractitionerNet HotTopic* on tobacco provides practitioners general and youth-specific information and resources.
Linkages and networks	• *Hot Talk*—provides youths with access to a network of youths.	• Practitioner discussion groups. • Links to on-line resources. • Updated listings of relevant events.
Information management	• The whole CyberIsle Website provides a vehicle for meeting the seven critical functions. As one teen said, *"You can find it somewhere else, but this is a huge package deal."*	• All the TeenNet Websites provide ways of delivering seven critical functions, easily accessible 24 hours, paced at user speed, and allowing for interaction among practitioners.
Professional development	• Not applicable.	• Discussion groups. • Resources—links to on-line resources and professional organizations. • Training modules—how to use technology for health promotion with youth (in particular TeenNet's Smoking Zine).

313

youths as a stand-alone self-directed intervention. Here are the key features:

Billboard: the starting point of the Zine. There are five steps to complete. As each step is finished, the cigarette shrinks on the billboard.

Quizzes: questions about smoking and individualized scores. For smokers who want to quit, there is a comprehensive quitting resource. Those who don't want to quit are encouraged to come back after some time and retake the quizzes to see if their scores change.

Note to self: youths can make personal notes for future reference. These notes can be added to or changed at any time when the youth is in the Zine.

Speak out: links youth directly to Hot Talk, a discussion forum in which teens can talk with each other about their experiences or just read what others have written.

The following overview is taken from the *Guide to Using the Zine* on the Website developed by TeenNet youth advisors:

• *Step 1: Makin' Cents* (consciousness raising) calculates how many cigarette packs a person smokes per year, and then takes him or her shopping with them. A user selects the number of packs smoked per month; nonsmokers just choose a number. When "continue" is selected, a shopping cart appears; clicking on it brings up the shopping district. Clicking once on a store brings up a list of products in the lower left side of the screen. The user chooses what he or she wants to buy, and the cost (in cigarette packs) is deducted from the total. When all the packs have been used, a table appears with all the things that were bought.

• *Step 2: It's My Life* (assessment) is a quiz to determine one's personal smoking level.

• *Step 3: To Change or Not to Change* (readiness or stages of change) helps smokers decide if they want to quit and nonsmokers consider whether they will start. The user's score in It's My Life (Step 2) determines which quiz will come up. The user selects an answer and hits the button for a score.

• *Step 4: It's Your Decision* (decision balance) helps a user identify concerns about smoking and not smoking, as well as how he or she feels about changing. The "OK" button displays the results of the quiz. At the bottom of the page is a section on how to interpret the results.

• *Step 5: What's Next* presents all the user's scores and recommendations about what can be done next. For smokers who are ready to quit, the next section helps them to determine a goal, to learn why they smoke, and to choose a quitting method; it suggests ways to avoid temptation and to identify their concerns about smoking. The Support page allows them to list people they can depend on for support. The last page offers the opportunity to print out any section on a personalized matrix.

PRACTITIONERNET

This Website (*www.practitionernet.org*) provides comprehensive resources, discussion groups, and continuing education modules for practitioners on how to effectively integrate the use of information technology (including CyberIsle's Smoking Zine and Teen Clinic Online) into clinical practice, prevention, and health promotion with youth. Each workshop consists of both on-line and face-to-face components. In particular, PractitionerNet addresses the critical functions of professional development, linkages and networks and information management (see Table 10.3).

ENGAGING HARD-TO-REACH POPULATIONS: STREET-INVOLVED YOUTH

TeenNet is examining use of the Web for drug education and prevention with street-involved and low socioeconomic status youths. This population has very high rates of substance abuse, sexually transmitted diseases, and related health conditions. "Street-involved" or "street-connected" youths are people under the age of 25 who participate in street life, that is, youths who spend a considerable part of the day on downtown streets. Many are homeless; but some may live in shelters, hostels, with friends or relatives, or still live at home, and all participate in street life.

To our initial surprise, many street-involved youths are active users of the Internet. For example, in one study conducted at Shout Clinic (a downtown Toronto clinic that provides comprehensive health services to street-involved youths), adolescents were asked about what drugs they took (both medical and recreational), what specific information they wanted to know about those drugs, where they currently obtained drug information, and questions related to Internet usage. The findings showed a willingness to use the Internet for accessing drug information. However, these youths wanted content that was more relevant to their needs and life conditions (Skinner, 1998):

95% of youths were currently receiving drug information.
70% disliked the information they received.

90% were willing to use the Internet for accessing drug information. 75% currently had Internet access through friends, cafés, schools, home, and public libraries.

CONCLUSION

This chapter began by posing the question, How do we engage teens in health promotion? The Internet offers an exciting and versatile way of attracting their attention, even that of hard-to-reach and high-risk populations such as street-involved youth. But information technology by itself is insufficient. Our experience on the TeenNet project underscores the value of having a high level of youth participation from day one! This participatory approach is critical if practitioners are to use information technology effectively for substance abuse prevention and brief treatment interventions. A sense of ownership and pride was expressed by two teens when asked about their experience in working with TeenNet:

> "It makes me as a teen feel good that people care about what teens think and what they have to say. Most of the time we are overlooked. Not many teens get the chance to actually be heard . . . thank you."

ACKNOWLEDGMENT

The research for this chapter was supported, in part, by a grant to Harvey Skinner (Principal Investigator) from the Hospital for Sick Children Foundation, Toronto.

REFERENCES

Abbate, J. (1999). *Inventing the Internet.* Cambridge, MA: MIT Press.

Abrams, M. (Ed.). (1998). *World Wide Web: Beyond the basics.* Englewood Cliffs, NJ: Prentice-Hall.

Adlaf, E., Ivis F., & Paglia, A. (1999). *Drug use among Ontario students 1977–1999: Finding from the OSDUS [Ontario Student Drug Use Survey].* Toronto, Ontario, Canada: Addiction Research Foundation

Argyris, C., Putnam, R., & Smith, D. (1985). *Action science.* San Francisco: Jossey-Bass.

Bandura, A. (1997). *Self-efficacy: The exercise of control.* New York: Freeman.

Botvin, G., & Botvin, E. (1997). School-based programs. In J. Lowinson, P. Ruiz, R. Millman, & J. Langrod (Eds.), *Substance abuse: A comprehensive textbook* (pp. 764–775). Baltimore: Williams & Wilkins.

Dusenbury, L., & Falco, M. (1997). School-based drug abuse prevention strategies: From research to policy and practice. In R. Weissberg, T. Gullotta, R. Hampton, B. Ryan, & G. Adams (Eds.), *Enhancing children's wellness* (pp. 47–75). Thousand Oaks, CA: Sage.

Ellickson, P. (1995). Schools. In R. Coombs & D. Ziedonis (Eds.), *Handbook on drug abuse prevention* (pp. 93–120). Toronto: Allyn & Bacon.

Erikson, P. G., Riley, D. M., Cheung, Y. W., & O'Hare, P. A. (Eds.). (1996). *Harm reduction: A new direction for drug policies and programs.* Toronto, Ontario, Canada: University of Toronto Press.

Johnston, L., Bachman, J., & O'Malley, P. (2000). *Monitoring the future: National results on adolescent drug use overview of key findings 1999.* Washington DC: National Institute on Drug Abuse.

Lynagh, M., Schofield, M., & Sanson-Fisher, R. (1997). School health promotion programs over the past decade: A review of the smoking, alcohol and solar protection literature. *Health Promotion International, 12*(1), 43–59.

Marlatt, G. A., & Gordon, J. R. (1985). *Relapse prevention: Maintenance strategies in the treatment of addictive behaviors.* New York: Guilford Press.

Martino, S., Grilo, C. M., & Fehon, D. C. (2000). Development of the Drug Abuse Screening Test for adolescents (DAST-A). *Addictive Behaviors, 25,* 57–70.

Miller, W. R., & Rollnick, S. (1991). *Motivational interviewing: Preparing people to change addictive behavior.* New York: Guilford Press.

Minkler, M., & Wallerstein, N. (1997). Improving health through community organization and community building. In K. Glanz, F. Lewis, & B. Rimer (Eds.), *Health behavior and health education: Theory, research and practice* (pp. 241–269). San Francisco: Jossey-Bass.

Pricewaterhouse Coopers. (2000). *Teen purchasing power weak in online shopping arena* [On-line]. Available: *http://www. pwcglobal. com/Extweb/ncpressrelease. nsf*

Prochaska, J., DiClemente, C., & Norcross, J. (1992). In search of how people change. Applications to addictive behaviors. *American Psychologist, 47*(9), 1102–1114.

Rollnick, S., Mason, P., & Butler, C. (1999). *Health behavior change: A guide for practitioners.* Edinburgh, Scotland: Churchill Livingstone.

Ryan, R. M., & Deci, E. L. (2000). Self-determination theory and the facilitation of intrinsic motivation, social development and well-being. *American Psychologist, 55,* 68–78.

Skinner, H. A. (1998). *TeenNet project overview* [On-line]. Available: *http://www. teennetproject.org*

Skinner, H. A. (1982). The Drug Abuse Screening Test. *Addictive Behaviors, 7,* 363–371.

Skinner, H. A. (2000). Assessment of substance abuse using the Drug Abuse Screening Test (DAST) In R. Carson-DeWitt (Ed.), *Encyclopedia of drugs, alcohol, and addictive behaviors* (Rev. ed., Vol. 1, pp. 147–148). New York: Macmillan.

Skinner, H. A. (2001). *Promoting health through organizational change.* Boston: Allyn & Bacon.

Skinner, H. A., & Bercovitz, K. L. (1997). *Person-centred health promotion* (Report

No. HP-10-0404). Toronto, Ontario, Canada: Centre for Health Promotion, University of Toronto and ParticipACTION.

Skinner, H. A., Morrison, M., Bercovitz, K., Haans, D., Jennings, M. J., Magdenko, L., Polzer, J., Smith, L., & Weir, N. (1997). Using the Internet to engage youth in health promotion. *International Journal of Health Promotion and Education, 4*, 23–25.

Teenage Research Unlimited. (2000). *Spring Update Wave* (Vol. 33.) [On-line]. Available: *http://www.teenresearch.com*

Tobler, N., & Stratton, H. (1997). Effectiveness of school-based drug prevention programs: A meta-analysis of the research. *Journal of Primary Prevention, 8*(1), 71–128.

III

Future Directions

11

Transdisciplinary Research to Improve Brief Interventions for Addictive Behaviors

DAVID B. ABRAMS and RICHARD R. CLAYTON

THE SCOPE OF TRANSDISCIPLINARY RESEARCH

This chapter selectively explores transdisciplinary research strategies that hold promise for improving brief interventions for addictive and risky behaviors. A transdisciplinary approach (Kahn & Prager, 1994; Stokols, 1998) can lead to innovative interventions by (1) bridging the latest discoveries in the basic biological, behavioral, sociological, and public health disciplines; (2) including a life-span developmental perspective on trajectories and transitions, from none to chronic debilitating addiction or risky behavior; and (3) developing a research agenda that ensures a seamless linkage between researchers and practitioners.

The transdisciplinary approach requires researchers from different disciplines to listen across the professional gulf that separates them (Kahn & Prager, 1994). The development of better interventions for behaviors as complex as the addictions and risk taking among adolescents calls for collaboration among researchers from domains as diverse as cellular biology, genetics, cognitive neuroscience, animal models, and cognitive theory. Levels of nested sociological and environmental contextual factors (such as family, school, and neighborhood), and socioeconomic forces must also be considered. Transdisciplinary research can also range in its focus from basic

321

science to clinical treatments, diffusion of best practices into the fabric of the community, and policy. Basic research identifies the biobehavioral and sociocultural mechanisms that underlie addictive and risky behaviors. Translational research focuses on developing more effective applications for intervention and policy formation (Abrams, 1999a, 1999b; Baer, 1993).

Research to Practice

Even more critical than the integration across research domains is the need to involve practitioners, policy makers, delivery system administrators, and adolescents and their families in the process of research, stimulating researchers to address the needs of individuals more directly. Practitioners can inform researchers about patterns of behavior that emerge from brief treatments (e.g., individual profiles that result in treatment nonresponsivity, or special populations whose subculture has not received sufficient research attention). Eventually, the dialogue between research and practice can identify useful new hypotheses. Teams of transdisciplinary collaborators can better advance science than traditional unidisciplinary research that is isolated from practice.

Until recently, the mechanisms and models of addiction have been derived from research with self-selected participants (volunteers)—typically clinical samples of adults in treatments for chronic addictive disorders (Shadel, Shiffman, Niaura, Nichter, & Abrams, 2000). Such samples are limited in generalizability because the mechanisms that maintain chronic addiction in adults are likely to be different from those that determine initiation and progression to dependence among youths. The bridging of research and practice shares a philosophical goal with "action" or "participatory" research. Participatory research includes the target audience and the intervention practitioners from the onset of a research project—in its earliest conceptualization (Abrams, Emmons, & Linnan, 1997). Participatory research ensures that interventions will be tailored to the unique needs of the target population and smoothly integrated into existing delivery systems. Participatory research strategies are especially important when the target audience is youth.

Many of the brief interventions described in this book employ some of the hallmarks of participatory research strategies (Brown & Lourie, Chapter 8, this volume). For example, conducting focus groups with the target audience of adolescents presenting in clinics and with the health care providers who treat them ensures that the brief motivational interventions are tailored to both the audience and the context of service delivery. This bridging of research and practice may have enhanced the efficacy of the interventions.

Clinical Efficacy to Community Dissemination and Policy Research

Brief motivational interventions conducted in circumscribed clinical settings (e.g., hospital emergency department) have to be viewed within the broader public health context. Research efficacy trials are usually conducted under ideal circumstances, with small samples, short-term followups of treatment outcomes, and a narrowly defined target audience. Efficacy trials must then be translated into longer term and more generalizable dissemination trials of efficiency and cost-effectiveness. Dissemination trials can help to answer questions such as, Would a motivational intervention delivered in an emergency room with adolescents involved in drunkdriving accidents work as well when modified for a classroom setting with adolescents, the vast majority of whom are at low risk and may never drive while intoxicated? Dissemination research can dramatically improve the potential for practitioners to make a larger scale and a longer lived impact on the whole community, in which the goal is to change the health status of an aggregate unit rather than an individual.

Dissemination trials ideally should be targeted prospectively to either (1) a whole population or (2) a high-risk subpopulation. The aggregate unit (audience) might be a whole community or an entire school district. By definition, targeting a whole population implies that the vast majority of individual members are not seeking treatment and may not be experiencing any problem behaviors. They are "nonvolunteers," and a dissemination trial must reach and engage them in the program. The members of the aggregate unit must be proactively recruited and represent the full continuum of risk from low to high. For population-based interventions, advantages must be weighed against disadvantages. Advantages include reaching all the members of the audience and preventing the onset of problems (primary prevention). Disadvantages include the risk of sensitizing those at low risk and stimulating their curiosity, as well as the excess costs of delivering an intervention to a large number of individuals who may not need it.

Interventions that involve a high-risk subpopulation would include a brief screening to identify those at high risk. For example, all schoolchildren who have smoked more than 100 cigarettes might be targeted because they are not only at unusual risk for progression to nicotine addiction but are also at risk for adopting other substance abuse or risky behaviors, as well as behavioral, school, and social problems.

Measuring the success of a dissemination trial must include an index of reach (degree of penetration into the population), as well as of the efficacy of the intervention. Dissemination trials address issues of efficiency, cost-effectiveness, and benefit to society at large in terms of their potential for making a community-wide (or public health) impact (Abrams et al.,

1996). Public health impact may be defined as reach × efficacy per unit cost. Dissemination trials give practitioners a broader range of tools to translate research into practice and policy and also give researchers the challenge of working with practitioners to make their research more valuable to society.

The most cost-effective (or efficient) interventions identified by dissemination research become the basis for evidence-based practice. Best practice guidelines can then be incorporated into the policies and procedures of organizations and agencies responsible for delivering services to local communities and at the state and national levels. Thus the concept of making a societal impact must include considerations such as training practitioners, as well as identifying the best modes and methods of delivery—so that interventions become part of the fabric of the community. Dissemination research should also address the short, medium, and longer term economic and other benefits to society (Chaloupka & Warner, in press). The end result of translating research from clinical trials to dissemination studies is to provide practitioners and policy makers with the tools to change sufficient absolute numbers of individual problem behaviors at the aggregate level of communities and society to shift the population prevalence curve of substance abuse and risky behavior.

Stepped Care to Bridge Prevention, Early Treatment, and Rehabilitation

The brief interventions described in this book bridge an important gap between the primary prevention programs that are typically directed to whole populations early in the life span and later abstinence-oriented clinical treatments that are directed at rehabilitating those who already manifest risky behaviors and associated comorbidities (e.g., conduct disorder, antisocial personality, affective and attention-deficit disorders). In general, adolescents with severe comorbid complications who are on rapidly accelerating trajectories toward addiction have not received the clinical or the research attention they deserve, and treatment is often "too little and too late." More detail on issues of comorbidity is provided by Winters (Chapter 3, this volume) and by Myers, Brown, Tate, Abrantes, and Tomlinson (Chapter 9, this volume). These adolescents seem to have slipped through the cracks between, on the one hand, less intensive primary prevention programs that are directed to the general population, and, on the other, more intensive clinical treatment programs designed for individuals in rehabilitation or psychiatric facilities who have manifested severe problems and chronic use (Baer, 1993; Pentz, 1993). From a public health perspective, we have failed so far to sufficiently reduce the overall population prevalence rates of tobacco, other substance abuse, and other risky behaviors. To achieve such a reduction requires an integration of prevention, early intervention, and rehabilitation models of care.

In order to make a significant public health impact, different research and practice agendas must be united into a comprehensive and integrated stepped-care approach to intervention and policy (Abrams et al., 1996; Abrams, Clark, & King, 1999). This coordination will require at least three steps. Less intensive interventions (Step 1) directed at primary prevention in whole populations may have to be coupled with screening for high-risk subgroups who receive moderate or brief motivational interventions (Step 2). Brief interventions may have to be stepped up to more intensive clinical interventions (Step 3) for the smaller but important subgroup with severe problems who continue to progress toward the patterns that are typical of older chronic adult populations (Abrams et al., 1996; Sobell & Sobell, 1999).

A stepped-care approach is also compatible with a harm minimization model of intervention. Miller, Turner, and Marlatt (Chapter 2, this volume) place harm minimization within a developmental framework. Marlatt and colleagues suggest that brief motivational interventions can be the starting point in minimizing the harmful consequences of substance abuse and can also be the entry point for delivery of more intensive levels of stepped-care interventions to adolescents and young adults (Marlatt et al., 1998).

With the revolution in informatics and computer-assisted communications, the tools of brief motivational interventions can be placed together with self-help or self-change programs on the Internet or other media (see Skinner, Maley, Smith, Chirrey, & Morrison, Chapter 10, this volume). Computer-tailored intervention can combine the advantages of less intensive prevention interventions that have broad reach into a population with the self-change and coping-skills training that is found in more intensive clinical rehabilitation programs (Abrams, Mills, & Bulger, 1999). Brief motivational interventions delivered by computer could have the potential to make a large and cost-efficient impact on a population level.

In summary, the scope of a transdisciplinary research agenda ranges along three broad dimensions (see Figure 11.1). First, more emphasis should be placed on transdisciplinary models of the clusters of etiological variables and processes that contribute to predisposing pathways of risk and protective factors. Such clusters range from familial genetic transmission and other molecular biological substrates to individual differences in cognitive–behavioral and other psychological factors to sociocultural–environmental contextual considerations. Second, a life-span developmental perspective is important. It includes longitudinal designs and trajectories and critical sensitive periods and transitions, ranging from parental–familial influence to prenatal environmental to early, middle, and late childhood, adolescence, and adulthood (Mayhew, Flay, & Mott, 2000; Schulenberg,

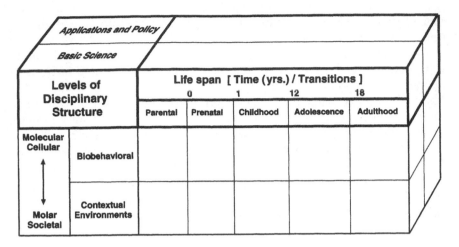

FIGURE 11.1. The three domains of transdisciplinary addiction research: (1) organizational structure of the disciplines from molecular to molar (biobehavioral mechanisms to contextual environments); (2) trajectories across time and across developmental transitions; and (3) from basic science to applications and policy formation.

Maggs, Steinman, & Zucker, Chapter 1, this volume). Different variables may predict poorer outcomes at different developmental stages (e.g., exposure to alcohol/cocaine/nicotine in utero versus exposure to the role modeling of older siblings and peers in late childhood). Moreover, short-term treatment studies and cross-sectional survey designs may lack sufficient sensitivity and specificity to distinguish a significant transition, reflecting a different trajectory (e.g., from several episodes of binge use of alcohol to a regular pattern of heavy alcohol use that indicates a transition from experimentation to serious dependence). Third, an explicit effort must be made to support translational research that bridges basic science, clinical treatment, and dissemination and that eventually also has policy implications. Participatory research must be given greater emphasis by including practitioners in setting the research agenda.

DEVELOPMENTAL TRAJECTORIES AND PATHWAYS

The recommendation made by Schulenberg and colleagues to consider a life-span developmental perspective as a central organizing construct (see Chapter 1, this volume) is compelling. A developmental perspective permits multiple opportunities to introduce brief motivational interventions that can alter the transitions, trajectories, and pathways toward undesirable outcomes. Such interventions could range from early primary prevention (e.g., preventing in utero exposure to nicotine, cocaine, or alcohol in a high-risk pregnancy) to identifying high-risk subgroups during early or middle childhood to treating adolescents who are still experimenting with addictive substances before the risky behaviors have become entrenched. The techniques of brief motivational interventions could be especially helpful when applied to all of these audiences because they address individuals or families who usually are unaware of the need to change and are therefore low in motivation.

As Schulenberg and colleagues (Chapter 1, this volume) appropriately note, etiological factors (and therefore opportunities for intervention) may be different in different developmental phases of the life span. Identifying critical transitions across developmental phases and better understanding the architecture of various trajectories can help us to discover individuals at higher risk for negative consequences. Brief motivational interventions may be inadequate or contraindicated for a subgroup of adolescents who have the highest profiles of genetic, biobehavioral, and familial susceptibility. More intensive levels of treatment, as in a stepped-care model, might be considered for such individuals.

This agenda will not be easy to implement because the phenomena of interest, sufficiently complex in themselves, are even more complex when mapped onto a myriad of modal transitions and trajectories (Chassin, Presson, Pitts, & Sherman, 2000). Chassin and colleagues (2000) and Schulenberg and colleagues (Chapter 1, this volume) have identified trajectories for both nicotine addiction and alcohol abuse that link predisposing predictor variables to different clusters of trajectories, such as early versus late onset, rapid versus slow uptake trajectories, and no-use and erratic-use patterns. Understanding the pathways of risk and protective factors that predict different trajectories could help scientists and practitioners design improved motivational interventions. For example, intervening early in a trajectory (e.g., just before onset of puberty) could alter cognitive–behavioral variables (e.g., positive outcome expectancies about substance use) during a "sensitive" period such that a small change results in dramatic alteration of the entire trajectory.

In examining pathways of risk and protective factors, the similarities, differences, and boundary conditions among nicotine, alcohol, marijuana, cocaine, heroin, and other substances must be considered, as well as their clustering with other risky behaviors (e.g., risky sex), psychiatric disorders (particularly conduct, mood, and attention disorders), and the environmental context (e.g., the "pockets of prevalence" in low-income inner-city neighborhoods; Abrams, 1995; Abrams, Marlatt, & Sobell, 1995; Merikangas, Avenevoli, Dierker, & Grillon, 1999; Monti, Rohsenow, Colby, & Abrams, 1995). One substance may potentiate the other (e.g., early smoking leads to later polysubstance abuse). Two chapters in this volume focus on innovative and practical approaches to the problems related to comorbidities and risky sex among youths. Myers and colleagues (Chapter 9, this volume) provide many examples of the potential value and the challenges involved in considering the comorbidity of psychiatric problems and substance abuse within the context of brief motivational interventions, and Brown and Lourie (Chapter 8, this volume) discuss the challenges of HIV prevention.

Biological mechanisms derived from cellular, molecular, genetic, and neuroscience disciplines have significantly advanced our understanding of some of the underlying neurochemical pathways (e.g., brain reward circuitry) that unfold over the human life span and that are implicated in the addictions and related disorders of behavioral control (Koob & LeMoal, 1997). We must recognize, however, that recent advances in biology and neurosciences have not been integrated with advances in the understanding of the influences of proximal and distal social and environmental contexts and other psychosocial factors (Abrams, 1999a, 1999b, 2000). Equally impressive is the heterogeneity of the nested contextual factors at the personal, proximal, distal, and environmental levels. These factors have been empirically mapped by Flay, Phil, Petraitis, and Hu (1995). Individuals are always nested in a variety of contexts (family, school, neighborhood, community), and the trajectories and pathways in addictive and risky behaviors are affected by the extraindividual contextual factors (discussed later). The site and circumstances in which interventions, whether brief or extensive, are delivered constitute another important nexus of contextual influences that may interact with and be influenced by not only the receptivity of the individual for the intervention but also the likelihood of its success (Stokols, 1992). Brief motivational interventions might have to be expanded so that they can be delivered in the context of family therapy or group therapy and in conjunction with pharmacological treatments.

Integrating basic biobehavioral mechanisms with contextual factors over the life span is likely to enhance clinical and public health interventions, ranging from earlier primary prevention to later treatment for chronic addictive and risky behaviors. Such approaches should explicitly search for and articulate interactions in biobehavioral and contextual domains over the developmental life course. Selected examples of individual (biobehavioral) and contextual (environmental) factors that could improve theories and interventions are presented in the following sections.

BIOBEHAVIORAL FACTORS AT THE INDIVIDUAL LEVEL

In this section, we explore selected examples of biobehavioral mechanisms across some of the major life-span developmental transitions, from parental transmission of genetic risk to early adulthood (see Figure 11.1). Etiological mechanisms can and should inform prevention and treatment interventions and public policies by helping to identify predictors and profiles of risk or susceptibility to future problems, to develop more effective screening instruments, and to improve tailoring of prevention, early treatment, and clinical interventions to specific subpopulations (Kellam & Anthony, 1998). Opportunities for intervention can occur at many points along the developmental continuum. Factors that are important prior to the initiation of addictive and other risky behaviors may be thought of as more distal or as predisposing factors. Factors that are closer to the initiation of use and to the progression from experimentation to regular use and dependence may be thought of as more proximal or precipitating factors (Flay et al., 1995).

Cognitive–Behavioral Factors

Bandura's (1997) cognitive social learning theory is one useful model that characterizes the emergence of self-control over individual behavior as a reciprocal interaction between proximal contextual and environmental variables and biobehavioral factors. Ultimately, it will be important to link more distal biobehavioral mechanisms and their interactions with environmental contexts to the proximal cognitive learning mechanisms or schemata in human memory that govern human choice and behavioral expression. Expectancy (outcome and efficacy), the central concept in explaining human behavior within social cognitive theory, may be especially important in understanding how brief motivational interventions produce their effects. Expectancy is a learned relationship between a stimulus, a response, and the outcome of the response. In outcome expectancies, therefore, the adolescent's subjective estimate of the likelihood of reinforcement determines the strength of the response (e.g., to seek out or use tobacco, other substances, or engage in risky behavior in order to obtain desired gratification).

Goldman, Del Boca, and Darkes (1999) point out that the concept of expectancy has expanded in the past decade to encompass transdisciplinary perspectives from cognitive neuroscience and information processing. Expectancy may be applied to memory functions or "cognitive schema" as an umbrella term for "a variety of neuro-cognitive processes that serve a common function, namely preparing the (person) to respond to future circumstances" (Goldman et al., 1999, p. 205). There is considerable evidence that expectancies mediate addictive behavioral outcomes. For example, in the alcohol literature, expectancies (1) correlate with alcohol use, (2) appear in children before actual drinking begins, (3) prospectively predict drinking, and (4) are modified by drinking experiences. Many laboratory experiments with humans (see Goldman et al., 1999, for details) demonstrate that changes in expectancies are associated with changes in drinking (both increases and decreases). Goldman and colleagues conclude that "the alcohol expectancy memory system is part of the causal pathway leading to alcohol use and alcoholism" (p. 224).

The expectancy schemata are important for understanding motivational interventions. For example, well before children enter adolescence, their beliefs and expectations about the effects of tobacco, alcohol, and other substances are already formed (Miller, Smith, & Goldman, 1990). These beliefs (outcome expectancies) are often of a very positive nature (smoking and drinking lead to positive social benefits and reduced anxiety). Role models and media portrayals are some of the sources of these early cognitive schemata about the positive outcome expectancies of substance abuse. Expectancies can be detected in preschool children (Zucker, Kincaid, Fitzgerald, & Bingham, 1996). As children mature toward actual drug use, expectancies change from primarily negative (unpleasant outcomes) to positive (social effects, mood, and arousal; Dunn & Goldman, 1996). In college students, expectancies predict future high-risk drinking behavior (Carey, 1995).

Coping Skills

The development of coping skills is another important consideration in the emergence of self-regulation over stressful environmental demands and in achieving positive social, mood, and arousal effects. The expectancies that come to guide the coping skills used by adolescents to manage stress, other moods, and social situations may be more or less adaptive. Less adaptive coping skills would include expectancies that the use of an addictive substance or behavior is the best way to achieve desired outcomes. If expectancies for alternative coping skills are not clearly apparent or available, then substance use may become the only way an individual knows how to cope with a particular social situation (e.g., shyness) or feeling (e.g., depression, anxiety, frustration). Substance abuse as a form of coping or self-medication may short-circuit the development of a broad repertoire of more adaptive coping skills, and confidence in one's ability to achieve desired outcomes (self-efficacy expectations) would be low, making it unlikely that the adolescent would try to use more adaptive coping skills.

The cognitive schemata for the self-regulation of individual behavior are likely to become more consolidated during adolescence, and this may be one reason that brief motivational interventions are effective. Brief interventions may be primarily directed at changing cognitive coping skills and the self-efficacy and outcome expectancies known to be important in the self-regulation of addictive and risky behaviors. The plasticity of cognitive schemata is such that relatively small changes in expectancies produced by a brief motivational intervention could produce large alterations in the future trajectories of addictive and risk-taking patterns. These cognitive expectancy schemata could well be altered by brief motivational interventions before they become entrenched as a result of actual substance usage. A transdisciplinary research agenda would address the mechanisms by which brief motivational interventions have their greatest impact in relation to sensitive developmental transitions (e.g., puberty) and in interaction with predisposing and precipitating biobehavioral and contextual factors that form the cognitive self-regulatory schemata. Such research is important, as it may result in improved brief motivational interventions or in helping to identify with which subgroups of adolescents and at what sensitive developmental life transitions we can intervene effectively.

Familial Transmission of Substance Abuse

There is growing evidence that substance use disorders and other psychiatric and behavioral problems (e.g., conduct disorder, sociopathy, attention-deficit/hyperactivity disorder) are familial. Genetic factors explain a significant degree of familial aggregation (Merikangas et al., 1998). The familial aggregation of alcoholism is well established, but an increasing number of studies suggest that other drug abuse and nicotine dependence may also be familial. Some studies have found greater levels of heritability for drug abuse and for nicotine dependence than for alcoholism (Swan, 1999). However, the nature and the scope of genetic mediators and how these might interact with various environmental exposures across the human life span provide rich opportunities for future research. Smith and Anderson (Chapter 4, this volume) point out the many ways in which personality and learning factors can combine to create additional risk for adolescent problem drinkers. Such risk factors create additional challenges for clinical and public health intervention.

Genetic susceptibility in parents can result in critical gene–environment interactions in offspring as early in the developmental life span as in utero. Evidence of the deleterious effects of alcohol and cocaine on the fetus is well known. There is new evidence that in utero exposure to nicotine also may alter neuroadaptive mechanisms, resulting in higher susceptibility to behavioral disorders of under- or overcontrol in early childhood and in risk of progression to nicotine dependence and alcohol and substance abuse and to criminality, violence, and sociopathy in adolescence and adulthood (Griesler, Kandel, & Davies, 1998). Preventing exposure or reducing harm during pregnancy can therefore become an important intervention opportunity for motivational enhancement and other treatments of the parents. Exposure during pregnancy may also be an important marker in developing screening instruments to identify children at high risk for addictive and other risky behaviors. Such a marker may reflect not only altered brain function as a result of exposure to toxins but also the likelihood of impaired family and parental controls following birth and possible genetic predisposition as well.

Merikangas and colleagues (1998) reported an eightfold increased risk of drug disorders among the relatives of probands with drug disorders across a wide range of substances, including opiates, cocaine, cannabis, and alcohol. Their results suggest that there may be risk factors that are specific to particular classes of drugs, as well as risk factors that underlie substance use disorders in general. Genetic factors can influence susceptibility to addictive behaviors through individual differences in the effects of the drugs themselves (e.g., regarding metabolism, sensitivity, tolerance, and side effects), as well as cognitive and other behavioral factors (e.g., the alteration of mood, stress reduction, depression, and anxiety).

Because the family plays a critical role in the etiology of drug abuse and risky behaviors, it is important that basic research continue to probe for a better understanding of the mechanisms through which family exerts its influence. Additional controlled family and twin studies are important to identify the horizontal and vertical transmission of gene and environment interactions. Such research has critical implications for prevention and other interventions, including the development and refinement of sensitive and specific screening instruments for risk susceptibility that may target families and their offspring at highest risk for early intervention (see, e.g., Kellam & Anthony, 1998).

CONTEXTUAL FACTORS

Although significant progress has been made in understanding the individual-level biological, psychological, and, to a certain extent, social aspects of substance abuse, large gaps still exist in understanding the influence of contextual factors in the shape of transitions and trajectories in substance abuse (see Wang et al., 1999). The same is clearly true with regard to the influence of contextual factors on the efficacy and effectiveness of prevention and treatment interventions. Context sometimes refers, at least partially, to where individuals and groups are located physically and to the extra-individual or group characteristics of those locations. The physical geographical context provides the setting influences on the behaviors that occur within it. The physical context is always integrally connected to and facilitative of the enactment of roles central to an institutional context.

Research to date has focused largely on identifying the importance of individual differences in explaining trajectories to initiation and maintenance of substance abuse and has largely ignored the potential influence of the heterogeneity of contextual factors in explaining outcomes. This situation is illustrated in a compelling fashion by a study conducted with mice in three laboratories.

Crabbe, Wahlsten, and Dudek (1999) used eight inbred strains of mice and one null mutant strain, all of which were the same age (77 days), all of which had been fed using the same brand of feed, and all of which had housing conditions similar across laboratories. The only thing the investigators varied systematically was whether the mice had been shipped for testing to one of three different laboratories or bred locally. In addition, they started their experiments on the same day and at the same time and used the same apparatus. The results are striking. "Despite our efforts to equate laboratory environments, significant and, in some cases, large effects of site were found for nearly all variables" (Crabbe, Wahlsten, Dudek, 1999, pp. 1670–1671). If context emerges as critically important in this kind of research study, imagine how important it is for researchers to understand contextual influences on the transitions and trajectories of substance abuse in adolescents. Imagine how important context may be with regard to brief interventions. There are undoubtedly many contextual treatment factors that may impinge on outcomes. Some of these are external to the intervention process itself, whereas others are more directly related to the context within which intervention delivery occurs.

A number of physical and institutional contexts are especially relevant with regard to understanding transitions and trajectories in substance abuse and efficacious and effective treatment interventions. The *family*, usually located physically within a house or apartment, contains a variety of statuses, roles, expectations, and norms that may be relevant to trajectories, as well as to treatment outcomes (see Distefan, Gilpin, Choi, & Pierce, 1998). Waldron, Brody, and Slesnick (Chapter 7, this volume) explore the use of family therapy for substance abuse. We know that social support within the context of family relations is predictive of positive outcomes in treatment. *Education* is typically tied to the physical location of schools and the accompanying statuses, roles, and norms that go with education. With expansions of school health clinics and an increasing recognition of the need for treatment interventions within the school context, this context takes on added significance. This is what Dryfoos (1994) calls full-service schools. The potential value of training school counselors and educational psychologists in the techniques of brief motivational interventions could significantly broaden the impact of these interventions. Evaluation of their efficacy and cost-effectiveness within school settings could inform health care policy.

The term *local institutions* refers to a variety of nonfamily and nonschool physical and social settings that may influence trajectories in substance abuse and treatment outcomes. Such local institutions might include voluntary organizations such as the Boys' and Girls' Clubs and the Boy Scouts and Girl Scouts. Organizations designed to provide and monitor sports activities, youth-focused organizations that are anchored in churches, workplaces, and medical and social service organizations located within subcommunities (see LaPrelle, Bauman, & Koch, 1992; Rountree & Clayton, 1999) are also considered in this category.

In this volume and in the existing literature, we pay close attention to the importance of teachable moments and motivational interviewing. Less attention has been paid to opportunistic interventions that may be geographically and temporally proximate to behaviors associated with substance abuse and offered within the context of established role relationships between the person exhibiting the problem and the person intervening. The comprehensiveness of the community prevention trial to reduce alcohol-involved trauma, described by Holder and colleagues (1997), provides compelling evidence of the value of mobilizing and facilitating the organization of community infrastructures to reduce the consequences of substance abuse.

The conceptual framework for this community trial is based on the premise that addictive problems arise through an interaction of individual, interpersonal, and social factors. The interaction warrants "community systems" interventions. Holder and colleagues (1997) identify five mutually reinforcing components of effective community-wide prevention: (1) community mobilization, (2) responsible beverage service, (3) reducing drinking and driving, (4) controlling underage drinking, and (5) limiting alcohol access. There are multiple leverage points within the community model at which brief motivational counseling interventions might be incorporated. For example, motivational factors could be combined with training bartenders in the "responsible beverage service" component, the "drinking and driving" component, and the focus on preventing underage drinking. Motivational technologies could be used to further strengthen community-based interventions designed to increase community awareness, create supportive infrastructures, and modify individual and collective beliefs, attitudes, and expectations—such as perceptions of risky consequences of drinking or the probability that behaviors that violate community norms (drunken drivers, underage drinkers) will be detected and that negative consequences will follow. The impact of brief interventions at the population level further underscores the importance of the types of interventions described in this volume (see Edwards, 1994; Sampson, 1997).

Peer contexts do not have an institutional-specific reference because peer networks and influences exist within and across schools, neighborhoods, and local institutional spheres. Conceptualization of peer contexts and influences have tended to focus on the *selection* and *socialization* of peers and so-called peer clusters (Sussman et al., 1990; Ureberg, Degirmencioglu, & Pilgrim, 1997), as well as on the structure of peer networks (Ennett & Bauman, 1994). A substantial amount of knowledge exists with regard to the influence of peers on transitions and trajectories in substance abuse. Far less is known about the role of peers as adjuncts to the therapeutic process, whether in brief or more extensive interventions.

The *policy* and *economic contexts* that exist at the societal and local levels probably have an indirect effect on trajectories and treatment outcomes. From a prevention perspective, some of the most powerful effects on initiation of tobacco and alcohol use come from increases in the prices of the commodities. The organizational entities that are responsible for providing treatment interventions are often driven more by concerns about the up-front costs of treatment delivery than they are about the long-term costs and benefits of the intervention. In the dynamically changing fiscal contexts of the health care industry, there will be a strong interest shown in the power of the brief interventions discussed in this volume.

As important as individual differences are in the etiology of substance abuse, it is our contention that they can best be understood only in context. This is certainly also true with regard to understanding how to make our treatments of substance abuse more effective. This requires new paradigms that bring together disciplines that cover the scientific territory from cells to society.

It is our assumption that an adequate understanding of transitions and trajectories and treatment outcomes requires seeing all individuals as nested in a variety of contexts. These contexts may directly influence trajectories and will likely illuminate the meanings associated with understanding these trajectories and outcomes. The leverage of brief motivational interventions could be enhanced by considering context and nested levels of environmental factors that interact with biological, cognitive–behavioral risk factors, and coping skills.

CONCLUSION

Brief interventions along the continuum from primary prevention in populations to high-risk subgroups to individual treatment and rehabilitation have the potential to provide the most efficient methods to benefit society and reduce the burden of many chronic diseases, disability, and premature death. A life-span developmental perspective permits both basic science research on etiological mechanisms and the translation of discoveries into clinical and public health practice to yield maximum leverage by identifying the critical transitions and pathways to addiction and risky behavior. For example, knowing that early exposure to tobacco, alcohol, and other drugs during pregnancy has serious and lifelong consequences permits a practitioner to use teachable moments for parents during prenatal visits that lend themselves to the techniques of brief motivational interviewing. The pubertal transition provides another potential point for intervention, a point at which tobacco and alcohol experimentation may begin within a context of biological, behavioral, and socioenvironmental stress and change.

In order to further develop and maximize the potential for brief motivational interventions, professionals can advance the field by using a transdisciplinary strategy that systematically includes key disciplines and dimensions that have previously been investigated within unidisciplinary frameworks. Integration of basic science and its applications to intervention and policy formation, within a life-span developmental perspective and across the biobehavioral and the nested contextual environmental domains, provides a template for the next decade to guide research that will inform practice and benefit society.

However, there are a large number of gaps in the scientific base and a myriad of unanswered questions. Most initial substance use occurs in adolescence, at least in the United States, and brief interventions designed to interrupt the trajectory toward more extensive and intensive use might benefit from knowledge about fundamental neurobiological processes in adolescence. Further, alcohol and nicotine are often used concurrently by both adolescents and adults, but little is known about the neurobiological mechanisms that operate when both are consumed. Although it is clearly possible and desirable to develop brief interventions for substance use during the earlier phases of development of consumption patterns, knowledge of the neurobiological mechanisms might provide important clues to improving both the efficacy and effectiveness of such interventions. Mapping out the brain's reward circuitry and linking this to cognitive–behavioral mechanisms (for instance, how motivational self-control mechanisms operate cognitive schemata such as expectancies within human memory) could provide new ideas to further enhance the effectiveness of motivational intervention techniques.

One critical task is to conduct research that considers the multiple pathways of mediating and moderating variables that result from the transdisciplinary integration of neurobiological factors and gene–environment interactions across the critical developmental transitions and the proximal and distal contextual factors. An individual's formation of outcome expectancies about the benefits and risks of substance abuse and his or her degree of self-efficacy in employing alternative coping responses in the face of tempting cues are likely to be important cognitive mechanisms that could predict risk and/or recovery. Such cognitive mediators could be modified by brief motivational interventions during "sensitive" developmental periods, resulting in powerful alterations in longer term trajectories toward healthier outcomes.

Current unidisciplinary models of addictive and risky behaviors have made incrementally important but necessarily limited contributions to effective interventions. Moreover, as the past three decades have revealed, from a unidisciplinary perspective, it has been extremely difficult to identify effective interventions (prevention or early treatment) that have a long-lived and population-wide impact (Flay et al., 1995). Primary prevention interventions have often produced modest to no effects on the longer term outcome of interest. Such interventions have generally not been designed to screen for high-risk individuals (who possibly need different and more intensive interventions) or to address the needs of those who have already progressed to regular use. Even in cases in which there is sufficient evidence, we have been relatively ineffective in disseminating evidence-based programs because of inadequate infrastructures and the lack of a good scientific base of research on dissemination and how to optimize program utilization. Thus evidence-based programs have not been effectively and efficiently disseminated to larger populations. The development of informatics and communications systems that can deliver tailored interventions to large numbers of individuals using a variety of media (computers, the Internet) may further enhance the societal impact of brief motivational interventions (Abrams, Mills, & Bulger, 1999; Skinner et al., Chapter 10, this volume).

If one could accurately map the scientific terrain concerning the epidemiology, etiology, prevention, and treatment of substance use and abuse, one might be impressed by the amazing progress that has been made despite major gaps in the foundational knowledge base. The appropriate conclusions drawn from the many excellent chapters in this volume are that the transitions, trajectories, and pathways to substance use and abuse are extremely complex. The factors that account for these transitions and trajectories, the pathways to substance use and progression within and across substances, and the contextual factors that impinge on and influence the efficacy and effectiveness of brief interventions are incredibly heterogeneous.

In this concluding chapter, we call for intensive and extensive *transdisciplinary* interaction and collaboration between researchers and practitioners as one strategy for making huge strides both in understanding the phenomena we are attempting to treat and in delving more efficiently into the underlying processes and mechanisms of substance use and abuse. It is also clear that we need a great deal more research on the treatment process itself—the message strategies that are at the basis of brief interventions, the influence of contextual factors on the delivery and receipt of these messages, and, as always, a better understanding of how to improve adherence with the regimen and discipline required for ensuring a higher probability of behavioral change. Each of us is more comfortable with our own approach to dealing with research and clinical issues—such is to be expected. However, if our goal is significant improvement in the efficacy and effectiveness of our interventions and reduction in the consequences of substance abuse at the individual, family, and societal levels, we must become more transdisciplinary. This will not be easy, but it is, in our opinion, essential. We consider this an inescapable conclusion of the papers in this volume.

ACKNOWLEDGMENTS

We thank Barbara Doll for manuscript preparation. This work was supported in part by funding from NIAAA Grant No. R01AA11211, NCI Grant No. 1P50 CA84719, and the Robert Wood Johnson Foundation's Tobacco Etiology Research Network (TERN).

REFERENCES

Abrams, D. (1999a). Transdisciplinary paradigms for tobacco prevention research. *Nicotine and Tobacco Research, 1*, S15–S23.

Abrams, D. (1999b). Nicotine addiction: Paradigms for research in the 21st century. *Nicotine and Tobacco Research, 1*, S211–S215.

Abrams, D. B. (2000). Interdisciplinary concepts and measures of craving: Commentary and future directions. *Addiction, 95*(Suppl. 2), S237–S246.

Abrams, D. B. (1995). Integrating basic, clinical, and public health research for alcohol-tobacco interactions. In J. B. Fertig & J. P. Allen (Eds.), *Alcohol and tobacco: From basic science to policy* (NIAAA Alcohol Research Monograph 30; NIH Publication No. 95-3931). Bethesda, MD: National Institute of Alcoholism and Alcohol Abuse.

Abrams, D. B., Clark, M. M., & King, T. K. (1999). Increasing the impact of nicotine dependence treatment: Conceptual and practical considerations in a stepped-care plus treatment-matching approach. In J. A. Tucker, D. M. Donovan, & G. A. Marlatt (Eds.), *Changing addictive behavior* (pp. 307–330). New York: Guilford Press.

Abrams, D. B., Emmons, K. M., & Linnan, L. A. (1997). Health behavior and health education: The past, present, and future. In K. Glanz, F. M. Lewis, & B. K. Rimer (Eds.), *Health behavior and health education: Theory, practice and research* (2nd ed., pp. 453–478). San Francisco: Jossey-Bass.

Abrams, D. B., Marlatt, G. A., & Sobell, M. B. (1995). Overview of section II: Treatment, early intervention, and policy. In J. B. Fertig & J. P. Allen (Eds.), *Alcohol and tobacco: From basic science to policy* (NIAAA Research Monograph No. 30, NIH Publication No. 95–3931). Bethesda, MD: National Institute of Alcoholism and Alcohol Abuse.

Abrams, D. B., Mills, S., & Bulger, D. (1999). Challenges and future directions for tailored communication research. *Annals of Behavioral Medicine, 21*(4), 299–306.

Abrams, D. B., Orleans, C. T., Niaura, R. S., Goldstein, M. G., Prochaska, J. O., & Velicer, W. (1996). Integrating individual and public health perspectives for treatment of tobacco dependence under managed health care: A combined stepped care and matching model. *Annals of Behavioral Medicine, 18*(4), 290–304.

Baer, J. S. (1993). Etiology and secondary prevention of alcohol problems with young adults. In J. S. Baer, G. A. Marlatt, & R. J. McMahon (Eds.), *Addictive behaviors across the life span* (pp. 111–137). Newbury Park, CA: Sage.

Bandura, A. (1997). *Self-efficacy: The exercise of control.* New York: Freeman.

Carey, K. B. (1995). Alcohol-related expectancies predict quantity and frequency of heavy drinking among college students. *Psychology of Addictive Behaviors, 9,* 236–241.

Chaloupka, F. J., & Warner, K. E. (in press). The economics of smoking. In J. P. Newhouse & A. Cuyler (Eds.), *The handbook of health economics.* New York: North-Holland.

Chassin, L., Presson, C. C., Pitts, S. C., & Sherman, S. J. (2000). The natural history of cigarette smoking from adolescence to adulthood: Multiple trajectories and their psychosocial correlates. *Health Psychology, 19*(3), 223–231.

Crabbe, J. C., Wahlsten, D., & Dudek, B. C. (1999, June 4). Genetics of mouse behavior: Interactions with laboratory environment. *Science, 284,* 1670–1672.

Distefan, J. M., Gilpin, E. A., Choi, W. S., & Pierce, J. P. (1998). Parental influences predict adolescent smoking in the United States. *Journal of Adolescent Health, 22,* 466–474.

Dryfoos, J. G. (1994). *The full-service school.* New York: Oxford University Press.

Dunn, M. E., & Goldman, M. S. (1996). Empirical modeling of an alcohol expectancy network in elementary-school children as a function of grade. *Experimental and Clinical Psychopharmacology, 4,* 209–217.

Edwards, G. (1994). *Alcohol policy and the public good.* New York: Oxford Medical Publications.

Ennett, S. T., & Bauman, K. E. (1994). The contribution of influence and selection to adolescent peer group homogeneity: The case of adolescent cigarette smoking. *Journal of Personality and Social Psychology, 67,* 653–663.

Flay, B. R., Phil, D., Petraitis, J., & Hu, F. B. (1995). The theory of triadic influence: Preliminary evidence related to alcohol and tobacco use. In J. Fertig & J. P. Allen (Eds.), *Alcohol and tobacco: From basic science to policy* (NIAAA Research Monograph No. 30, NIH Publication No. 95-3931, pp. 37–57). Bethesda, MD: National Institute of Alcoholism and Alcohol Abuse.

Goldman, M. S., Del Boca, F. K., & Darkes, J. (1999). Alcohol expectancy theory: The application of cognitive neuroscience. In K. E. Leonard & H. T. Blane (Eds.), *Psychological theories of drinking and alcoholism* (2nd ed., pp. 203–246). New York: Guilford Press.

Griesler, P. C., Kandel, D. B., & Davies, M. (1998). Maternal smoking in pregnancy, child behavior problems, and adolescent smoking. *Journal of Research on Adolescence, 8*(2), 159–189.

Holder, H. D., Salz, R. F., Grube, J. W., Boas, R. B., Gruenwald, P. J., & Treno, A. J. (1997). A community prevention trial to reduce alcohol-involved accidental injury and death: Overview. *Addiction, 92*(Suppl. 2), S155–S172.

Kahn, R. L., & Prager, D. J. (1994, July 11). Interdisciplinary collaborations are a scientific and social imperative. *The Scientist,* p. 12.

Kellam, S. G., & Anthony, J. C. (1998). Targeting early antecedents to prevent tobacco smoking: Findings from an epidemiologically based randomized field trial. *American Journal of Public Health, 88,* 1490–1495.

Koob, G.F., & LeMoal, M. (1997). Drug abuse: Hedonic homeostatic dysregulation. *Science, 278,* 52–58.

LaPrelle, J., Bauman, K. E., & Koch, G. G. (1992). High intercommunity variation in adolescent cigarette smoking in a 10-community field experiment. *Evaluation Review, 16,* 115–130.

Marlatt, G. A., Baer, J. S., Kivlahan, D. R., Larimer, M. E., Quigley, L. A., Somers, J. M., & Williams, E. (1998). Screening and brief interventions for high-risk college student drinkers: Results from a two-year follow-up assessment. *Journal of Consulting and Clinical Psychology, 66*(4), 604–615.

Mayhew, K. P., Flay, B. R., & Mott, J. A. (2000). Stages in the development of adolescent smoking. *Drug and Alcohol Dependence, 59*(Suppl. 1), S61–S81.

Merikangas, K. R., Avenevoli, S., Dierker, L., & Grillon, C. (1999). Vulnerability factors among children at risk for anxiety disorders. *Biological Psychiatry, 46,* 1523–1535.

Merikangas, K. R., Stolar, M., Stevens, D. E., Goulet, J., Preisig, M. A., Fenton, B., Zhang, H., O'Malley, S. S., & Rounsaville, B. J. (1998). Familial transmission of substance use disorders. *Archives of General Psychiatry, 55,* 973–979.

Miller, P. M., Smith, G. T., & Goldman, M. S. (1990). Emergence of alcohol expectancies in childhood: A possible critical period. *Journal of Studies on Alcohol, 51,* 343–349.

Monti, P. M., Rohsenow, D. J., Colby, S. M., & Abrams, D. B. (1995). Smoking among alcoholics during and after treatment: Implications for models, treatment strategies and policy. In J. B. Fertig & J. P. Allen (Eds.), *Alcohol and tobacco: From basic science to policy* (NIAAA Alcohol Research Monograph No. 30, NIH Publication No. 95–3931, pp. 187–206). Bethesda, MD: National Institute of Alcoholism and Alcohol Abuse.

Pentz, M. A. (1993). Comparative effects of community-based drug abuse prevention. In J. S. Baer, G. A. Marlatt, & R. J. McMahon (Eds.), *Addictive behaviors across the life span* (pp. 69–87). Newbury Park, CA: Sage.

Rountree, P. W., & Clayton, R. R. (1999). A contextual model of adolescent alcohol use across the rural-urban continuum. *Substance Use and Misuse, 34,* 495–519.

Sampson, R. J. (1997). The embeddedness of child and adolescent development: A community-level perspective on urban violence. In J. McCord (Ed.), *Violence and childhood in the inner city* (pp. 31–77). New York: Cambridge University Press.

Shadel, W. G., Shiffman, S., Niaura, R., Nichter, M., & Abrams, D. B. (2000). Current models of nicotine dependence: What is known and what is needed to advance understanding of tobacco etiology among youth. *Drug and Alcohol Dependence, 59*(Suppl. 1), S9–S21.

Sobell, M. B., & Sobell, L. C. (1999). Stepped care for alcohol problems: An efficient method for planning and delivering clinical services. In J. A. Tucker, D. M. Donovan, & G. A. Marlatt (Eds.), *Changing addictive behavior* (pp. 331–343). New York: Guilford Press.

Stokols, D. (1992). Establishing and maintaining health environments: Toward a social ecology of health promotion. *American Psychologist, 47,* 6–22.

Stokols, D. (1998, May). *The future of interdisciplinarity in the school of social ecology*. Paper presented at the Annual Awards Reception, Social Ecology Associates, University of California, Irvine.

Sussman, S., Dent., C. W., Stacy, A. W., Burciaga, C., Raynor, A., Turner, G. E., Charlin, V., Craig, S., Hansen, W. B., Burton, D., & Flay, B. R. (1990). Peer group association and adolescent tobacco use. *Journal of Abnormal Psychology, 99*, 349–352.

Swan, G. E. (1999). Implications of genetic epidemiology for the prevention of tobacco use. *Nicotine and Tobacco Research, 1*(Suppl. 1), S49–S56.

Ureberg, K. A., Degirmencioglu, S. M., & Pilgrim, C. (1997). Close friend and group influence on adolescent cigarette smoking and alcohol use. *Developmental Psychology, 33*, 834–844.

Wang, M. Q., Fitzhugh, E. C., Green, B. L., Turner, L. W., Eddy, J. M., & Westerfield, R. C. (1999). Prospective social-psychological factors of adolescent smoking progression. *Journal of Adolescent Health, 24*, 2–9.

Zucker, R. A., Kincaid, S. B., Fitzgerald, H. E., & Bingham, R. C. (1996). Alcohol schema acquisition in preschoolers: Differences between children of alcoholics and children of nonalcoholics. *Alcoholism: Clinical and Experimental Research, 19*, 1011–1017.

Index

CPSIA information can be obtained at www.ICGtesting.com
Printed in the USA
BVOW08s0640090116

432204BV00001B/3/P